Neurological
Differential Diagnosis

Neurological Differential Diagnosis

an illustrated approach
with 288 figures

JOHN PATTEN

HAROLD STARKE LIMITED
LONDON

SPRINGER-VERLAG
NEW YORK · HEIDELBERG · BERLIN

First published October 1977

John P. Patten, BSc., M.B., M.R.C.P., is Consultant Neurologist at the Regional
Neurological Unit, Guildford, Surrey; formerly Resident Medical Officer, The National
Hospital for Nervous Diseases, London; and has been Visiting Assistant Professor of
Neurology in the University of Texas Medical Branch, Galveston, Texas

Library of Congress Cataloging in Publication Data

Patten, John, 1935–
    Neurological differential diagnosis.

    Includes index.
    1. Nervous system—Diseases—Diagnosis.
    2. Diagnosis, Differential. I. Title

RC348.P37   616.8'04'75   77–6897
ISBN 0–387–90264–3 (Springer)

ISBN 0–287–66988–2 Harold Starke Ltd., United Kingdom
ISBN 0–387–90264–3 Springer-Verlag New York Inc.
ISBN 3–540–90264–3 Springer-Verlag Berlin Heidelberg

Harold Starke Limited, 14 John Street, London WC1N 2EJ, England
Springer-Verlag New York Inc., 175 Fifth Avenue, New York 10010, U.S.A.
Springer-Verlag Heidelberger Platz 3, D-1000 Berlin 33, Germany
Springer-Verlag D-6900 Heidelberg 1, FRG.

Printed in Great Britain at the University Press, Oxford
by Vivian Ridler, Printer to the University

CONTENTS

PREFACE

The majority of doctors are ill at ease when confronted by a patient with a neurological problem. Candidates for qualifying examinations and higher diplomas dread that they will be allocated a neurological "long case".

This is a serious reflection on the adequacy of training in neurology. It is still possible in some medical schools for a student to go through his entire clinical course without an attachment to the neurological unit. Increasing competition for teaching time has led to the situation where in most U.S. medical schools and at least one new medical school in the U.K., a two-week clinical attachment to the neurology service is considered adequate. Those fortunate enough to attend a post-graduate course find a minimum of three months' intensive training is necessary before any confidence in tackling a neurological problem is achieved.

Unfortunately, neurological textbooks seldom seem to recognise the intensely practical nature of the subject. There are many short texts that achieve brevity by the exclusion of explanatory material; these are difficult to read and digest. At the opposite extreme are the neurological compendia, often unbalanced by excessive coverage of rare diseases and all based on the assumption that patients announce on arrival that they have a demyelinating, heredo-familial, neoplastic, etc., etc., disorder. These texts are useful only to those who already have a good working knowledge of neurological diseases.

Patients present with symptoms that need careful evaluation before physical examination which in turn should be firmly based on the diagnostic possibilities suggested by the history. Understanding neurological symptoms and signs requires a good knowledge of the gross anatomy of the nervous system, its blood supply and supporting tissues; and yet an almost universal feature of neurological texts is the paucity of instructive diagrams. Most students readily admit that this is an insoluble problem as their poorly remembered neurological anatomy is often both inadequate and inappropriate to the clinical situation.

The present text is a personal approach to this complex and fascinating subject and basically reflects the way the author coped with this difficulty. The subject matter is dealt with in two ways:

(1) A symptomatic, regional anatomical basis for those areas where local anatomy determines symptoms and signs, allowing what might otherwise be regarded as "small print" anatomy to be understood and appreciated.

(2) A full discussion of the historical diagnostic clues in those conditions that are diagnosed almost exclusively on symptoms such as headache, face pain and loss of consciousness.

Throughout, an attempt has been made to preserve the "common things are common" approach which is widely rumoured to be the secret of passing examinations, and is also the basis of good clinical practice. Rare disorders are discussed briefly, but it is important that beginners realise that rare diseases are usually diagnosed when it becomes apparent that the disorder does *not* fit into any of the common clinical pictures. The first aim therefore should be to gain a very good grasp of the common disorders rather than attempting to learn long lists of very rare diseases.

The text is profusely illustrated by the author and although anatomical accuracy has been preserved, artistic licence has been taken whenever necessary to illustrate an important point. Each diagram is drawn from a special angle of view that enables the reader to visualise the area under discussion *in situ* in the patient. It is easy to construct a "diagram" so remote from actual anatomy that it becomes incomprehensible. It is hoped that this problem has been avoided.

Neurological terms are defined whenever they occur and neurological "jargon" is explained, although the beginner is well advised to keep to factual statements until he is very sure of himself. As an example of the incorrect use of jargon the following is abstracted from a report by a physician. The patient actually had a left sixth nerve palsy and a mild hemiparesis due to cerebal metastases.

He has the spastic dystonic gait of the multiple sclerotic. Also he has a third nerve paraplegia with ocular movements to the left and with nystagmus. He has cogwheel rigidity of the upper extremities and an absence of patellar reflexes. His speech is beginning to slur and there is the mask facies of the multiple sclerotic . . . I do not believe . . . further studies to be necessary as the clinical signs are all too obvious!

Specific references are not given; this book is intended for the novice who wishes to develop a "feel" for the subject and in the author's opinion references are unnecessary. This is not intended to indicate that the writer claims originality for all the information provided. The knowledge contained in this text is a distillate of wisdom gained from many teachers and, indeed, generations of teachers who have passed on their own observations. The personal part of this text is the attempt to organise this information around the anatomy of the nervous system to reinforce this knowledge and make the subject less intimidating to the beginner. In particular I would like to acknowledge my debt to my first teacher, Dr. Swithin Meadows, who aroused my enthusiasm for the subject and then inspired me to attempt to emulate his skill as a clinical neurologist.

I am also indebted to many undergraduate students at Westminster Medical School, University College Hospital and the University of Texas Medical Branch, and post-graduates at the National Hospital for Nervous Diseases whose questions, suggestions and enthusiasm originally encouraged me to bring this approach to a wider audience.

Dr. John R. Calverley, M.D., Associate Professor of Neurology in the University of Texas Medical Branch at Galveston, provided enormous encouragement in the early development of this project and allowed me to try the format on several generations of post-graduate students in his Department.

I would like to express my thanks to him and his colleagues for making my stay in his Department so instructive and enjoyable. Dr. M. J. Harrison read the original manuscript and made many useful suggestions which have been incorporated into the text. I am very grateful for his help and encouragement.

I would like to thank my wife and family for their continued support during the years this text has been in preparation and Miss Gillian Taylor for typing the often illegible manuscript.

John Patten

Guildford, 1977

Chapter 1

HISTORY-TAKING AND PHYSICAL EXAMINATION

By tradition the first chapter in any textbook of C.N.S. diseases deals with history-taking, and this necessity appears inescapable. Yet in neurology the history is so critical, in indicating both the site and the nature of the lesion, that adequate coverage is impossible in a single chapter. The features of the clinical history appropriate to each region will form a major part of each of the subsequent chapters. At this stage discussion will be confined to some broad generalisations.

The secret of good history-taking is to be a good listener. However rushed the doctor may be, it is vital that the patient feels that he has the whole of the doctor's time and attention during the interview. The doctor must also be constantly aware that the majority of patients are extremely frightened, even though their actual behaviour may range from tongue-tied, tremulous anxiety to the blustering type of patient who insists that he came only because his wife was worried about him! The patient requiring most care, attention and caution is the one who is self-effacing and apologetic for wasting your time; with remarkable regularity these are the patients who have a serious disease.

Every effort should be made to put the patient at ease. Several minutes spent discussing inconsequential subjects such as the weather may seem to be time-wasting to the uninitiated but the relaxation and the insight gained into the patient's mood, his reaction to his disease and his intellectual ability is often greater than one can obtain with several minutes of formal testing, or more direct questioning.

As soon as the patient is talking freely the subject of his symptoms should be introduced. Although a referring letter may be of help in guiding the questioning, it is always important to ask the patient to relate the *entire* history again. Otherwise, half-digested views expressed by other doctors, relatives or workmates may intrude into the history as facts rather than supposition. The importance of cross-checking the history with a relative or friend is vital. In diseases affecting the patient's consciousness or intellect the history may be confused or impossible to obtain without the help of a third party. In other conditions patients frequently understate the duration and severity of their disability and again a completely different story may emerge from enquiries made of a relative. In general these supplementary interviews are best conducted in another room while the patient is undressing, particularly in the case of epileptic attacks in children, where the parents are often loath to reveal any of the details of ictal behaviour in front of the child. Peculiar behaviour traits at any age clearly cannot be discussed easily in front of the patient and a private interview with relatives, fellow-employees and others in contact with the patient is vital.

In all cases an accurate history of the entire course of the illness is essential. The diagnostic differences between weakness of an arm coming on overnight, over a week or over several months are so important that vague statements such as "gradually" should not be accepted at face value. A clerk with a radial nerve palsy present on waking one Sunday morning was cautiously asked if he had been drinking. With considerable reluctance, anxiety and embarrassment he admitted that he had become drunk for the first time in his life the night before. Yet with a single question one could exclude a stroke (the diagnosis made elsewhere) and explain both the aetiology and excellent prognosis of a "Saturday night radial nerve palsy" to the relieved patient.

In many patients bizarre historical events may be deliberately concealed for fear of embarrassment or of moral judgements made by the doctor. The onset of symptoms during sexual activity or alcohol indulgence are frequently suppressed for this reason. The family of an elderly patient with periodic confusion and amnesia (who had been extensively investigated elsewhere) were asked about her drinking habits. An initial angry denial was later retracted following a family conference, with the admission that her wardrobe was full of empty sherry bottles! Considerable tact is called for in these instances and yet the matter must be pursued if unnecessary investigations and incorrect diagnoses are to be avoided.

In neurological medicine, in addition to the importance of making the diagnosis, in many instances the doctor's subsequent role will be to help the patient accept and cope with what may prove to be a lifelong disability. The establishment of an easy confident relationship at the first interview will help ensure a useful supportive role in the future.

When one sees the comment "hopeless historian" on the notes it is really as much a comment on the doctor taking the history! The doctor must tailor the interview to suit the patient and the skill to do this can only be acquired; it cannot be taught. The ability to sit back and listen does not come easily to many, but it is only the eventual realisation that one cannot force the pace of an interview without losing much of value that leads to the ability to take a good history.

The circumlocutory historian and the patient who insists on including irrelevant detail can be the most trying of all. Any attempt to alter the line of questioning will start another sequence of irrelevances. It is best to sit and listen and wait for the useful pieces of information to emerge. These are often the facts regarded as the least important by the patient! Considering how infinitely variable symptoms could be, it is amazing how often patients eventually describe their feelings and symptoms in almost identical phrases. The diagnosis of several classical syndromes depends on typical symptom descriptions. For example, the "red hot needle" jabs of pain in tic douloureux; the feeling of "déjà vu" often associated with temporal lobe attacks, or the "icy cold bandage around the waist or legs" described by patients with spinal cord lesions. Some of the feelings are so bizarre that the patient hesitates to describe them for fear of being accused of imagining things. A useful rule in neurology is that the more bizarre and unusual a symptom, the more likely it is to be organic. An arrogant approach—assuming that a symptom which is not known to the examiner must be functional or imaginary—is very likely to lead to misdiagnosis. It is dangerous to presume universal knowledge.

The above suggestions may not appeal to those who think that a doctor ought not to adopt a passive role and who see themselves as too busy and too important to be slowed down by vague patients. Such a person would be ill advised to embark on a career in neurology.

The usual sequence of a medical consultation is that the history leads on to the physical examination. It is only at this stage that the full value of the history becomes apparent. If a *full* neurological examination were performed on each patient it would take up to an hour for its completion and would prove extremely boring. The history serves to indicate those parts of the examination that should be performed with special care, skill and finesse. Few would perform exactly the same physical examination on a patient with headache as they would on a patient with pain in the leg, and yet the ability to tailor the examination to the situation is based entirely on the history. If a confident diagnosis of the site and probable nature of the lesion has not been made by the completion of the history it is very unlikely that the diagnosis will suddenly become apparent during the physical examination.

Having made a provisional diagnosis based on the history, the physical examination should be performed in the same relaxed way. A warm room with reasonable privacy is essential for a neurological examination. Although the doctor is accustomed to the sight of a tendon hammer and tuning fork, he must remember that the patient may not have seen either previously. He should always explain what he is about to do *before* doing it. Suddenly flashing a light in the patient's eyes or sticking a pin into a limb without warning hardly inspires patient confidence or patient co-operation. When attempting to elicit the plantar responses the examiner should warn the patient that it will hurt. Patients will tolerate considerable discomfort if invited to do so, but do not take kindly to unannounced aggression! Elicitation of both the supinator and ankle jerks is quite painful for the patient and yet one sees doctors repeatedly striking the tendon and wondering why the patient will not relax. Notes such as "patient will not relax" or "plantars impossible" can usually be regarded as due to poor examination technique rather than an adverse comment on the patient's co-operation.

The correct method of performing the various parts of the neurological examination will be detailed in the following chapters. This will always be in the setting of diseases that actually cause abnormalities.

In the author's view the only way to understand the mechanism and correct elicitation of physical signs is in relation to the situation where correct technique actually matters. For example, in a patient with backache, correct testing of the corneal response may not be critical, but in a patient with a giddy attack, facial weakness or face pain, the sign must be understood and elicited correctly, as the depression or absence of a corneal response may be the only physical sign of an underlying lesion in the cerebellopontine angle.

Throughout this book the emphasis is on the recognition of the diagnostic features in the history, and the planning of the clinical examination to confirm or refute the provisional diagnosis *at the bedside*. The ultimate objective is to arrive at the correct diagnosis in the least number of moves and at the least risk to the patient; this must always be the overriding consideration.

Chapter 2

THE PUPILS AND THEIR REACTIONS

Due to the long intracranial and extracranial courses of the nerve pathways controlling the size and reactions of the pupils, lesions in many areas may cause pupillary abnormalities. Important differential diagnostic information may easily be overlooked by a cursory examination of the pupils or unnecessary investigations may be performed when a physiological inequality in pupil size is mistaken for a physical sign. In the unconscious patient the size and reactions of the pupils are of paramount importance in both diagnosis and minute-to-minute management of the patient.

BASIC EXAMINATION TECHNIQUE

1. The size, shape and symmetry of the pupils in moderate lighting conditions should be noted.

2. The direct and indirect responses of the pupils to a bright light should be elicited. An inadequate light source is the most frequent cause of absence of the light reflexes. The direct light reflex is the constriction of the pupil that occurs when it is directly illuminated. The indirect response or consensual light reflex is the simultaneous constriction of the opposite pupil.

3. The accommodation reaction should be tested. This reaction is the constriction of the pupil that automatically occurs as the patient attempts to converge the eyes. Failure to elicit this response is usually due to the patient's failure to converge the eyes. Convergence is most easily achieved if the patient tries to look at the end of his own nose, or at the examiner's finger brought in from below the line of the nose. The majority of people find it much easier to converge while looking downwards. It is helpful if the examiner holds the patient's eyelids up so that the pupils can be easily observed.

General Considerations

1. It is essential to establish whether any drops have been put in the patient's eyes. Many patients have been investigated for what later proved to be pharmacological pupillary inequality because of a failure to observe this simple rule.

2. If the pupils are unequal it is important to decide *which* is abnormal. A frequent mistake is to investigate for the cause of a dilated pupil on one side when the patient actually has a constricted pupil on the other side due to a Horner's syndrome!

3. If the pupils are unequal in size there are two additional features that may help establish the cause. If there is ptosis of the eyelid on the side of the *small* pupil the patient has a Horner's syndrome on that side. If there is ptosis on the side of the *large* pupil the patient has a partial third nerve lesion on that side. The light reflex and accommodation reflexes will be normal in Horner's syndrome and impaired in a partial third nerve lesion. In the absence of ptosis if both pupils react normally to light and accommodation the patient has "physiological anisocoria" (i.e. he has probably always had pupillary inequality). Many normal people have slight asymmetry in the size of the pupils.

4. Whenever a patient is found to have a widely dilated pupil that is fixed to light and accommodation without ptosis, the possibility that the patient has deliberately instilled atropine drops into the eye should always be considered. The writer has encountered this situation twice; both the patients were nurses.

5. Pupils are usually small in infancy, become larger in adolescence and are "normal" size in adulthood. In old age they again become small and the light reaction is accordingly difficult to see. Many elderly patients are incorrectly suspected of having Argyll–Robertson pupils because of this normal change in pupil size with age which is called "senile miosis" (miosis—pupillary constriction; mydriasis—pupillary dilation).

6. The pupils of many patients show a phasic constriction and dilation to light of constant intensity. This phenomenon is called "hippus" and has no definite pathological significance.

PUPIL SIZE AND REACTIONS

Pupil size is controlled by a ring of constrictor fibres innervated by the parasympathetic nervous system and a ring of radially arranged dilator fibres controlled by the sympathetic nervous system.

The resting size of the pupil is governed by the amount of light falling on either eye and depends on the integrity of the parasympathetic nerves. Increased activity in the sympathetic is reflected in slight pupillary dilation as occurs in an anxiety state. It is unusual for changes in pupil size to affect vision so that the majority of pupillary abnormalities are asymptomatic.

Parasympathetic Pathways (Figure 2.1)

The intensity of light falling on the retina is conveyed in the optic nerve to the optic chiasm. The impulses are then split and conveyed in *both* optic tracts to *both* lateral geniculate bodies. Some ten per cent of the fibres reaching the geniculate bodies subserve the light reflex and are relayed in the periaqueductal grey to both Edinger—Westphal nuclei and therefore light falling on *either* eye inevitably excites *both* nuclei and causes constriction of *both* pupils—the anatomical basis of the consensual light reflex.

The Edinger—Westphal nuclei are also stimulated by activity in the adjacent third nerve nuclear mass which controls the medial rectus muscles. therefore when both medial rectus muscles are activated in an attempt to converge the eyes, the Edinger—Westphal nuclei become active and constrict the pupils, this being the suggested basis of the accommodation reflex.

The parasympathetic fibres are carried in the third nerve to the orbit; and lie in a superficial and dorsal position which may explain the variable abnormalities of the pupil in third nerve palsies to be discussed later (Figure 2.1A).

The final relay of the pathway is in the ciliary ganglion in the posterior orbit, which gives origin to eight to ten short ciliary nerves, which sub-divide into sixteen to twenty branches, that pass around the eye to reach the constrictor muscle of the pupil.

Clinical Lesions affecting the Parasympathetic Control of the Pupil

1. The light reflex and the resting size of the pupil depend on adequate light perception by at least one eye. There is *no* direct light reaction in a completely blind eye, but the resting pupil size will be the same as the pupil size in the intact eye. If both eyes are blind both pupils will be dilated and fixed to light *if* the cause is located anterior to the lateral geniculate bodies. If, however, bilateral blindness is the result of destruction of the occipital cortex the light reflex pathways will be intact. Therefore, it is possible for a patient to be completely blind with preserved light reflexes in both eyes. Furthermore, if there is *any* perception of light in an eye that is for practical purposes blind, the light reaction may well be intact.

Lesions in the retina, optic nerve and chiasm and the optic tract of minimal degree, in particular optic nerve damage due to multiple sclerosis, cause what is known as an "afferent pathway lesion". This results in an abnormal pupillary response known as the Marcus Gunn pupil. When the normal eye is stimulated by a bright light there is no abnormality. When the affected eye is stimulated the reaction is slower, less complete, and so brief that the pupil may start to dilate again (the pupillary escape phenomena). The reaction is best seen if the light is rapidly alternated from one eye to the other, each stimulus lasting about a second with two or three seconds between. The reaction is thought to be due to a reduction in the number of fibres subserving the light reflex on the affected side.

2. A lesion of one optic tract does not affect the resting size of the pupil due to the consensual light reflex. In this situation a better light reflex may be seen if the light is shone on the intact half of the retina (see Chapter 3 for details of the field defect). This is called the Wernicke pupil reaction. It is very difficult to elicit this sign due to dispersion of light in the eye.

3. Lesions compressing or infiltrating the tectum of the mid-brain (the area of the superior collicular bodies) will interfere with the decussating light reflex fibres in the periaqueductal area. This results in pupils that are dilated and fixed to light. This is often coupled with loss of upward gaze and is known as the Parinaud syndrome (see Chapter 7).

4. The Argyll—Robertson pupil is also traditionally ascribed to damage in the periaqueductal area. The typical Argyll—Robertson pupil is small, irregular and fixed to light, but reacts to accommodation. It is the latter feature that suggests that the light pathways leading to the Edinger—Westphal nuclei are damaged, but this cannot explain the small size of the pupil or its irregularity. It is also worth noting that accommodation is a much stronger stimulus to pupillo-constriction than light and the apparent dissociation may merely reflect very minimal pupil reactivity. It has been suggested that a local lesion of the iris must be responsible. (The Argyll—Robertson pupil reaction is a classical sign of meningo-vascular syphilis.) Other causes of Argyll—Robertson pupils are pinealomas, diabetes and brain stem encephalitis. These conditions usually cause fixed *dilated* pupils; a *small* irregular fixed pupil is usually due to neurosyphilis. The Argyll—Robertson pupil cannot be dilated by atropine (Figure 2.2). Other causes of small pupils that are apparently fixed to light include senile miosis and the instillation of pilocarpine drops in the treatment of glaucoma.

5. Epidemic encephalitis lethargica, which last occurred in the 1920s, caused many cases of Parkinsonism associated with loss of the ability to converge the eyes. This disability produced pupils that reacted to light but not to accommodation. This "reversed" Argyll—Robertson pupil has become a clinical rarity.

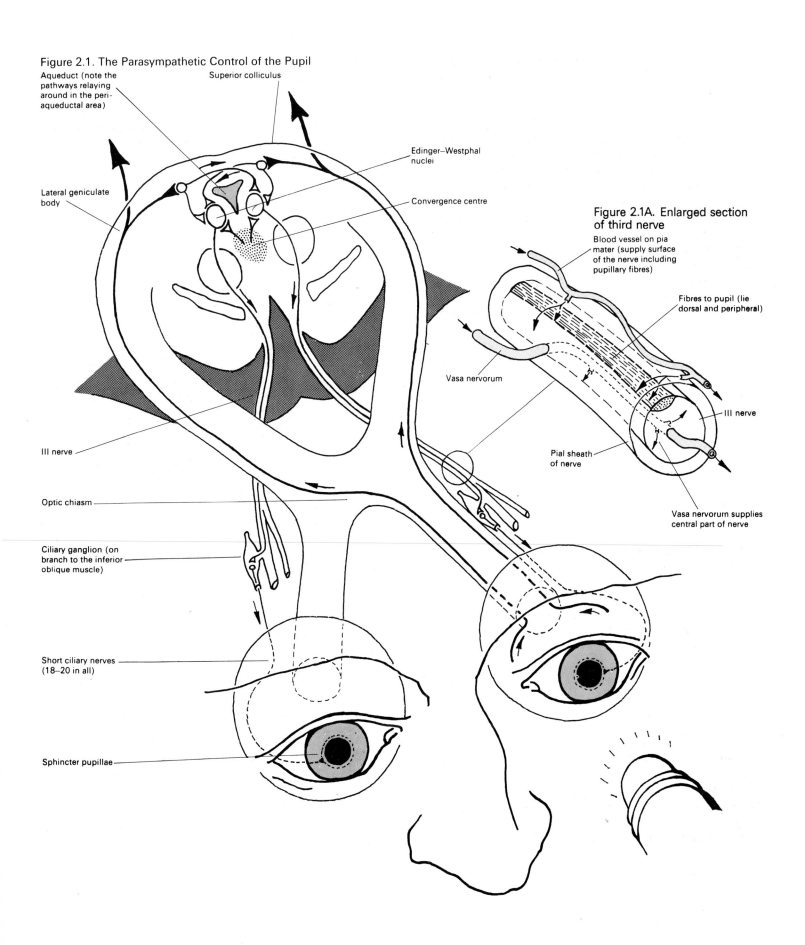

Figure 2.1. The Parasympathetic Control of the Pupil

Aqueduct (note the pathways relaying around in the peri-aqueductal area)

Superior colliculus

Edinger–Westphal nuclei

Lateral geniculate body

Convergence centre

Figure 2.1A. Enlarged section of third nerve

Blood vessel on pia mater (supply surface of the nerve including pupillary fibres)

Fibres to pupil (lie dorsal and peripheral)

Vasa nervorum

III nerve

III nerve

Pial sheath of nerve

Vasa nervorum supplies central part of nerve

Optic chiasm

Ciliary ganglion (on branch to the inferior oblique muscle)

Short ciliary nerves (18–20 in all)

Sphincter pupillae

Figure 2.2. Argyll—Robertson Pupil

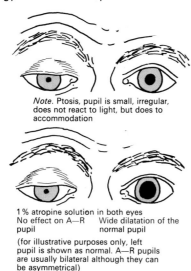

Note. Ptosis, pupil is small, irregular, does not react to light, but does to accommodation

1 % atropine solution in both eyes
No effect on A—R pupil   Wide dilatation of the normal pupil

(for illustrative purposes only, left pupil is shown as normal. A—R pupils are usually bilateral although they can be asymmetrical)

Figure 2.3. Holmes—Adie Pupil

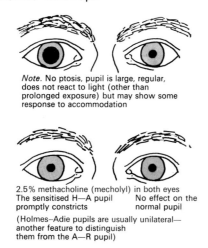

Note. No ptosis, pupil is large, regular, does not react to light (other than prolonged exposure) but may show some response to accommodation

2.5% methacholine (mecholyl) in both eyes
The sensitised H—A pupil promptly constricts   No effect on the normal pupil

(Holmes—Adie pupils are usually unilateral— another feature to distinguish them from the A—R pupil)

6. Lesions affecting the third nerve may or may not involve the pupillary fibres. This is of great differential diagnostic value and will be discussed in detail in Chapter 5. At this point it is sufficient to note that if the nerve trunk is infarcted the superficial pupillary fibres may well be spared. As a general rule, if the pupil is affected the cause is surgical (i.e. compressive); and, if spared, the cause is medical (either diabetes, meningovascular syphilis or arteriosclerosis). The whole investigative approach to the patient with a third nerve lesion is influenced by the state of the pupil.

7. Degeneration of the nerve cells in the ciliary ganglion causes a Holmes—Adie or "tonic" pupil. The cause of this condition is unknown but it is often associated with loss of knee jerks and impairment of sweating. The Holmes—Adie pupil is a widely dilated, circular pupil that may react very slowly to very bright light, and shows a more definite response to accommodation. This dissociation again probably demonstrates the greater constrictive effect of accommodation. Both reactions are minimal and thought to be produced by slow inhibition of the sympathetic and *not* by any residual parasympathetic activity. The Holmes—Adie pupil is usually unilateral and more frequently found in females. It is often unnecessarily confused with Argyll—Robertson pupils which are small, irregular and usually bilateral. Congenital syphilis can cause fixed dilated pupils, but these are bilateral and other signs of congenital neurosyphilis will usually be found.

Confirmation of the diagnosis is best made by the pupillary response to $2\frac{1}{2}$ per cent methacholine drops. This chemical is too rapidly hydrolysed by acetylcholine-esterase to have any effect in the normal eye. In the denervated pupil, post-denervation hypersensitivity (due to enzyme depletion) allows the pupillo-constrictor effect to be seen. It has recently been shown that 80 per cent of diabetic patients react to methacholine in this way and 8 per cent of normal subjects also show a response. Therefore the test cannot be regarded as entirely specific for the Holmes—Adie pupil (Figure 2.3).

8. Blunt trauma to the iris may disrupt the fine short ciliary nerve filaments in the sclera causing an irregularly dilated pupil with impairment of the light reaction. A history of trauma is diagnostic. This is called post-traumatic iridoplegia (paralysis of the iris).

9. Diphtheria is a rare cause of pupillary dilatation due to damage to the ciliary nerves. It usually occurs in the second and third weeks of the illness and is often combined with the palatal paralysis. The pupillary abnormality usually recovers.

Sympathetic Pathway

The course of the cervical sympathetic pathway is shown in Figure 2.4. Although the pathway apparently starts in the hypothalamus there is a considerable degree of *ipsilateral* cortical control (see Chapter 10). A lesion anywhere in the pathway on the right side will affect the right pupil. There are three neurones. The first passes from the hypothalamus to the lateral grey in the thoracic spinal cord; the second from the spinal cord to the superior cervical ganglion and the third from the superior cervical ganglion to the pupil and blood vessels of the eye.

Figure 2.4. Horner's Syndrome

(showing the complete course of the sympathetic and pathological lesions and their sites of occurrence)

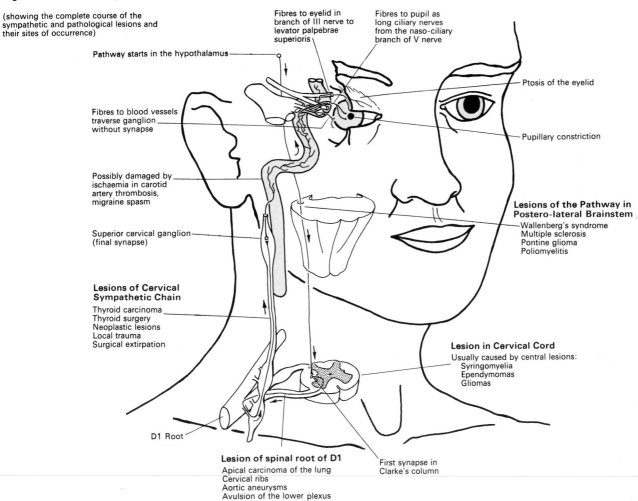

Fibres to eyelid in branch of III nerve to levator palpebrae superioris

Fibres to pupil as long ciliary nerves from the naso-ciliary branch of V nerve

Pathway starts in the hypothalamus

Ptosis of the eyelid

Fibres to blood vessels traverse ganglion without synapse

Pupillary constriction

Possibly damaged by ischaemia in carotid artery thrombosis, migraine spasm

Lesions of the Pathway in Postero-lateral Brainstem
Wallenberg's syndrome
Multiple sclerosis
Pontine glioma
Poliomyelitis

Superior cervical ganglion (final synapse)

Lesions of Cervical Sympathetic Chain
Thyroid carcinoma
Thyroid surgery
Neoplastic lesions
Local trauma
Surgical extirpation

Lesion in Cervical Cord
Usually caused by central lesions:
Syringomyelia
Ependymomas
Gliomas

D1 Root

Lesion of spinal root of D1
Apical carcinoma of the lung
Cervical ribs
Aortic aneurysms
Avulsion of the lower plexus

First synapse in Clarke's column

The third neurone enters the cranial cavity on the surface of the carotid artery and reaches the eye and eyelid as follows:

1. Fibres carried in the third nerve innervate the levator muscle of the eyelid.
2. Fibres in the nasociliary nerve traverse the ciliary ganglion without synapse to supply the blood vessels of the eye.
3. Other fibres branch from the nasociliary nerve as the long ciliary nerves to innervate the pupil by passing around the eye.

Abnormalities of the Sympathetic Pathway

Wherever the site of the lesion, a single physical sign results from damage to the sympathetic pathway and is known as Horner's syndrome. Associated physical signs allow the location of the causative lesion to be identified in some cases.

Horner's syndrome can be extremely subtle and the sign is easily overlooked by the less than obsessional examiner.

The features are as follows:

1. The affected pupil is slightly smaller than its fellow, due to reduced pupillodilator activity. This asymmetry is minimal in a bright light and exaggerated in darkness. The pupil reacts *normally* to light and accommodation but over a reduced range.
2. There is a variable degree of ptosis of the eyelid. In severe cases the lid may reach to the edge of the pupil, in other patients the ptosis may be barely detectable; and may vary from time to time during the day.

3. The conjunctiva may be slightly bloodshot (loss of vasoconstrictor activity).
4. Sweating over the forehead may be impaired, depending on the site of the lesion (see later).
5. In congenital Horner's syndrome the iris on the affected side fails to become pigmented and remains a blue-grey colour.
6. Enopthalmos (sunken eye) is not an easily detected feature of Horner's syndrome in man.

Causes of Horner's Syndrome

1. *Hemisphere Lesions*

Hemispherectomy or massive infarction of one hemisphere may cause a Horner's syndrome on the same side.

2. *Brain Stem Lesions*

The sympathetic pathways in the brain stem lie adjacent to the spinothalamic tract throughout its course. Hence Horner's syndrome due to a brain stem lesion is often associated with pain and temperature loss on the opposite side of the body. Vascular lesions, multiple sclerosis, pontine gliomas, and brain stem encephalitis may all cause a Horner's syndrome at this level (see Chapter 11).

3. *Cervical Cord Lesions*

Due to the central position of the pathway in the lateral column at D1 level the sympathetic is often involved in central cord lesions. Syringomyelia, cord gliomas or ependymomas will usually cause loss of pain sensation in the arms, loss of arm reflexes and often a *bilateral* Horner's syndrome. This can be very hard to detect as it is only the ptosis that draws attention to the condition—the pupils being small, but symmetrical and reactive! (see Chapter 15).

4. *D1 Root Lesions*

The D1 root is rarely affected by simple disc lesions, or degenerative disc disease. The root lies on the apical pleura where it may be damaged by primary or metastatic malignant disease. The classical syndrome of Pancoast, usually due to a cancer of the lung apex, consists of pain in the axilla, wasting of the small hand muscles and a Horner's syndrome, all on the same side. Other causes include cervical rib (usually in young females) and avulsion of the lower brachial plexus (Klumpke's paralysis). (See Chapter 18.)

5. *The Sympathetic Chain*

Throughout its course in the neck the sympathetic may be damaged by neoplastic infiltration, during surgical procedures on the larynx or thyroid, or surgically extirpated for a

Figure 2.5. Horner's Syndrome

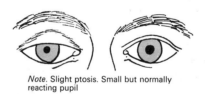

Note. Slight ptosis. Small but normally reacting pupil

Peripheral Lesion
(above superior cervical ganglion)

Cocaine 4% in both eyes

No effect as amine oxidase depleted due to post-ganglionic denervation

Dilates the normal pupil

Adrenaline 1:1000 in both eyes

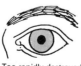

Marked effect as adrenaline is not destroyed by amine-oxidase. Even the lid will elevate

Too rapidly destroyed by amine-oxidase to have any effect

Central Lesion
(below superior cervical ganglion)

Cocaine 4% in both eyes

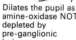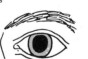

Dilates the pupil as amine-oxidase NOT depleted by pre-ganglionic lesion

Dilates the normal pupil

Adrenaline 1:1000 in both eyes

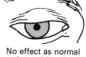

No effect as normal amine-oxidase levels still present

No effect on the normal pupil

number of indications. Malignant disease in the jugular foramen at the skull base causes various combinations of Horner's syndrome and lesions of cranial nerves IX, X, XI and XII (see Chapter 6).

6. *Miscellaneous*

Congenital Horner's syndrome is not rare and has been mentioned previously. Horner's syndrome may occur during migraine headache. Lesions in the cavernous sinus or orbit usually damage both the sympathetic and the parasympathetic leading to a semi-dilated pupil that is fixed to light combined with other extra-ocular nerve palsies (see Chapter 5).

Other Features of Horner's Syndrome

The associated physical signs or history usually leave little doubt as to the site and cause of Horner's syndrome. There are some other useful diagnostic pointers.

Central lesions usually affect sweating over the entire head, neck, arm and upper trunk on the same side. Lesions in the lower neck affect sweating over the entire face. Lesions above the superior cervical ganglion may not affect sweating at all, as the main outflow to the facial blood vessels and sweat glands is below the superior-cervical ganglion.

The presence of three neurones in the pathway leads to some useful pharmacological tests based on the phenomenon of denervation hypersensitivity.

The decrease in amine-oxidase caused by a lesion at or beyond the superior cervical ganglion, sensitises the pupil to adrenaline 1:1,000, which has no effect on the normal pupil.

Conversely, the effect of cocaine on the pupil *depends* on its blocking effect on amine-oxidase, therefore cocaine has no effect on a distally denervated pupil. It will only dilate the pupil in a Horner's syndrome if the lesion is below the superior cervical ganglion and there is amine-oxidase at the nerve endings for it to block.

These tests may be useful in the absence of other localising neurological signs in indicating the approximate site of the lesion. The pattern of responses are summarised in Figure 2.5.

PUPILLARY ABNORMALITIES IN THE UNCONSCIOUS PATIENT

The management of head injuries and the unconscious patient are discussed in Chapter 23.

1. *Normally Reacting Equal Pupils*

In an unconscious patient normal pupils are a reassuring sign indicating that no immediate surgical action is necessary. In the absence of a history of head trauma an immediate search for metabolic causes of coma should be initiated. Seventy per cent of unconscious patients have *not* had an intra-cranial catastrophe, but are in diabetic coma, hypoglycaemic coma, other metabolic coma, or have taken a drug overdose. Normal pupillary reactions are an important pointer to these possibilities. Only glutethamide and amphetamine (dilated pupils) or opiates (constricted pupils) cause misleading pupillary changes.

Table 1

PUPILLARY ABNORMALITIES		
Reaction to Light	*Small Pupils*	*Large Pupils*
Non-reactive	A–R pupil	Holmes–Adie pupil
	Pontine haemorrhage	Post-traumatic iridoplegia
	Opiates	Mydriatic drops
	Pilocarpine drops	Glutethamide overdose
		Cerebral death
		Atropine poisoning
		Amphetamine overdose
Reactive	Old age	Childhood
	Horner's syndrome	Anxiety
		Physiological anisocoria

2. *Unequal Pupils*

This is the single most important physical sign in the unconscious patient. Until proved otherwise a dilated pupil indicates that a herniated temporal lobe is stretching the third nerve on that side and prompt surgical action is required. Problems occur if the eye was directly damaged in the injury, or if someone has put mydriatic drops in the eye in the pointless search for papilloedema (pointless because patients with acute head injury will die long before papilloedema can appear).

3. *Bilateral Dilated Pupils*

The final stage of progressive tentorial herniation is heralded by progressive dilatation of the previously unaffected pupil. The chances of the patient recovering from this stage are remote. This is also used as one of the signs of irreversible cerebral damage in cardiac arrest. Glutethamide, atropine (mushroom) and amphetamine poisoning are the only metabolic causes of bilateral dilated pupils.

4. *Bilateral Pin-point Pupils*

This situation is the hall-mark of another lethal neurological situation; a massive intra-pontine haemorrhage which is usually accompanied by pin-point pupils, deep coma and a spastic tetraparesis with brisk reflexes. Opiates produce similar pupillary abnormalities but depressed reflexes. In the elderly unconscious patient the possibility that pilocarpine drops have been instilled for glaucoma should be considered in view of the hopeless prognosis if intrapontine haemor-rhage has occurred. Other causes of coma should be rapidly excluded if this is the case.

The pupils should always be examined with the special problems of that particular patient in mind. In this way there is less risk of a subtle abnormality being overlooked and the risk of unnecessary investigation of physiological variations is greatly reduced.

Chapter 3

THE VISUAL FIELDS

The visual pathways extend from the retina to the occipital pole. Part of their course is extra-cerebral and part in the substance of the hemisphere.

Due to the complex but constant decussations and rotations of nerve fibres in the visual pathways, visual field defects can provide very accurate localising information.

Patients tend to notice abrupt visual deterioration and may present with a detailed description of their defect whereas defects of slow onset may develop unnoticed by the patient. A routine examination of the optic fundus, visual acuity and visual fields should be made in all patients with neurological disease. It is unwise to assume that the patient's visual fields are normal because he has no visual symptoms. At the opposite extreme patients with seriously impaired vision require very careful field testing however difficult this may be to perform.

Often in the neurological examination signs are more easily detected if the examiner has some idea as to what he might find, or what he must exclude. The technique and use of confrontation field testing at the bedside is described in detail in relation to the various clinical situations in which field defects may be encountered.

CONFRONTATION TESTING OF THE VISUAL FIELDS

The results of confrontation testing are often recorded in clinical notes somewhat disparagingly as 'fields grossly normal'; as if the test were a poor substitute for more accurate testing. In skilled hands confrontation testing can be as accurate as screen or perimeter testing and in some situations may be the only way that the fields can be tested.

These situations include the examination of patients with a seriously disturbed mental state, physical disability preventing the patient from sitting at the apparatus or a dense central field defect that prevents the patient fixing his eyes on a target object, which is necessary to keep the eye still during testing.

In patients with greatly reduced visual acuity qualitative tests of the fields using hand movements and finger counting can only be performed by confrontation methods.

The Technique (Figure 3.1)

For accurate field testing red and white hatpins of 2 mm. and 5 mm. diameter should be used. Routine screening is usually performed with a 5 mm. white pin. The smaller pins are useful for detecting small scotomata (small field defects in the centre of the visual fields). The red pins are especially useful in testing the visual fields where a compressive lesion of the optic nerve, optic chiasm or optic tract is suspected. In these situations the ability to count fingers (marked CF on a field chart) and to detect hand movements (marked HM on the chart) are also of value.

1. The examiner should sit opposite the patient, ideally in a chair but where circumstances demand one may lean across the bed in front of the patient. Each eye is tested individually and if the examiner routinely holds the patient's other eye shut with his hand held at arm's length, a constant examiner-patient distance is established. An idea of the size of the normal field at this distance is easily acquired and skill in detecting early peripheral field defects is quickly achieved.

2. Throughout the test the patient is asked to look straight at the examiner's eye (the right eye when testing the patient's left eye and vice versa). This ensures that the patient holds his eye still during testing. If the patient cannot see the examiner's eye, he is asked to stare in the direction of the examiner's face while an assessment of the peripheral visual field is made. The examiner is in an ideal position to see if the patient has to move his eye to find the test object.

3. The test pin (usually the 5 mm. white) is brought in along a series of arcs to a point some 18 inches in front of the patient's eye. If an arc from behind were not used the patient's temporal field would extend to infinity if the test object was large enough. The pin should be brought in from "round the corner" of the patient's field—from four directions, NE., SE., SW. and NW. This will be bound to pick up any field defect in either the upper or lower temporal or nasal fields.

4. The close control that the examiner has over the whole proceedings enables quick repeat testing to be performed and "pseudo" field defects due to bushy eyebrows or a large nose are quickly detected. Quite often field defects due to these problems are accidentally recorded on a standard perimeter. Merely tilting the patient's head from the line of the obstructing organ will solve the problem.

5. If any defect is difficult to interpret, on an organic basis, as a cross check on the patient's reliability the patient's blind spot should be found and compared with the examiner's own blind spot.

Figure 3.1. Visual Field Testing by Confrontation

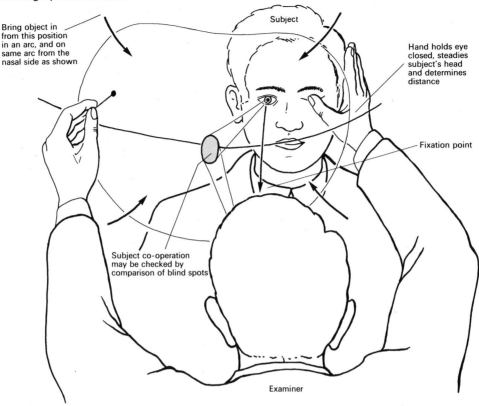

Bring object in from this position in an arc, and on same arc from the nasal side as shown

Subject

Hand holds eye closed, steadies subject's head and determines distance

Fixation point

Subject co-operation may be checked by comparison of blind spots

Examiner

The results should be recorded *as seen by the patient* which means reversing the defect as seen by the examiner during confrontation testing. To further avoid confusion the right and left fields should be clearly indicated and a factual note added as to the nature of the field defect made; i.e. right homonymous hemianopia, or bitemporal upper quadrantic hemianopia etc. The different terms are illustrated in Figure 3.2.

APPLICATION OF CONFRONTATION TESTING TO SPECIFIC CLINICAL SITUATIONS

1. The Patient who has Noticed a "Hole" in his Vision

Small scotomas are often noticed by accident while the patient is reading a notice or looking at a clock (a scotoma is a small patch of visual loss in the visual field). The onset always appears to be abrupt as it is invariably *noticed* suddenly by the patient. An exception occurs when an embolus impacts in the central retinal artery and then moves peripherally. Abrupt blindness followed by a diminishing

deficit can usually be described on a minute-to-minute basis by an intelligent patient and leaves no doubt as to both the acuteness of onset and the nature of the problem.

Faced with this symptom it is best to allow the patient to find the defect himself by moving the white pin about in his own visual field. Once the position is found the size and shape of the defect can be established by moving the pin in and out of the blind area. Special attention should be paid to whether: (1) the defect crosses the horizontal meridian (retinal lesions due to a vascular occlusion do not do so), (2) the defect extends to the blind spot (defects due to B_{12} deficiency, toxins, or glaucoma usually extend into it), (3) the defect crosses the vertical meridian (organic visual field defects due to pathway damage usually show a sharp vertical edge).

2. The Patient with "Blurred Vision in One Eye"

The examiner should ask the patient to look in the general direction of his eye if the patient's visual acuity is too poor to actually see it. Then, working outwards from the defect with a 5 mm. white pin, the examiner should try to establish the size and shape of the scotoma. If the pin is not seen at all, two

Figure 3.2. Field Defect Nomenclature

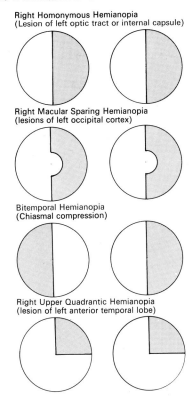

Right Homonymous Hemianopia
(Lesion of left optic tract or internal capsule)

Right Macular Sparing Hemianopia
(lesions of left occipital cortex)

Bitemporal Hemianopia
(Chiasmal compression)

Right Upper Quadrantic Hemianopia
(lesion of left anterior temporal lobe)

or three fingers held still should be tried and finally, if all else fails, a moving hand should be brought in from the periphery. If the examiner can establish that there is a rim of intact peripheral vision, however poor it is, then the patient has a central scotoma, usually implying either retrobulbar neuritis or optic nerve compression (see below). Once a central scotoma in one eye is detected it is essential to test the peripheral field of the *good* eye, looking for a defect in the upper temporal field. If such a defect is present, it is highly likely that the optic nerve is compressed, (see Figure 3.11 for explanation). This is known as a junctional scotoma.

3. The Patient with Sudden Visual Deterioration in Both Eyes

Acute *bilateral* inflammation of the optic nerve (retrobulbar neuritis) may occur but is unusual. The two important conditions to be excluded are severe bilateral papilloedema due to any cause or the rapidly progressive phase of visual deterioration in a patient with optic chiasmal compression.

Papilloedema alone does not affect central vision but when a haemorrhage or exudate occurs into the macula area of the retina rapid visual failure will occur. This possibility can be readily excluded by fundal examination. If sudden deterioration occurs in the course of an ongoing visual failure ophthalmoscopy will often reveal the presence of optic atrophy. If optic atrophy is found, however poor the visual acuity, the fields *must* be tested. Chiasmal compression may be misdiagnosed as retrobulbar neuritis or tobacco amblyopia if the fields are *not* tested. Patients with chiasmal compression often develop severe but unrecognised bitemporal field defects and seek advice only when central vision becomes acutely impaired. If a bitemporal field defect is detected urgent investigation to exclude a lesion compressing the optic chiasm is mandatory.

CASE REPORT

A 36-year-old patient had been investigated for infertility and subsequently became pregnant following the use of Clomiphen. During the pregnancy she became toxaemic with a blood pressure as high as 200/120. In the 34th week she developed rapidly progressive visual failure initially thought to be due to the hypertension. On neurological examination both optic discs were pale but there was no suspicion of papillaedema or haemorrhage into the maculae. Although visual acuity was less than 6/60, using hand movements and finger counting it was obvious that she had a dense bitemporal hemianopia due to chiasmal compression. The child was delivered by caesarean section immediately and the chiasm explored the next day. The remnants of a pituitary tumour were found admixed with blood clots. Following this her vision became normal and the premature infant developed normally. Any delay in recognition of the clinical situation could have resulted in permanent blindness.

Testing for a bitemporal field defect involves the standard routine except that the red pin is particularly helpful. The typical defect resulting from damage to the chiasm is a bitemporal hemianopia. In the early stages this may be a defect to a *red* object only. The patient may describe the red pin as appearing to be grey in the affected half field changing to red as it crosses into the intact nasal half field. Many normal people notice that the red pin is a duller red in the temporal field and that it is appreciably brighter in the nasal field; this is a physiological variation without significance. Later in the course of the disease the defect extends to cause complete loss of recognition of a white pin in the temporal fields and finally finger and even hand movements will not be detected as the defect becomes complete.

Even at this late stage if the chiasm is compressed from below, (by a pituitary lesion) the upper half of the temporal field may be completely lost but some hand movements may be detected in the lower half field, or vice versa in the case of chiasmal compression from above and behind (by a cranio-pharyngioma), (see Figures 3.6 and 3.13 for explanation).

4. The Patient who Complains of "Difficulty in Reading" or "Bumps Into Things On One Side"

Quite often patients attend hospital, aware that something is wrong with their vision but unaware that they have a dense homonymous field defect. Some patients insist they are blind in one eye because they cannot see to that side. Blindness in one eye causes impairment of distance perception but the good eye provides a full field of vision to both sides. Patients complain bitterly that they cannot read if the visual defect splits the midline. If they have a left-sided field defect they cannot find the beginning of the next line, or if the defect is on the right side, reading may prove impossible as they cannot scan to the next word.

In general, if the patient *is* aware of his visual defect the defect is macular splitting (i.e. bisects the central field). If the patient is unaware of a deficit and merely bumps into things, he may have a macular sparing hemianopia or an attention hemianopia. The latter defect is not an absolute defect but an inability to see in one half field vision when vision is distracted by an object in the other half field (see below).

Testing for an homonymous hemianopia should involve three phases:

1. The examiner should test for an attention field defect. The examiner sits in front of the patient, who should keep both his eyes open; each of the examiner's hands should be held about one foot to the side and eighteen inches in front of each of the patient's eyes. The patient is then asked to point to either hand when he sees the fingers move. At first just one hand should be moved. If the patient consistently fails to see the hand on one side he may well have a full hemianopia, *but* if he sees the fingers move on one hand when they are moved alone but *cannot* see them when both hands are moved simultaneously he has an "attention hemianopia" The anatomical basis for this finding is shown in Figure 3.3.
2. Then formal testing of the whole field in each eye by the standard confrontation technique should be performed to establish whether the patient has a field defect on one or other side.
3. The field must then be evaluated to see if the defect is "macula splitting" or "macula sparing". This is of considerable diagnostic and prognostic importance. Basically, one is looking for a small 5° circle of retained vision in the centre of the hemianopic field. The pin is brought across the midline above and below the centre of vision to detect the midline of the field. Then the pin is brought across on the central meridian. If the pin is detected on the same line as the first two points then the defect splits the macula. If it is about $1\frac{1}{2}$ to 2 inches

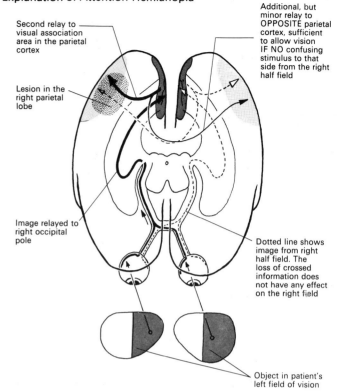

Figure 3.3. Diagram to show the Possible Explanation of Attention Hemianopia

Second relay to visual association area in the parietal cortex

Additional, but minor relay to OPPOSITE parietal cortex, sufficient to allow vision IF NO confusing stimulus to that side from the right half field

Lesion in the right parietal lobe

Image relayed to right occipital pole

Dotted line shows image from right half field. The loss of crossed information does not have any effect on the right field

Object in patient's left field of vision

to the side of the midline then the macula is spared (Figure 3.4). The importance of this distinction is discussed later.

Confrontation testing will establish the basic defect. If there is any doubt about the central field further field testing using the Tangent Screen or an arc or bowl perimeter is necessary.

Visual Evoked Responses (VER)

In the last few years an important advance in the investigation of visual pathway disease has been provided by studying the visual evoked responses.

The technique involves subjecting the eye to a flickering chequer board pattern on an illuminated screen while recording the activity in the visual cortex with occipital surface electrodes. The apparatus is standardised and differences in the latency, size and shape of the potentials recorded indicates damage to one or other optic nerve. It is also a useful test in suspected hysterical blindness. If a patient stares in the direction of the screen a response can be detected indicating intact visual pathways.

Figure 3.4. Diagram to Show the Detection of "Macular-Sparing" During Confrontation Field Testing

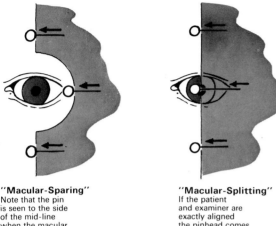

"Macular-Sparing"
Note that the pin
is seen to the side
of the mid-line
when the macular
is spared

"Macular-Splitting"
If the patient
and examiner are
exactly aligned
the pinhead comes
into view exactly
in the midline of
the pupil as shown

The pin is brought in from the blind field.
This prevents the patient shifting gaze to
follow the pin—making it difficult to detect
the midline position

THE ANATOMY OF THE VISUAL PATHWAYS

To understand field defects one must understand the apparently intricate anatomy of the pathways. Yet the course of the pathways make considerable sense when understood and the details become easy to remember.

1. The macula of the retina (the most important group of retinal cells, responsible for central vision) is situated to the side of the optic nerve head (it is *not* the nerve head itself which is a popular misconception). The fibres have to shift sideways *en masse* to get into the appropriate position in the optic nerve. This causes the macular fibres to crowd into the temporal half of the disc (see Figure 3.5).

2. The macular fibres complete the shift to the centre of the optic nerve as it joins the chiasm. The nerve is then effectively split down the middle. The lateral fibres go straight back into the optic tract on the same side and the medial fibres cross (decussate) to the other side. They do so in important positions which are fully discussed later in the text. The function of the chiasm is to bring the information from the halves of each retina that look to the right and the halves that look to the left together in the same optic tract (Figure 3.6).

3. When information derived exclusively from the left or right side of vision arrives in the optic tract the information is initially conveyed in the inner and outer halves of the tract. Subsequently information from the same point on each retina must be relayed to immediately adjacent parts of the

visual cortex. This process starts with the rotation of the fibres in the optic tract through 90°. This brings the fibres from the lower and upper fields together in the medial and lateral halves of the tract respectively. Then in the posterior tract the fibres fan out towards the six layers of the geniculate body as shown, allowing the adjacent fibres from each retina to interdigitate. The macula fibres occupy a big central wedge of the geniculate body with the lower fields represented medially and the upper fields laterally.

4. The fibres then sweep out into the hemisphere as two diverging fans, which later rejoin to reach the occipital cortex as shown in Figure 3.7. Although this course is almost impossible to indicate diagrammatically the fibres all sweep back into the cortex deep in the substance of the hemisphere; they do not run straight back just under the medial surface. Therefore a lesion at area 5 in Figure 3.7 does *not* damage the fibres to the macular area which lie deep in the substance of the brain at this point.

5. The calcarine or occipital cortex lies astride the calcarine fissure. The cells subserving the peripheral fields lie anteriorly, and those subserving macular vision are concentrated at the extreme tip: the upper fields represented in the lower half and the lower fields in the upper half of the cortex.

VISUAL DEFECTS DUE TO LESIONS AT VARIOUS SITES

1. Retinal Lesions

The retina consists of the retinal nerve cells lying on the choroid at the back of the eye. The nerve fibres from these cells come straight forward and then angle sharply to run on the surface of the retina towards the optic nerve head. They do so in an orderly way as shown in Figure 3.5. The most critical part of the retina is the very densely packed mass of cells known as the macular. The fibres from this area form the papillomacular bundle as they enter the optic nerve. These nerve cells are those most sensitive to a variety of toxins and if damaged a caeco-central scotoma results (see Figure 3.8). The commonest toxin is tobacco. Alcohol, some drugs and Vitamin B_1 and B_{12} deficiencies also cause caeco-central scotomas. Many neurological disorders are associated with retinitis pigmentosa (see Chapter 4). This usually begins as a peripheral retinal cell degeneration, often sparing a ring of peripheral vision. Choroido-retinitis, due to local patches of inflammation of the retina, causes scotomas of shape and size appropriate to the area of damage. A very severe form is juxta-papillary choroido-retinitis in which the damage occurs adjacent to the optic disc and damages incoming

Figure 3.5. Schematic Diagram to Show the Optic Nerve Head and Macula Lutea

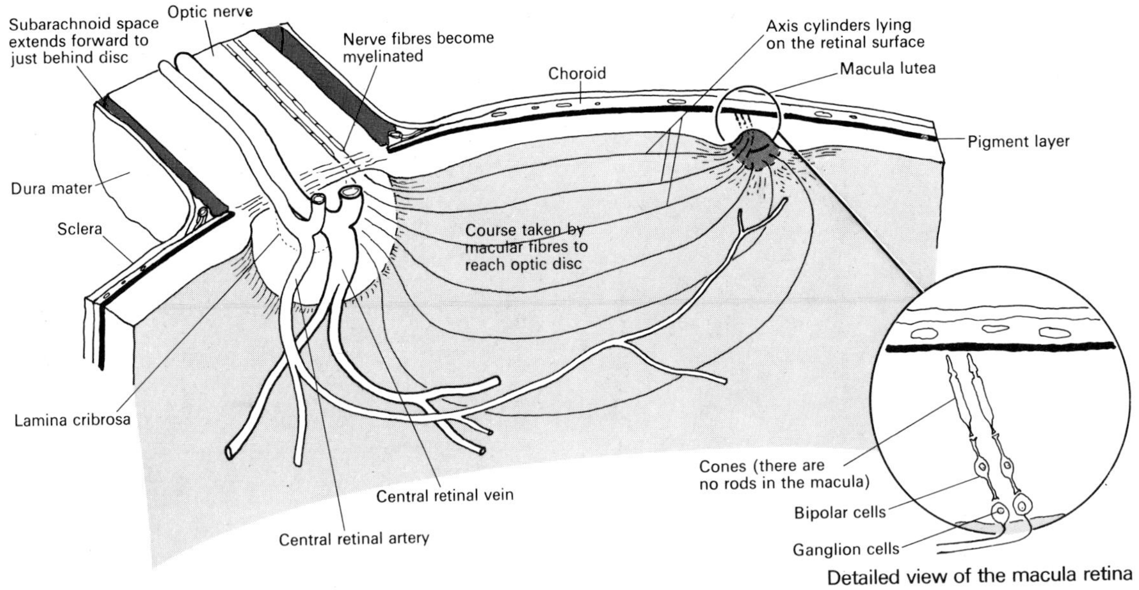

Detailed view of the macula retina

nerve fibres leading to a more serious field defect with an arcuate scotoma typical of nerve bundle damage.

The circulation of the retina is provided by the central retinal artery which divides into upper and lower branches supplying the retina above and below the horizontal median of the eye. Occlusion of a branch, usually by an embolus, causes a defect in the appropriate area that extends only to the horizontal meridian (Figure 3.9).

2. Optic Nerve Head Lesions

Development defects of the disc (colobomata) and hyaline masses that develop during life (drusen) may cause central scotomas or arcuate scotomas if they damage nerve fibre bundles. Glaucoma damages retinal nerve fibres on the disc margins causing arcuate scotomas radiating from the blind spot often initially extending upwards (a Seidel scotoma). This later extends from below the blind spot until complete (a Bjerrum scotoma) (Figure 3.10).

Papilloedema (swelling of the optic nerve head) *may* cause field defects in several ways.

  a. Enlargement of the blind spot due to oedema of adjacent retinal cells directly involved in the disc swelling.

  b. Haemorrhage or exudate into the macula which may cause abrupt visual failure.

  c. Chronic papilloedema may cause progressive gliosis (scarring) of the optic nerve head. Eventually progressive visual failure occurs often starting as per-

ipheral field constriction due to damage to fibres crossing the swollen disc margins.

  d. A dilated third ventricle may splay the chiasm causing a binasal hemianopia (see later).

  e. If the cerebral hemisphere herniates on one side the posterior cerebral artery may be stretched across the tentorial edge—causing a macular sparing hemianopia. This can be a false localising sign (see Chapter 23).

3. Optic Nerve Lesions

a. *Acute Retrobulbar Neuritis*

This is really the universal response of the optic nerve to a variety of toxic and metabolic insults. An attack of retrobulbar neuritis is *not* necessarily synonymous with an attack of multiple sclerosis. The number of patients with retrobulbar neuritis who go on to get other manifestations of multiple sclerosis ranges from fifteen to fifty per cent. In young females the birth control pill has been implicated as a cause of retrobulbar neuritis in some cases.

Symptomatically the patient complains that central vision is impaired by a "fluffy ball", a "puff of smoke", a "steamed up window" or a sensation as if "looking through ground glass", and often claims that if he could "see round it", vision would be normal. The visual acuity is usually impaired down to 6/60 or 6/36 (20/200 in U.S.A.). There may be some discomfort in the eye, especially provoked by movement but this is rarely severe.

Figure 3.6. The Functional Anatomy of the Optic Nerves, Chiasm and Tracts to the Geniculate Body

(It is suggested that the reader starts by reading all the captions to get a general idea of what happens and why. Then individual quadrants of vision, and their pathways should be followed right through from retina to geniculate body. Finally an attempt to work out the effect of lesions at different points can be made and checked against the field defects shown in subsequent figures)

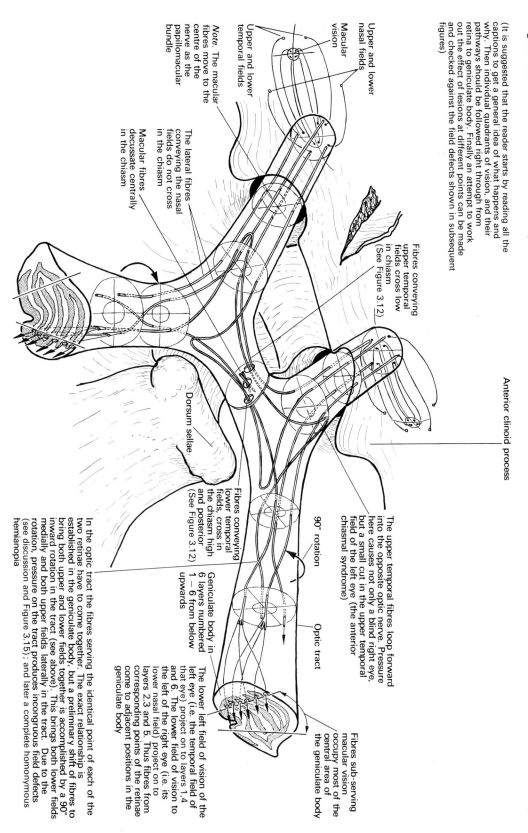

Upper and lower nasal fields

Macular vision

Upper and lower temporal fields

Note. The macular fibres move to the centre of the nerve as the papillomacular bundle

The lateral fibres conveying the nasal fields do not cross in the chiasm

Macular fibres decussate centrally in the chiasm

Fibres conveying upper temporal fields cross low in chiasm (See Figure 3.12)

Dorsum sellae

Fibres conveying lower temporal fields, cross in the chiasm high and posterior (See Figure 3.12)

Anterior clinoid process

The upper temporal fibres loop forward into the opposite optic nerve. Pressure here causes not only a blind right eye, but a small cut in the upper temporal field of the left eye (the anterior chiasmal syndrome)

90° rotation

Optic tract

Fibres sub-serving macular vision occupy most of the central area of the geniculate body

Geniculate body in 6 layers numbered 1 — 6 from below upwards

The lower left field of vision of the left eye (i.e. the temporal field of that eye) project on to layers 1,4 and 6. The lower field of vision to the left of the right eye (i.e. its lower nasal field) project on to layers 2,3 and 5. Thus fibres from corresponding points of the retinae come to adjacent positions in the geniculate body

In the optic tract the fibres serving the identical point of each of the two retinae have to come together. The exact relationship is established in the geniculate body, but a preliminary shift of fibres to bring both upper and lower fields together is accomplished by a 90° inward rotation in the tract (see above). This brings both lower fields medially and both upper fields laterally in the tract. Due to the rotation, pressure on the tract produces incongruous field defects (see discussion and Figure 3.15); and later a complete homonymous hemianopia

Figure 3.7. The Visual Radiations and Field Defects

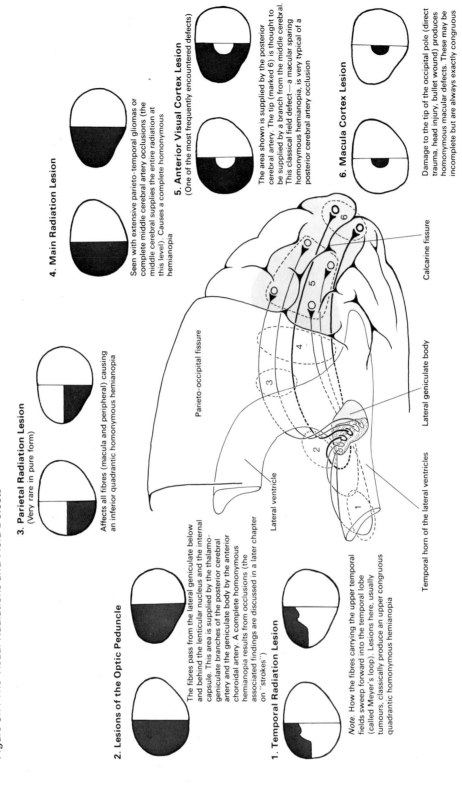

3. **Parietal Radiation Lesion**
(Very rare in pure form)

Affects all fibres (macula and peripheral) causing an inferior quadrantic homonymous hemianopia

2. **Lesions of the Optic Peduncle**

The fibres pass from the lateral geniculate below and behind the lenticular nucleus and the internal capsule. This area is supplied by the thalamo-geniculate branches of the posterior cerebral artery and the geniculate body by the anterior choroidal artery. A complete homonymous hemianopia results from occlusions (the associated findings are discussed in a later chapter on "strokes").

1. **Temporal Radiation Lesion**

Note. How the fibres carrying the upper temporal fields sweep forward into the temporal lobe (called Meyer's loop). Lesions here, usually tumours, classically produce an upper congruous quadrantic homonymous hemianopia

4. **Main Radiation Lesion**

Seen with extensive parieto-temporal gliomas or complete middle cerebral artery occlusions (the middle cerebral supplies the entire radiation at this level). Causes a complete homonymous hemianopia

5. **Anterior Visual Cortex Lesion**
(One of the most frequently encountered defects)

The area shown is supplied by the posterior cerebral artery. The tip (marked 6) is thought to be supplied by a branch from the middle cerebral. This classical field defect—a macular sparing homonymous hemianopia, is very typical of a posterior cerebral artery occlusion

6. **Macula Cortex Lesion**

Damage to the tip of the occipital pole (direct trauma, head injury, bullet wound) produces homonymous macular defects. These may be incomplete but are always exactly congruous

Parieto-occipital fissure

Calcarine fissure

Lateral ventricle

Lateral geniculate body

Temporal horn of the lateral ventricles

Figure 3.8. Toxic Amblyopia

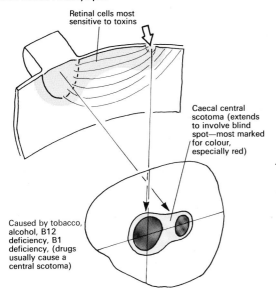

Retinal cells most sensitive to toxins

Caecal central scotoma (extends to involve blind spot—most marked for colour, especially red)

Caused by tobacco, alcohol, B12 deficiency, B1 deficiency, (drugs usually cause a central scotoma)

Figure 3.10. Glaucoma

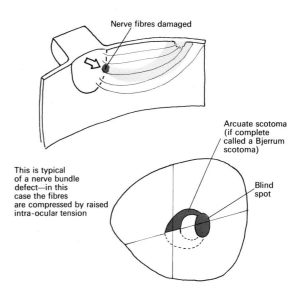

Nerve fibres damaged

Arcuate scotoma (if complete called a Bjerrum scotoma)

This is typical of a nerve bundle defect—in this case the fibres are compressed by raised intra-ocular tension

Blind spot

The majority recover within ten to fourteen days, especially those cases due to multiple sclerosis. In cases due to toxic causes recovery may not occur.

The field defect is a central scotoma most marked to a red pin, but a full recovery of the visual field to all colours usually occurs.

Figure 3.9. Retinal Artery Branch Occlusion

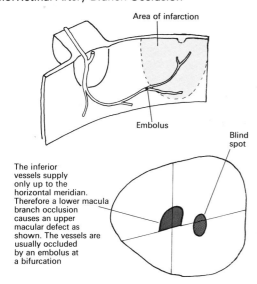

Area of infarction

Embolus

Blind spot

The inferior vessels supply only up to the horizontal meridian. Therefore a lower macula branch occlusion causes an upper macular defect as shown. The vessels are usually occluded by an embolus at a bifurcation

In the acute stage the optic disc appears normal unless the inflammation is just behind the nerve head when "papillitis" with swelling of the nerve head is seen. This is distinguished from papilloedema by the severe loss of visual acuity, as vision remains normal in the case of papilloedema unless special complications occur (see above).

b. *Optic Nerve Compression* (Figure 3.11)

The papillo-macular bundle conveying central vision is the part of the optic nerve that is most vulnerable to extrinsic compression. Hence a compressive lesion tends to cause a central scotoma and not a field defect spreading in from the periphery as might be anticipated on purely anatomical grounds.

The central defect may develop so slowly that the patient discovers the loss of vision by accident when grit or soap gets into the good eye. A useful distinction from retrobulbar neuritis is that on fundal examination in such a case, there is often well-marked optic atrophy present when the visual deficit is first discovered, whereas in acute retrobulbar neuritis, optic atrophy usually takes several weeks to appear.

CASE REPORT

A 28-year-old Italian chef in London went to Italy on holiday. He borrowed a friend's motor scooter and was riding along without protective goggles. Some grit flew into his left eye. He put his hand

Figure 3.11. Intracranial Optic Nerve Compression

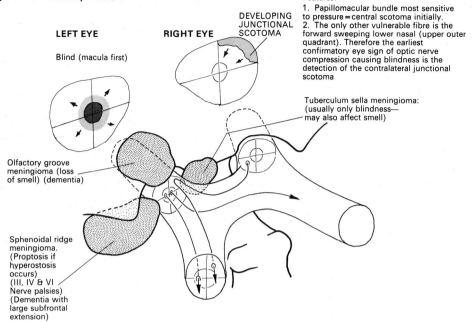

LEFT EYE   RIGHT EYE

DEVELOPING JUNCTIONAL SCOTOMA

Blind (macula first)

Features:
1. Papillomacular bundle most sensitive to pressure = central scotoma initially.
2. The only other vulnerable fibre is the forward sweeping lower nasal (upper outer quadrant). Therefore the earliest confirmatory eye sign of optic nerve compression causing blindness is the detection of the contralateral junctional scotoma

Tuberculum sella meningioma: (usually only blindness— may also affect smell)

Olfactory groove meningioma (loss of smell) (dementia)

Sphenoidal ridge meningioma. (Proptosis if hyperostosis occurs) (III, IV & VI Nerve palsies) (Dementia with large subfrontal extension)

up to his eye and discovered he could not see. He had accidentally discovered he had become blind in the right eye. This proved to be due to optic nerve compression by a meningioma.

Any central scotoma that is discovered accidentally or any "acute retrobulbar neuritis" that does not recover should be regarded as due to optic nerve compression until proved otherwise.

An important part of the initial and follow-up examinations is a search for an early field cut in the opposite eye due to damage to the decussating fibres that loop forward into the optic nerve. This is known as the anterior chiasmal Syndrome of Traquir.

In all cases the sense of smell and the functioning of cranial nerves III, V, VI and the corneal reflex should be carefully tested.

c. *Optic Nerve Glioma*

Malignant gliomas in the optic nerve, optic chiasm or optic tract mainly occur in children or in patients with neurofibromatosis. The visual defect produced by a glioma in the optic nerve is usually a "hole" in vision which may occur anywhere in the field. Optic atrophy is usually well established by the time that the defect is noticed and x-rays may reveal evidence of enlargement of one or both optic foraminae. Gliomas in the optic chiasm or optic tract produce the typical field defects of lesions in these areas.

d. *Metastatic Disease*

The optic nerve may be secondarily involved by local or remote malignant disease including the malignant lymphomas.

4. Optic Chiasm Lesions

The anatomy of the chiasm has already been indicated in detail in Figure 3.6. From a practical point of view four anatomical features are important.

a. The optic chiasm does not lie on the tuberculum sellae as is often thought but is usually situated above and behind the pituitary gland and the dorsum sellae (Figure 3.12). There is some anatomical variation in the exact position which may cause variations in the field defect. The position described and discussed is that most frequently reported.

b. The central papillo-macular bundle is less vulnerable to compression in the chiasm and visual defects usually spread in from the periphery to involve macular vision late in the course of the disease.

c. The lower nasal fibres (upper temporal fields) cross low and anteriorly in the chiasm and are damaged by lesions arising in the pituitary fossa.

d. The upper nasal fibres (lower temporal fields) cross high and posteriorly in the chiasm and are damaged by lesions damaging the chiasm above and behind— notably craniopharyngiomas.

a. *Anterior Chiasmal Lesions* (Figure 3.11)

The junction of the optic nerve and the chiasm may be damaged from any direction. Meningiomas commonly arise from the densely adherent dura mater in this region and cause progressive visual failure in one eye with loss of sense of smell and/or lesions of cranial nerves III, IV, V and VI. The visual field loss includes a peripheral defect in the opposite eye (the anterior chiasmal syndrome of Traquir).

b. *Chiasmal Lesions*

The basic field defect is a bitemporal hemianopia—the patient is in effect wearing "blinkers". The defect may develop very insidiously with later abrupt visual failure as the presenting symptom. In both sexes endocrine dysfunction usually antedates visual symptoms by many years. In the male impotence and in the female secondary amenorrhoea are the main endocrine symptoms.

In addition to chromophobe adenomas (non-functioning pituitary tumours), eosinophil adenomas (secreting growth hormone and causing acromegaly), aneurysms of the carotid syphon, and chordomas arising from notochord remnants in the dorsum sella may all produce identical syndromes. It is always wise to perform full plain x-rays, angiography and pneumo-encephalography *before* surgical exploration to exclude these other lesions. All cause a bitemporal hemianopia, that spreads down from *upper* field into the lower field (Figure 3.13).

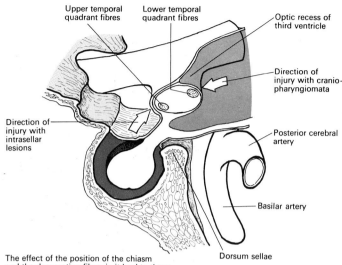

Figure 3.12. Relationship of the Optic Chiasm to the Third Ventricle and Hypophysis Cerebri

The effect of the position of the chiasm and the decussating fibres in it lead to three general points of great clinical importance:
1. Pressure causes bitemporal defects in vision
2. Lesions arising in the sella cause a defect starting in upper quadrants
3. Lesions arising behind or above the sella cause defects starting in lower quadrants

Figure 3.13. Chiasmal Compression from below

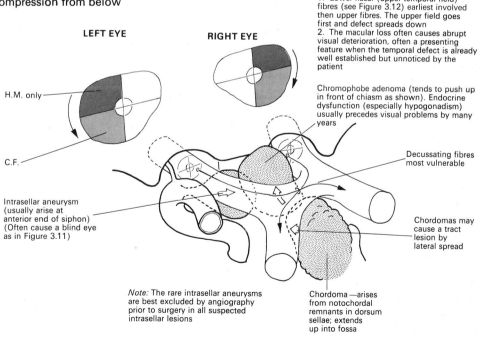

Features:
1. Lower nasal (upper temporal field) fibres (see Figure 3.12) earliest involved then upper fibres. The upper field goes first and defect spreads down
2. The macular loss often causes abrupt visual deterioration, often a presenting feature when the temporal defect is already well established but unnoticed by the patient

Chromophobe adenoma (tends to push up in front of chiasm as shown). Endocrine dysfunction (especially hypogonadism) usually precedes visual problems by many years

Decussating fibres most vulnerable

Chordomas may cause a tract lesion by lateral spread

LEFT EYE

RIGHT EYE

H.M. only

C.F.

Intrasellar aneurysm (usually arise at anterior end of siphon) (Often cause a blind eye as in Figure 3.11)

Note: The rare intrasellar aneurysms are best excluded by angiography prior to surgery in all suspected intrasellar lesions

Chordoma—arises from notochordal remnants in dorsum sellae; extends up into fossa

Craniopharyngiomas which press on the chiasm from above and behind cause three distinct syndromes in addition to the visual problem, which consists of a bitemporal hemianopia spreading up from the *lower* fields into the upper fields (Figure 3.14).

These are:

a. In infancy the tumour may cause pituitary dwarfism.
b. In adulthood progressive visual failure occurs with variable pituitary dysfunction.
c. In old age a craniopharyngioma may block the third ventricle causing hydrocephalus, and producing dementia and progressive visual failure secondary to papilloedema.

c. *Lateral Chiasmal Compression* (Figure 3.15)

Lateral compression of the chiasm is relatively rare. The most frequent cause is dilatation of the intra-cavernous part of an arterio-sclerotic carotid artery. This condition occurs more frequently in females.

The defect is usually unilateral but may become bilateral if the chiasm is pushed across against the opposite carotid artery. If the onset is abrupt the visual problem is usually combined with a blood-shot eye and extra-ocular nerve palsies (Chapter 5). Another possible mechanism is dilatation of the third ventricle in association with chronic aqueductal stenosis or blockage of the fourth ventricle outflow. The chiasm is splayed laterally by the dilating third ventricle and is damaged by the pulsatile carotid arteries pressing against its lateral edges.

5. Optic Tract Lesions (Figure 3.15)

Optic tract lesions produce incongruous homonymous hemianopias, (incongruous defects are those in which the shape of the defect is different in the two half fields (see Figure 3.2). Although incongruity can usually be established on confrontation testing, minor degrees are best demonstrated by formal screen testing. The importance of demonstrating incongruity is that a tract lesion is almost invariably the cause if incongruity is marked. Pituitary tumours, craniopharyngiomas, chordomas and meningiomas may all produce tract lesions. Often the cerebral peduncle on the same side is damaged and mild pyramidal signs in the opposite limb may be detected. Multiple sclerosis can produce a tract lesion but this is quite rare.

All pre-geniculate visual pathway lesions cause variability in the density of the defect with the possibility of progression from a simple field defect to a red pin, to a defect also to a white pin, and finally to the inability to detect even hand movements as the defect becomes complete. Detecting early defects requires considerable knowledge and some degree of skill but is extremely rewarding as early diagnosis really does have value in these situations.

When we come to consider lesions affecting the postgeniculate visual pathways, the situation is quite different. With the exception of attention hemianopias the defects are absolute and variable degrees of loss of vision are not seen. Therefore a 5 mm. white pin is all that is necessary to document the defect.

LESIONS AFFECTING THE VISUAL RADIATIONS

1. Optic Peduncle Lesions

Because the fibres emerging from the lateral geniculate body sweep over the trigone of the lateral ventricles, lying below and behind the capsular region (see also Chapter 9), field defects are *not* a feature of a simple capsular cerebral vascular accident. This region of the visual radiation is most often damaged by occlusion of one of the thalamogeniculate arteries arising from the posterior cerebral artery. This produces a clinical picture which includes an homonymous hemianopia with hemi-sensory loss (posterior thalamic damage) and a very mild motor deficit which usually recovers, presumably due to oedema of the adjacent motor pathways in the internal capsule (see Chapter 9).

2. Temporal Lobe Lesions

The fibres carrying visual information from the upper temporal fields sweep forwards and downwards into the temporal lobe in what is known as Meyer's loop. In the anterior loop there is some splaying of the fibres so that an incongruous defect can be produced but this is usually of minimal degree and once the fibres have looped round to pass posteriorly, congruous defects are the rule. (A congruous defect is one which however bizarre the shape, the defect is identical in both eyes.) In patients suspected of harbouring a temporal lobe lesion careful evaluation of the upper visual fields is indicated.

3. Parietal Lobe Lesions

The part of the visual radiation lying in the anterior part of parietal lobe is carrying information from the lower visual fields. Therefore a lesion in the anterior parietal part of the radiation will produce a lower quadrantic hemianopia. This is an extremely rare field defect only encountered on one occasion by the writer, the patient being an eight-year-old boy with a cerebral abscess. These fibres are quickly rejoined

Figure 3.14. Chiasmal Compression from above

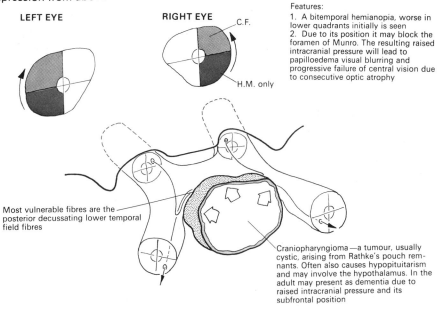

LEFT EYE

RIGHT EYE

C.F.

H.M. only

Features:
1. A bitemporal hemianopia, worse in lower quadrants initially is seen
2. Due to its position it may block the foramen of Munro. The resulting raised intracranial pressure will lead to papilloedema visual blurring and progressive failure of central vision due to consecutive optic atrophy

Most vulnerable fibres are the posterior decussating lower temporal field fibres

Craniopharyngioma—a tumour, usually cystic, arising from Rathke's pouch remnants. Often also causes hypopituitarism and may involve the hypothalamus. In the adult may present as dementia due to raised intracranial pressure and its subfrontal position

Figure 3.15. Lateral Chiasmal and Optic tract Compression

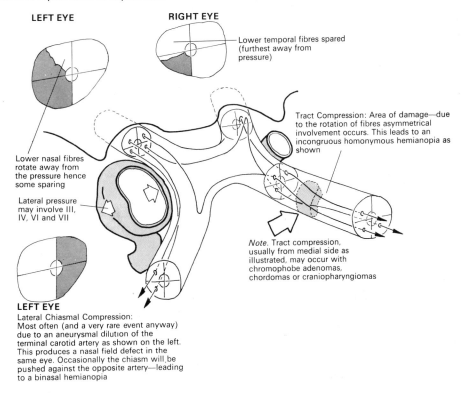

LEFT EYE

RIGHT EYE

Lower temporal fibres spared (furthest away from pressure)

Tract Compression: Area of damage—due to the rotation of fibres asymmetrical involvement occurs. This leads to an incongruous homonymous hemianopia as shown

Lower nasal fibres rotate away from the pressure hence some sparing

Lateral pressure may involve III, IV, VI and VII

Note. Tract compression, usually from medial side as illustrated, may occur with chromophobe adenomas, chordomas or craniopharyngiomas

LEFT EYE

Lateral Chiasmal Compression:
Most often (and a very rare event anyway) due to an aneurysmal dilution of the terminal carotid artery as shown on the left. This produces a nasal field defect in the same eye. Occasionally the chiasm will be pushed against the opposite artery—leading to a binasal hemianopia

by the upper field fibres sweeping up from the temporal lobe and more typically a parietal lesion damages *all* the fibres causing a complete homonymous hemianopia.

Attention hemianopias are due to peripheral parietal lesions and have been fully discussed earlier in this chapter.

4. Lesions of the Anterior Visual Cortex

The peripheral visual fields are represented in the most anterior part of the calcarine cortex. The blood supply of this area is derived from the posterior cerebral artery. Occlusion of this vessel causes infarction of this area and produces a macular sparing hemianopia. The other rare cause of this particular field defect is a meningioma of the tentorium cerebelli pressing against this area of the cortex. Vascular occlusions in this area occur quite commonly in migraine and in general a macular sparing hemianopia does not require extensive investigation. Bilateral infarction of this area leads to tunnel vision with a small ring of two to five degrees of intact vision. This is extremely disabling as patients can see only objects in the direct line of vision and cannot scan to an object in the peripheral fields, even though the visual acuity is quite normal. This may follow cerebral air or fat embolism. Non-organic tunnel vision is occasionally encountered in hysteria and is discussed below.

5. Lesions of the Macular Cortex

If the tip of one occipital pole is damaged a congruous, homonymous and extremely small hemianopia is produced. It is thought that the occipital pole has an independent blood supply from the middle cerebral artery and that this accounts for macular sparing in the posterior cerebral arterial occlusions discussed in section 4. For the same reason occasionally small hemianopic field defects may result from failure of this separate blood supply.

NON-ORGANIC VISUAL FIELD DEFECTS

The most frequently encountered field defect due to malingering or hysteria is tunnel vision or a generalised constriction of the visual field. This may vary in size during testing to the extent of producing a spiral field loss which is diagnostic of hysteria. The defect is best evaluated by using different test objects at different distances. In an organic field defect the size of the intact field increases as the distance increases. In nonorganic loss the defect remains the same size and could perhaps be more accurately called tubular vision (see Figure 3.16).

VISUAL HALLUCINATIONS

Damage to the visual pathways may cause irritative phenomena, appreciated by the patient as flashes of light or colour. More complicated visual images are usually the result of abnormal activity in visual association areas, in particular in the temporal lobes.

Retinal damage is perhaps the most familiar, as in the universal experience of "seeing stars" after a blow to the eye. Damage or ischaemia of the retina causes hallucinations confined to one eye, consisting of unformed "flashes" or "speckles" of light, like stars on a dark background. This is often the last phase of a syncopal attack before loss of consciousness and gives rise to the term "black-out". Similar disturbances of vision in one eye also occur at the onset of a migraine headache. Oedema of the retina due to central serous retinitis causes metamorphopsia (an undulating shape) and alterations in colour perception, but this is a visual aberration rather than an hallucination. Jaundice and digitalis overdose may alter colour perception so that everything appears yellow.

Optic nerve, chiasm and tract lesions do *not* cause visual hallucinations. Although complex visual hallucinations have been reported in patients with chiasmal lesions due to tumours it seems likely that these were due to simultaneous damage to the hypothalamus or medial temporal lobes caused by the same lesion.

Visual hallucinations due to occipital pole ischaemia, or due to seizures originating in this area consist of unformed blobs of colour—usually in the red-orange end of the spectrum. Undoubtedly the most common cause is ischaemia of the occipital poles occurring during or preceding a migraine attack. It is also quite possible for a patient to have repeated attacks of this sort without necessarily developing the headache and patients in this category should be kept

Figure 3.16. Diagram to illustrate Non-Organic Tunnel Vision

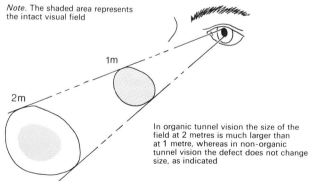

Note. The shaded area represents the intact visual field

1m

2m

In organic tunnel vision the size of the field at 2 metres is much larger than at 1 metre, whereas in non-organic tunnel vision the defect does not change size, as indicated

under careful review. The hallucination may be hemianopic or bilateral and consist of zig-zag lines or circular lines on a dark background, like a plan of a castle, the hallucination that is also called "fortification spectra". Red and orange blobs that may alter in size and seem to explode are often described. Another variant is a sensation as if rain were running down a window pane in one half of vision. This may persist for several hours.

Formed visual images, still pictures like a tableaux, or micropsia or macropsia, where the surroundings seem to get very small or very large, are a feature of temporal lobe epileptic phenomena or occur during migrainous vascular spasm, in which there is ischaemia of the medial temporal lobe. It has been suggested that the idea for "Alice in Wonderland" was the result of macropsia during a migraine attack experienced by Lewis Carroll. One patient seen recently by the writer suffered an episode of this type as she arrived at a cross roads. The distance to the other side seemed vast and she sat in the car too frightened to move until the hallucination passed off. The static tableaux type of hallucination is known as "déjà vu". These are extremely brief and consist of a feeling of familiarity with a scene that is abruptly "frozen". Typical attacks last a split second only and occur occasionally in normal people. In some patients with temporal lobe epilepsy they may occur many times a day and sometimes culminate in a seizure. More complicated and persisting visual hallucinations may occur as part of a temporal lobe attack, but occur more frequently in toxic confusional states or schizophrenia.

A feature of visual hallucinosis is that there is no detectable field defect even during the attack. However, if the hallucinations occur during the onset of ischaemic damage a defect may be detectable after the episode.

Chapter 4

EXAMINATION OF THE OPTIC FUNDUS

A complete discussion of abnormal fundal appearances is beyond the scope of the present text. However, it is essential that students examine the optic fundus in as many patients as possible to get a good idea as to the range of normal appearances and that every opportunity is taken to examine abnormal fundi. This is very much an acquired skill and so often fundal appearances are not clearly seen by students because of poor technique. We will therefore limit discussion to technique and a description of some of the appearances that may be encountered in patients with neurological disorders.

Hints on Fundal Examination

1. Ideally the fundus should be examined in a darkened room, but complete darkness may make it difficult to find the patient's eyes! There is no need to dilate the pupil routinely. This might cause subsequent diagnostic confusion and there is a definite risk of precipitating glaucoma in the elderly.

2. The patient should be asked to fix his gaze on a *distant* object, straight ahead at eye level, both to help him hold the eye still and to dilate the pupil. He should be told to keep his gaze fixed on that point, even when the examiner's head gets in the way of vision, as it inevitably does. Most problems are caused by the patient trying to follow the ophthalmoscope light.

3. The ideal line of approach should bring the optic disc straight into view. The examiner should look through the hole in the ophthalmoscope and then move in from about a foot away from the patient, keeping the pink-glowing pupil in view all the time. He should aim the light beam so that it would emerge from the back of the patient's head in the *midline* at eye level. He should immediately see the pale circle of the optic nerve head come into view *if* the patient continues looking straight ahead with his eye held still.

4. If only blood vessels are seen they should be followed backwards (i.e. against the angle of any branches that are seen) and the disc will eventually come into view (Figure 4.1).

As a general hint on fundal examination once some degree of skill has been achieved—if the disc is found with great difficulty, the patient may well have papilloedema (the pink disc has merged into the retina and the vessels end suddenly

Figure 4.1. Horizontal Section of the Eye to show Relative Positions of the Pupil, Macula and Optic Disc and the Pupillary Muscle Fibres

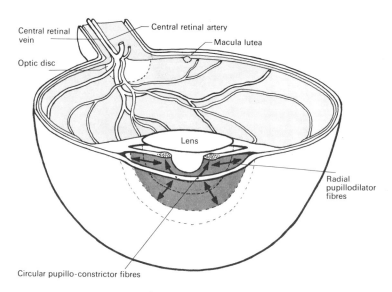

in oedema instead of on the disc), or if the disc flashes into view like a new tennis ball, the patient probably has primary optic atrophy, the disc pallor being accentuated against the normal retina. This simple rule can be extremely useful during the anxiety of the clinical examination for degrees and diplomas.

COMMON FUNDAL ABNORMALITIES

1. Papilloedema

To many doctors, a neurological examination of the optic fundus purely involves the exclusion of papilloedema. To others the absence of papilloedema is believed absolutely to exclude raised intracranial pressure. Neither view is correct.

Papilloedema due to raised intracranial pressure takes several weeks to develop and a patient with rapidly rising intracranial pressure may die long before any disc swelling is apparent. In any clinical situation, if the history suggests rising intracranial pressure, a normal disc does *not* mean that a lumbar puncture is without hazard (see also Chapter 25). Because of the slow development of disc changes there is a

Figure 4.2. The Sequence in Developing Papilloedema

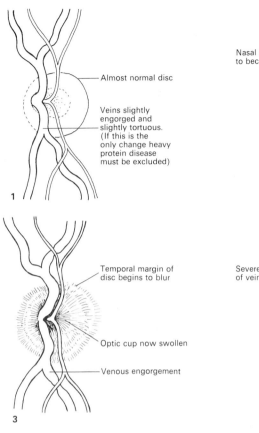

1 — Almost normal disc

Veins slightly engorged and slightly tortuous. (If this is the only change heavy protein disease must be excluded)

2 — Nasal edge starts to become indistinct

Optic cup fills and lamina cribrosa cannot be seen

Venous engorgement increases and A—V nipping may appear

3 — Temporal margin of disc begins to blur

Optic cup now swollen

Venous engorgement

4 — Severe engorgement of veins

Haemorrhages appear around the disc

Disc so swollen vessels "disappear" into or "emerge" from the oedema

The final appearance is identical with that of a central retinal vein thrombosis but the latter is unilateral and haemorrhages are usually a prominent feature

sequence of findings that may indicate incipient papilloedema.

The sequence may be as follows (Figure 4.2).

1. Some increase in venous calibre and tortuosity. If this change is very marked without other abnormality, heavy protein disease such as macroglobulinaemia should be excluded.

2. The central area of the disc (the optic cup) is usually slightly pale compared to the rest of the disc and the vessels are usually seen to plunge into it. In early papilloedema this area becomes pinker and less distinct, the vessels seeming to disappear suddenly on the surface of the disc.

3. The disc margins start to blur. It is essential to be aware from the examination of many normal discs that the nasal edge is *always* less distinct than the temporal edge, and this blurring and even slight heaping is accentuated in those patients whose retinal vessels

enter more to the nasal side than usual. Nevertheless, in true papilloedema the earliest swelling is seen at the nasal edge. One of the most frequent "false positive" signs in neurology is questionable blurring of the nasal disc margins.

4. Finally the whole disc becomes suffused and slightly elevated. The margins may disappear and the swelling completely conceals the vessel origins—the vessels seeming to emerge from a mushy swelling. Streaky perivenous haemorrhages occur but exudates are unusual in papilloedema due to raised intracranial pressure.

Conditions simulating Papilloedema

An exceptionally deep optic cup or medullated nerve fibres are common disc appearances simulating papilloedema. These are illustrated in Figures 4.3 and 4.4.

Figure 4.3. Deep Optic Cup simulating Papilloedema

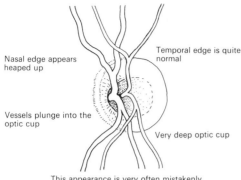

Nasal edge appears heaped up

Temporal edge is quite normal

Vessels plunge into the optic cup

Very deep optic cup

This appearance is very often mistakenly described as papilloedema. In papilloedema the cup is the first part of the disc to fill and become abnormal

Figure 4.4. Medullated Nerve Fibres

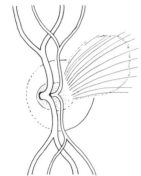

Normally nerve fibres are bare beyond the lamina cribrosa. Sometimes they are myelinated on the disc or even on to the retina as in this case

The appearance is typically flared and careful focusing will usually reveal the fibres traversing the area. This abnormality will produce a field defect as it obscures the retinal cells. The patient is unaware of the defect as it is present from birth

Papilloedema is often suspected but seldom confirmed. The early changes are very subjective, but the recent advent of fluoroscein retinal angiography has enabled the problem to be resolved in many cases. One should never rely on the absence of papilloedema as an absolute indication that intracranial pressure is not raised.

Causes of Papilloedema

Although a full discussion of the causes of papilloedema is inappropriate to the discussion of fundal appearances, a list of common causes is given in Table 2.

It should be noticed that the causes are not exclusively neurological. Raised intracranial pressure due to any mass lesion in the brain is the main cause, but conditions interfering with the circulation of the C.S.F., such as aqueductal stenosis and congenital anomalies in the posterior fossa, should always be considered.

There are a variety of other causes in many of which the mechanism of the papilloedema is obscure. In some cases a high C.S.F. protein or altered blood products block C.S.F. reabsorption by the arachnoid granulations. In some instances diffuse brain swelling is responsible and in others impaired venous drainage of the brain or of the retina itself is the cause. The common causes of central retinal vein thrombosis are therefore included in the table.

Table 2

CAUSES OF PAPILLOEDEMA:

1. Raised intracranial pressure due to mass lesions.
2. Raised intracranial pressure due to circulatory block
   —aqueductal stenosis.
   —intraventricular tumours.
   —fourth ventricle outflow block.
3. Due to cerebral oedema—post-head-injury.
   —post-cerebral anoxia.
   —benign intracranial hypertension
   —lead poisoning
   —steroid withdrawal
   —Vitamin A intoxication.
4. Due to raised C.S.F. protein or altered blood products
   —post-subarachnoid haemorrhage
   —post-meningitis
   —Guillain–Barre syndrome
   —hypertrophic polyneuritis
   —spinal cord tumours
5. The malignant phase of hypertension.
6. Metabolic disorders—hypercapnia.
   —hypocalcaemia in childhood in particular.
   —malignant thyrotoxic exopthalmos.
7. Disorders of the circulation including central retinal vein thrombosis
   —lateral sinus thrombosis.
   —jugular vein thrombosis.
   —superior vena caval obstruction.
   —polycythaemia rubra vera.
   —multiple myelomatosis.
   —macroglobulinaemia.
   —diabetes mellitus.
   —hyperlipidaemia.
   —arteriosclerotic vessels in the retina.
   —vasculitis, including temporal arteritis.

2. Secondary Optic Atrophy

If the patient survives the cause of his papilloedema, further changes may appear in the optic disc following subsidence of the papilloedema which may take six to ten weeks. Occasionally general physicians may seek neurological advice if papilloedema has not resolved within a few days of a patient receiving effective anti-hypertensive therapy. This concern is quite unnecessary: at least six weeks may elapse before significant resolution is apparent.

Even while disc swelling is still obvious, the nerve head may start to become a greyish white colour and the patient may notice decreasing visual acuity. Finally as the swelling subsides the patient is left with a flat greyish-white nerve head with very indistinct edges. This scarring process in the nerve head may lead to further serious deterioration of vision long after raised intracranial pressure has subsided. The earliest possible relief of raised pressure is therefore indicated, but no confident prognosis for vision can be given to a patient who has evidence of optic atrophy or decreased acuity when first seen. This is called consecutive or secondary optic atrophy.

3. Primary Optic Atrophy

Following any toxic insult, injury, occlusion of the central retinal artery, compressive, infiltrative or demyelinating process affecting the optic nerve, the patient may develop primary optic atrophy. The nerve head becomes extremely pale and the lamina cribosa becomes very distinct. Again, this is an extremely subjective impression and doubtful cases are often recorded as "slight pallor of discs". Many patients incorrectly suspected of suffering from multiple sclerosis have been diagnosed using this highly subjective sign as corroboratory evidence—a very unwise policy.

The normal variation in disc colour is considerable. The temporal edge of the disc is relatively avascular and always looks pale compared with the nasal half of the disc. The lamina cribrosa is often well marked and forms a very pale central area of the disc. The pallor of a normal disc may be accentuated by the rim of pigment that is often seen at the temporal edge of the disc caused by the slight retraction of the retina that occurs developmentally (Figures 4.5 and 4.6).

The visual acuity and the visual field to red are often normal and do not alone disprove the diagnosis of primary optic atrophy. The diagnosis remains an extremely subjective one although recent advances using visual evoked responses provide additional evidence of optic nerve damage.

4. Miscellaneous

1. Patients with decreasing visual acuity may have macular degeneration and a close inspection of the macular (to be

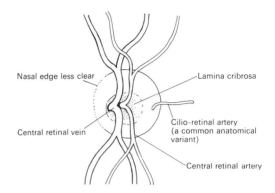

Figure 4.5. Normal Optic Disc

Nasal edge less clear

Lamina cribrosa

Central retinal vein

Cilio-retinal artery (a common anatomical variant)

Central retinal artery

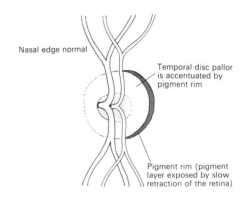

Figure 4.6. Pigment Rim simulating Optic Atrophy

Nasal edge normal

Temporal disc pallor is accentuated by pigment rim

Pigment rim (pigment layer exposed by slow retraction of the retina)

found two disc diameters from the temporal edge of the disc) is necessary. This requires dilatation of the pupil in most instances. The normal macular is a small pale yellow spot in a slightly darker area of the retina and expert opthalmological advice is necessary for full evaluation of this region.

2. Patients with transient ischaemic attacks may have evidence of embolisation of the retinal vessels. Small highly refractile fragments of cholesterol may be seen blocking arterioles usually at the bifurcations. Distally the vessels appear pale and empty.

3. Patients with night blindness, children with epilepsy and patients with several inherited neurological disorders may have retinitis pigmentosa. This consists of spiderlike nets of pigment that are initially seen at the periphery of the retina. They may be associated with a degree of primary optic atrophy secondary to destruction of the retinal cells in these pigmented areas. Later peripheral constriction of the fields occurs with optic atrophy. Marked narrowing of the arterioles is an important diagnostic feature.

4. Rapid loss of central vision, often described by the patient as if a red or orange ball were present in front of the eye with persistent after images, metamorphopsia or micropsia, are features of a disease known as central serous retinopathy. In this condition there is marked oedema and heaping up of the retina, causing the distortion of vision. The condition occurs mainly in young males and responds to steroids. Very brief attacks of metamorphopsia are usually due to temporal lobe disorders.

Ophthalmoscopy requires a certain amount of skill. Once the skill is acquired a considerable degree of familiarity with normal fundal appearances is necessary to detect minor but possibly significant abnormalities. In many instances the interpretation of appearances is highly subjective and it is wrong to place too much reliance on disputed appearances unless corroboratory evidence using flouroscein angiography or visual evoked potentials confirms the suspected abnormality.

Chapter 5

THE THIRD, FOURTH AND SIXTH CRANIAL NERVES

These three cranial nerves control the upper eyelid, eye movements and pupils and have long intracranial courses. Due to the latter feature they are subject to damage by a wide range of disease processes at various sites. A careful history and clinical examination usually provides all the information necessary for accurate diagnosis. Difficulty in remembering the actions of the various extraocular muscles and their nerve supply is a universal problem and therefore these features are covered extensively in this chapter.

THE EXTRA-OCULAR MUSCLES

The names, positions and actions of the extra-ocular muscles are illustrated and discussed in Figures 5.1–5.4.

The main points to note are:

1. The medial rectus muscle of one eye and the lateral rectus muscle of the other work as a pair to produce lateral eye movements. The central mechanism responsible for synchronising these actions is fully discussed in Chapter 7.

2. The vertically acting rectus muscles are most effective when the eye is abducted (i.e. looking outwards) as in this position the line of pull of the muscles is along the vertical axis of the eye.

3. In the same way the oblique muscles are maximally effective when the eye is adducted (i.e. looking inwards) as their line of pull is then along the vertical axis of the eye.

These are the only important points to remember when evaluating eye movements from a neurological standpoint. All the muscles have secondary actions and some have torsional effects. It is probably because these other movements are given such emphasis in anatomical textbooks that so few can understand or remember the simple facts needed for an adequate neurological examination!

DIPLOPIA

The single symptom that indicates damage to one or other of the three nerves under discussion is diplopia. This should not be taken to imply that diplopia is *always* due to a nerve lesion. A discussion of other causes of diplopia will be found at the end of this chapter.

Explanation of Diplopia

The eyes are normally positioned so that the image falls on exactly the same spot on the retina of each eye. The slightest displacement of either eye causes diplopia as the image is

Figure 5.1. The Actions of the Extraocular Muscles

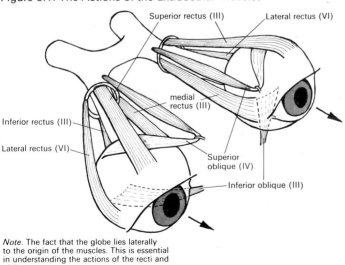

Note. The fact that the globe lies laterally to the origin of the muscles. This is essential in understanding the actions of the recti and obliques

Figure 5.2. The Actions of the Medial and Lateral Recti (lateral gaze to R side)

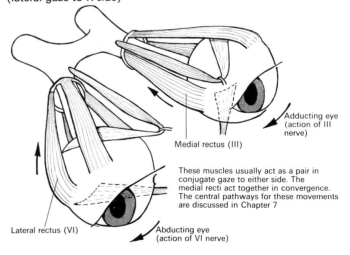

These muscles usually act as a pair in conjugate gaze to either side. The medial recti act together in convergence. The central pathways for these movements are discussed in Chapter 7

Figure 5.3

When the eye is adducted by the medial rectus the line of pull of the superior oblique becomes ideal to pull the globe up and over from behind. It is the main depressor of the adducted eye

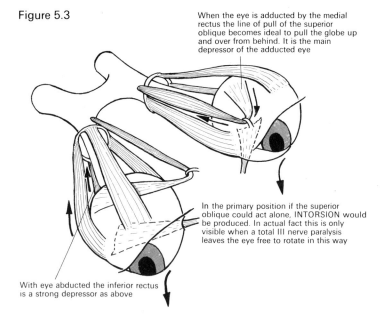

In the primary position if the superior oblique could act alone, INTORSION would be produced. In actual fact this is only visible when a total III nerve paralysis leaves the eye free to rotate in this way

With eye abducted the inferior rectus is a strong depressor as above

Figure 5.4

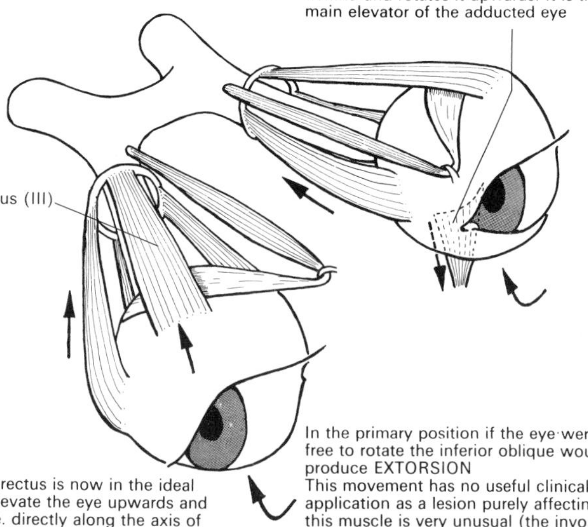

With the eye adducted the inferior oblique pulls the eye from below and behind and rotates it upwards. It is the main elevator of the adducted eye

Superior rectus (III)

In the primary position if the eye were free to rotate the inferior oblique would produce EXTORSION
This movement has no useful clinical application as a lesion purely affecting this muscle is very unusual (the involvement of the other III nerve innervated muscles dominating the signs)

The superior rectus is now in the ideal position to elevate the eye upwards and outwards (i.e. directly along the axis of the muscle). It is therefore the main elevator of the abducted eye

Figure 5.5. Diagram to show the Mechanism of Diplopia
(a L VI nerve palsy is illustrated)

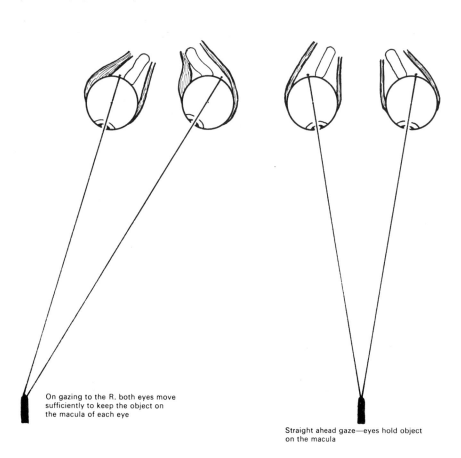

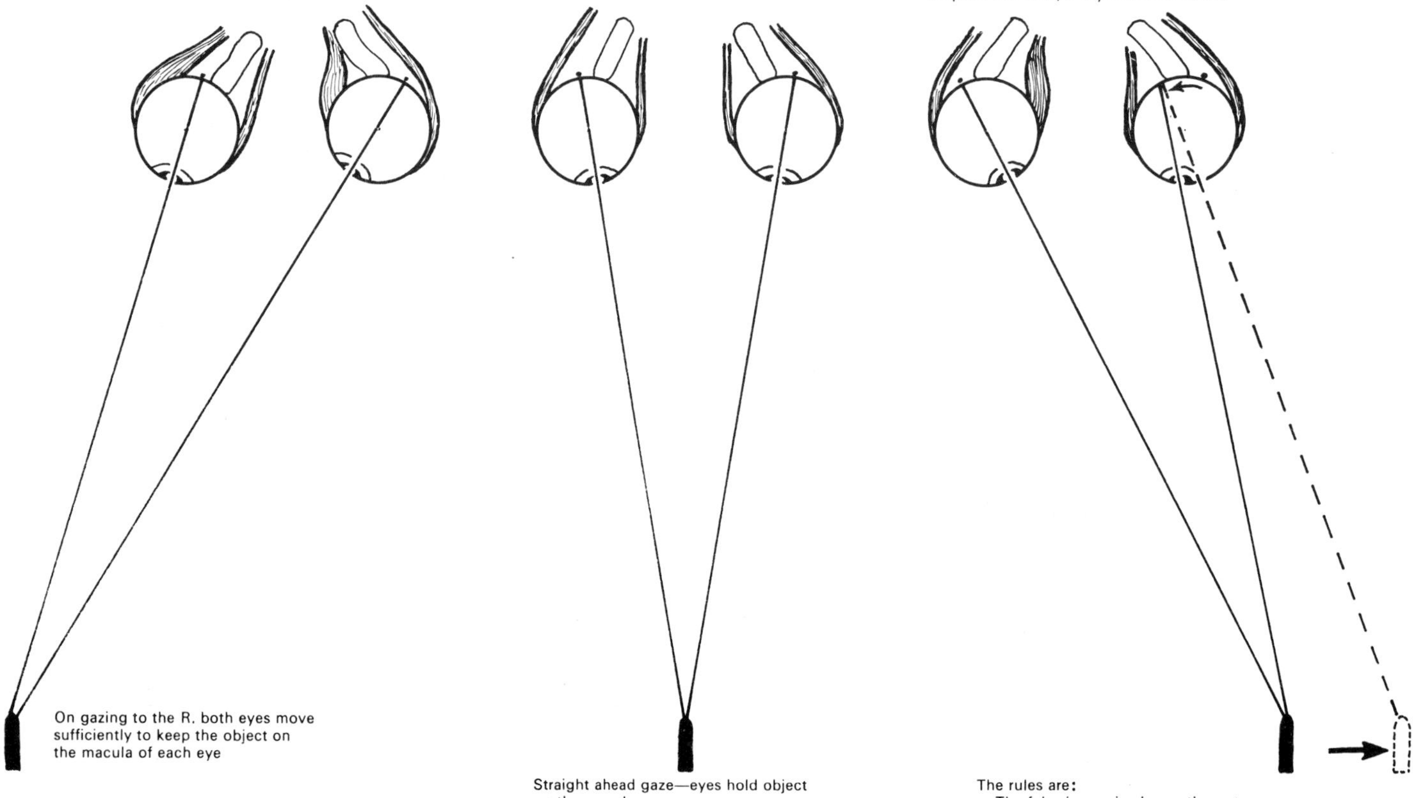

On looking to the L. the L. eye remains static. As the object moves the image falls on the retina to the nasal side and is projected further and further into the temporal half field, away from the macula

On gazing to the R. both eyes move sufficiently to keep the object on the macula of each eye

Straight ahead gaze—eyes hold object on the macula

The rules are:
The false image is always the outer one
The false image always comes from the affected eye

shifted to a different position on the retina of the displaced eye (confirm this by displacing one eye by gently pressing it through the eyelid).

In the case of nerve lesions the weak muscle or muscles can usually be detected by direct observation of the eye movements. Occasionally, mild lesions or other diseases may cause diplopia in which the degree of weakness is too slight to be observed. In these situations the *cover test* is useful. This test is based on the fact that the separation of the two images becomes greatest as the eyes attempt to look in the direction of the weak muscle, because the disparity in eye movements is then maximal. The false image falls progressively further away from the macula of the lagging eye and the false image is therefore *always* the *outer* image of the two. If the examiner asks the patient to follow a stick until double vision is maximal and then determines which eye he must cover to obliterate the outer image, the affected eye is identified. From the direction of the gaze the weak muscle can be determined (see Figure 5.5).

1. Third Nerve Palsy (Figure 5.6)

A complete third nerve lesion causes total paralysis of the eyelid, and diplopia *only* when the lid is held up. Severe diplopia then occurs in all directions *except* on lateral gaze to the side of the third nerve lesion (because the lateral rectus muscle is intact).

When the lid is lifted the eye will be found deviated outwards (lateral rectus action) and downwards (secondary depressant action of the superior oblique muscle). The integrity of these muscles and hence their nerve supply should be carefully evaluated to be certain that the third nerve is the only nerve affected.

To do this the examiner should test lateral gaze in the affected eye and note the disappearance of diplopia in that direction. The normal downward movement produced by the superior oblique muscle *cannot* be tested because the paralysed medial rectus does not allow the eye to adduct. Instead the secondary action of the muscle is observed. The depression of the eye is usually already apparent. If the patient makes a further effort to look downwards the eye will rotate inwards (intorsion) as the superior oblique muscle pulls sideways across the eye when it is in this position. Observation of this movement is the best evidence of an intact superior oblique muscle and hence the integrity of the IVth nerve.

The pupil may be normal or dilated and fixed to light. This important feature is fully discussed later.

2. Fourth Nerve Palsy (Figure 5.7)

A fourth nerve lesion causes weakness of the superior oblique muscle with very subtle diplopia. The weakness of the muscle in the primary position (looking straight ahead) allows the eye to rotate slightly outwards (extorsion). The very slight slant of the image will make the patient tilt his head slightly away from the side of the affected eye to line up the image from the normal eye. In children this head tilt may be misdiagnosed as torticollis. Frank diplopia occurs when the patient looks down and away from the side of the affected eye. This often leads to trouble going downstairs as two treads are seen when the patient looks downwards and sideways, as one normally does while descending stairs. Similarly, diplopia may occur while reading a newspaper or a book.

Figure 5.6. To show ptosis in complete III nerve palsy
(The eyelid sags passively—the eye can be shut tightly via the VII nerve)

Figure 5.7. To show the compensatory head tilt in a patient with a superior oblique paralysis of the right eye

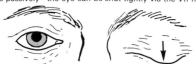

To show the position of the eye when the lid is lifted
The eye is abducted (intact VI) and slightly depressed (intact IV). The pupil is dilated

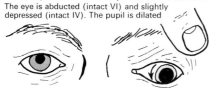

To confirm intact IV nerve; note the inward rotation (intorsion) of the eye when the patient attempts to look down. This is the rotary action of the superior oblique that occurs when the eye cannot be abducted

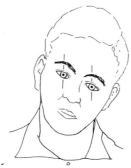

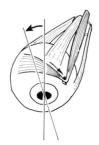

The patient has tilted his head to the L. to line up the image from the good eye with the outwardly rotated R. eye

Normally the superior oblique, by pulling across the top of the eye, slightly rotates it inwards
If paralysed the eye will rotate slightly outwards causing a slightly oblique image

Figure 5.8. To show voluntary eye closure to obliterate double vision with a VI nerve palsy of the left eye

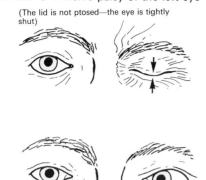

(The lid is not ptosed—the eye is tightly shut)

To show the position of the eye when open
The affected eye is deviated towards the nose.
To prevent diplopia the patient may turn the
head until the right eye is sufficiently
abducted to give a single image

3. Sixth Nerve Palsy (Figure 5.8)

A sixth nerve palsy causes the greatest problem as there is no ptosis to obliterate the false image. Occasionally patients will deliberately shut the affected eye to prevent the diplopia and this can be misinterpreted as ptosis. If the examiner closes the normal eyelid, the lid on the side of the "pseudo-ptosis" will revert to a normal position. At rest the affected eye is pulled medially by the unopposed action of the medial rectus muscle. The patient may compensate by turning his head towards the weak muscle.

INTRACRANIAL ANATOMY OF THE THIRD, FOURTH AND SIXTH CRANIAL NERVES
(Figure 5.9)

Note: The nerves run a generally converging course towards the apex of the orbit from widely separate origins in the brain stem.

1. The Third Nerve (Occulomotor Nerve)

The two third nerves emerge together between the cerebral peduncles. They then splay out as they pass anteriorly lying between the posterior cerebral arteries and the superior cerebellar arteries, and then run parallel to the posterior communicating arteries until they enter the cavernous sinus. They then lie between the two layers of dura that form the lateral wall of the sinus. The nerve enters the orbit through the superior orbital fissure and divides into two main branches. The upper branch supplies the eyelid and superior rectus muscle. The lower branch supplies all the other muscles and the pupil.

2. The Fourth Nerve (Trochlear Nerve)

This nerve has several unique features. Its nucleus lies in the dorsum of the brain stem and the fibres decussate (cross over) in the substance of the superior medullary velum so that the right nerve originates in the left trochlear nucleus and vice versa. The nerve runs a very long course leaving the posterior fossa and encircling the brain stem to enter the cavernous sinus. It enters the roof of the orbit and actually crosses the third nerve in order to do so. It derives its name from the fact that the muscle it supplies (the superior oblique) passes round a trochlear (pulley) in the anterior orbital roof.

3. The Sixth Nerve (Abducens Nerve)

This nerve emerges from the front of the brain stem at the ponto-medullary junction, deep in the posterior fossa. It ascends on the front of the brain stem and then angles sharply forwards over the tip of the petrous bone to enter the back of the cavernous sinus. It lies free in the sinus, enters the orbit through the superior orbital fissure, and passes laterally to reach the lateral rectus muscle.

CAUSES OF EXTRA-OCULAR NERVE LESIONS

There are five main sites of potential damage to these nerves as indicated in Figure 5.10.

1. Nuclear and Fascicular Lesions

These will be considered in detail in the chapter on brain stem lesions (Chapter 11). There are usually other evidences of brain stem damage to confirm that this is the site of the lesion and several named syndromes involving these nerves have been described. Causes include brain stem vascular disease, multiple sclerosis, pontine gliomas, poliomyelitis, Wernicke's encephalopathy and congenital maldevelopment of the cranial nerve nuclei.

2. Lesions in the Basilar Area

All three nerves are subject to damage by basal meningeal disease processes. These include tuberculous, fungal and bacterial meningitis, carcinomatous meningitis, direct neoplastic invasion from the sinuses and nasopharynx, meningovascular syphilis, sarcoid, Guillain–Barré syndrome and Herpes Zoster. In many of these conditions there are multiple or bilateral nerve lesions to indicate a diffuse pathological process.

Aneurysmal dilation of the upper basilar artery may also cause multiple nerve palsies and in particular bilateral third nerve lesions.

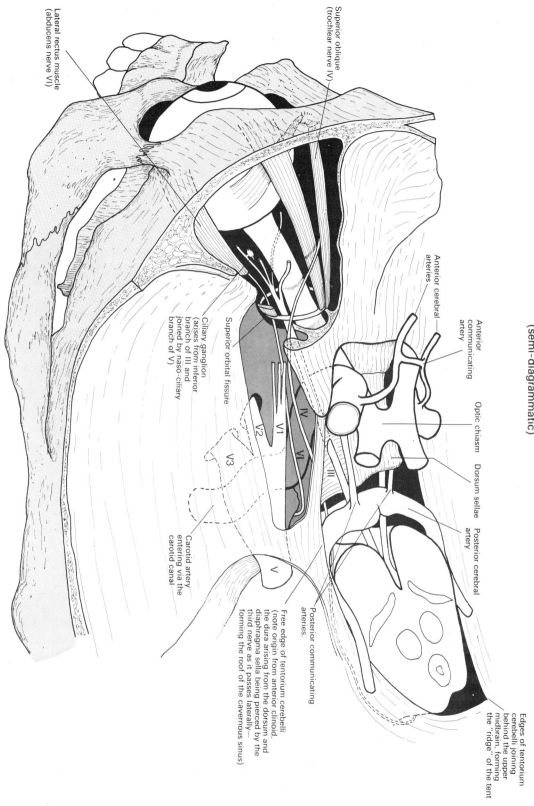

Figure 5.9. The Intracranial Course and Relations of Cranial Nerves III, IV, V, VI (semi-diagrammatic)

Lateral rectus muscle (abducens nerve VI)

Superior oblique (trochlear nerve IV)

Anterior cerebral artery

Anterior communicating artery

Optic chiasm

Dorsum sellae

Posterior cerebral artery

Edges of tentorium cerebelli joining behind the upper midbrain, forming the "ridge" of the tent

Superior orbital fissure

Ciliary ganglion (arises from inferior branch of III and joined by naso-ciliary branch of V)

V2

V1

V3

IV

VI

III

V

Posterior communicating arteries.

Carotid artery entering via the carotid canal

Free edge of tentorium cerebelli (note origin from anterior clinoid, the dura arising from the dorsum and diaphragma sella being pierced by the third nerve as it passes laterally—forming the roof of the cavernous sinus)

Figure 5.10. The Anatomical Basis of the various Lesions
Lesions as defined by sites in the text

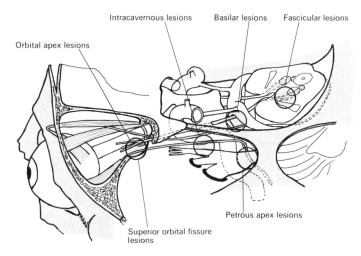

Orbital apex lesions

Intracavernous lesions Basilar lesions Fascicular lesions

Superior orbital fissure lesions

Petrous apex lesions

Figure 5.11. Posterior communicating artery aneurysms

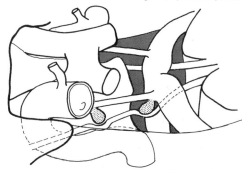

Aneurysms at either end (they typically occur at these sites) are likely to damage III nerve as the artery is immediately adjacent to it

Specific involvement of the third nerve in this area occur in two ways:

1. Direct compression by a posterior communicating artery aneurysm. The onset is usually acute with severe pain and the pupil is almost always affected, and is dilated and fixed to light (Figure 5.11).

2. The nerve may be progressively damaged by the prolapsing temporal lobe, when the hemisphere is displaced by a mass. This is called a tentorial pressure cone.

The patient becomes drowsy and the pupil on the affected side becomes dilated, ptosis develops and finally a complete third nerve palsy ensues. (Figure 5.12). A third nerve palsy in this situation is very rarely false-localising (discussed fully in Chapter 23), and urgent surgical intervention is indicated.

The sixth nerve may also be affected in the basal area by increased intracranial pressure but by a different mechanism. This is a situation usually encountered in children and is often false-localising. A tumour in the posterior fossa causes hydrocephalus (dilatation of the ventricles) and the *whole* brain tries to squeeze down through the tentorium. This pushes the brain stem downwards and the sixth nerve becomes stretched over the petrous tip. One or both nerves may be affected in this way by a lesion quite remote from the nerve itself (see Figure 5.12).

Figure 5.12. Diagram to show the different mechanisms underlying III and IV nerve palsies in patients with raised intracranial pressure (seen from front)

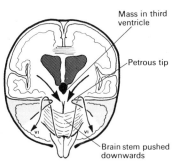

III nerve palsy (usually unilateral)

Extradural haematoma

Midbrain pushed across to L. side

Prolapsing temporal lobe

Edge of tentorium

VI nerve palsy (unilateral or bilateral)

Mass in third ventricle

Petrous tip

Brain stem pushed downwards

A large extradural haematoma pushes the hemisphere sideways under the falx and downwards through the tentorium. This stretches the third nerve over the edge of the tentorium. This is a very *reliable* localising sign

A mass in the third ventricle has caused symmetrical dilatation of both lateral ventricles. The entire brain stem is pushed downwards—pulling the VI nerve where it angulates over the petrous tip to enter the cavernous sinus. This is a very *unreliable* sign

3. Lesions at the Petrous Tip

The sixth nerve is clearly the only vulnerable nerve in this area and there are four main causes of damage.

1. Mastoiditis or middle ear infection may cause diffuse inflammation of the petrous bone and thrombosis of the overlying petrosal sinuses. This causes severe ear pain and a combination of sixth, seventh, eighth and occasionally fifth nerve lesions and is known as Gradenigo's syndrome. This must be differentiated from Ramsay-Hunt's syndrome (Geniculate Herpes Zoster) in which there is a vesicular eruption in the ear and a seventh nerve palsy and occasionally other cranial nerve lesions (see also Chapter 6).

2. Lateral sinus thrombosis secondary to mastoiditis may lead to rapidly rising intracranial pressure due to impaired cerebral venous drainage. This may cause a direct or indirect sixth nerve palsy as discussed above. To differentiate this situation from a posterior fossa abscess can be very difficult.

3. Carcinomas of the naso-pharynx or the para-nasal sinuses tend to infiltrate through the fissures of the skull base and a sudden painless sixth nerve palsy may be the first evidence of malignant disease in these tissues.

4. Benign transient sixth nerve palsies may occur in children following mild infections. This diagnosis is difficult to make and only really confirmed by the subsequent recovery, which may take several weeks.

4. Lesions in the Region of the Cavernous Sinus

1. Cavernous sinus thrombosis remains a very serious condition usually occurring as a complication of sepsis of the skin over the upper face or in the paranasal sinuses. As the sixth nerve lies free in the sinus it is the most vulnerable nerve. The sixth nerve palsy is coupled with severe pain, exophthalmus and oedema of the eyelids and later this involves the opposite eyelid as an extension of the thrombosis to the opposite cavernous sinus is almost inevitable.

2. Intrasellar tumours such as chromophobe adenomas may extend laterally into the sinus and then usually damage the third nerve (Figure 5.13).

3. Aneurysmal dilatation of the intracavernous portion of the carotid artery usually occurs in elderly hypertensive females. If the swelling of the artery is at the anterior end of the sinus, oedema of the eyelid, exophthalmos, blindness and a third nerve lesion may occur simultaneously heralded by quite severe pain. If the dilatation is at the posterior end of the sinus, the first division of the fifth nerve may be irritated with severe pain over the fifth nerve distribution (ophthalmic division) and a sixth nerve palsy. Again the eye becomes suffused and proptosed (Figures 5.14, 5.15). If the vessel actually ruptures into the sinus it is rarely fatal as the

Figure 5.13. Intrasellar mass spreading laterally

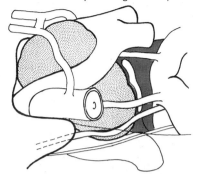

Optic chiasm compressed. Carotid siphon and nerves displaced laterally—
III nerve especially vulnerable

Figure 5.14. Intracavernous aneurysm (anterior type)

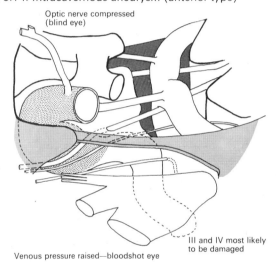

Optic nerve compressed (blind eye)

III and IV most likely to be damaged

Venous pressure raised—bloodshot eye

Figure 5.15. Intracavernous aneurysm (posterior type)

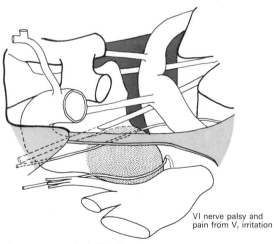

VI nerve palsy and pain from V₁ irritation

Venous pressure raised—bloodshot eye

cavernous sinus will contain the haemorrhage, but a severe unilateral and later bilateral pulsatile exophthalmos occurs. This is called a carotico-cavernous fistula and may also follow a head injury if a basal fracture tears the carotid artery at its point of entry into the sinus.

5. Lesions at the Superior Orbital Fissure and Orbital Apex

There are numerous neoplasms that may arise in the posterior orbit and a fairly well-defined syndrome results. These are listed in Table 3. Because all the nerves are relatively close together palsies of the third, fourth and sixth nerves in various combinations may occur. Involvement of the fifth nerve may cause pain and later numbness in the distribution of the first division of the fifth nerve, with depression of the corneal response.

Table 3

TUMOURS ARISING IN THE ORBIT AND OPTIC FORAMINA	
Meningiomas	40%
Haemangiomas	10%
Gliomas	5%
Pseudo-tumour of the orbit	5%
Carcinoma of the lacrimal duct	
Neurofibroma	
Fibrous dysplasia of bone	
Sarcoma	
Epidermoid	
Melanoma	40%
Lipoma	
Hand–Schuller–Christian Disease	
Tolosa–Hunt Syndrome	
Arterio-venous malformations	

Some generalisations are possible:

1. Malignant infiltration of the orbit (by direct spread of carcinoma of the nasopharynx or remote spread from carcinomas in other sites) produces rapidly evolving extra-ocular nerve palsies and exophthalmos.

2. Benign tumours in the orbit may cause very slowly progressive but quite marked exophthalmos with remarkably little visual loss or nerve palsies until quite late in the course of the disease. The diplopia is often purely the result of mechanical displacement of the globe.

3. Lesions in the superior orbital fissure or intracranial lesions just behind the fissure cause nerve palsies with little or no exophthalmos.

4. Lesions in the orbit tend to cause exophthalmos as an early sign. If, in addition, there is considerable pain and redness of the eye the condition known as "pseudo-tumour

of the orbit" must be considered. This is usually associated with a high E.S.R. and responds to steroids. It may well be a mild variant of the rare Tolosa–Hunt syndrome in which a mass of granulomatous tissue is found behind the eye and in the orbital fissure. The possiblity of unilateral exophthalmos with superior rectus muscle weakness being due to endocrine disease must always be excluded. Even in the absence of frank thyrotoxicosis, hyperthyroidism is the most common cause of unilateral exophthalmos.

5. Vascular tumours and arterio-venous malformations in the orbit may only cause proptosis when the patient is lying, bending forwards or performing the valsava manoeuvre.

Miscellaneous Disease Processes Causing Extra-ocular Nerve Lesions

1. There are three medical diseases that may cause acute extra-ocular nerve palsies. These are diabetes mellitus, meningo-vascular syphilis and arteriosclerosis. With the exception of diabetes the onset is usually painless (and in the writer's experience many diabetic palsies are also painless). The presumed pathology is infarction of the nerve trunk and hence in third nerve lesions due to these causes the pupil is usually spared. The prognosis in all instances is for complete recovery of function over some four to eight weeks. If recovery does not occur the diagnosis must be reconsidered. Compare this with an extra-ocular palsy due to a surgical cause which is usually painful, and in the case of a third nerve lesion *does* affect the pupillary response. Another rare "vascular" cause of extra-ocular nerve palsy is temporal arteritis; a condition confined to the elderly (over sixty years of age) (see also Chapter 20).

2. During the course of acute migraine headaches transient extra-ocular nerve palsies or a Horner's syndrome may occur. An incomplete third nerve palsy is the usual finding but less typically a sixth nerve palsy may be seen. The transience of the palsy, repeated identical attacks and the characteristics of the headache should suggest the diagnosis. The first episode may require angiographic exclusion of an aneurysm. A long history of repeated attacks may allow a confident diagnosis to be made without further investigations.

3. Third and sixth nerve lesions may occur during acute Herpes Zoster Ophthalmicus. The diagnosis is usually very obvious with an extensive vesicular eruption over the forehead preceded by severe pain. The prognosis for recovery is good.

4. Fourth nerve lesions in isolation are quite rare. Diabetes is probably the most frequent medical cause. In children

tumours infiltrating the superior medullary velum may produce bilateral fourth nerve palsies, and a similar picture occasionally follows severe head trauma, possibly due to haemorrhage into the same area. Unilateral weakness of the superior oblique commonly follows damage to the trochlear itself by injuries to the upper orbital margin.

Other Conditions Simulating Nerve Lesions

In general extra-ocular nerve palsies are "all or none"; partial palsies are relatively rare and usually *all* muscles supplied by the nerve show some degree of weakness. In the case of a fourth or sixth nerve palsy only one muscle can be affected, therefore if *two* muscles are affected the following conditions should be considered.

1. *Thyrotoxicosis*

Weakness of the superior rectus muscle and/or the lateral rectus muscle commonly causes diplopia in thyrotoxicosis irrespective of the presence of exophthalmos. The pathological changes in the muscles suggest that an inflammatory myopathic process is responsible.

2. *Myasthenia Gravis*

Diplopia and ptosis of the eyelid are the most common presenting symptoms of myasthenia gravis, and varying eye signs or fatigueability of eye movements should always raise this possibility. Many patients have had ophthalmological operations for squints later proven to be due to myasthenia gravis!

3. *Latent Strabismus*

Diplopia under conditions of fatigue, drowsiness or following impairment of vision in either eye is often due to the breaking down of a lifelong squint. A history of a childhood squint or previous orthoptic exercises usually establishes the cause. If there is no history the cover test may be useful. The examiner covers one of the patient's eyes and asks him to fix his gaze on a finger held about 18 inches away. When the other eye is uncovered it will be seen deviated inwards or outwards and will quickly pull back to line up with the other eye. This unmasks a latent deviation requiring positive muscle action to keep it compensated. Fatigue allows the eye to drift, resulting in diplopia usually in the evenings while watching TV!

4. *Progressive Ocular Myopathy*

This is a relatively rare form of muscular dystrophy in which the main muscle weakness occurs in the extra-ocular muscles and eyelids causing ptosis and diplopia. Careful examination usually discloses weakness of the facial and limb girdle muscles (also see Chapter 19). Familial ptosis is probably a mild variant of this condition that usually starts in late adulthood and may be associated with impaired upward gaze. Ptosis props fitted to the spectacle frames may be required to push the lid up off the pupil.

5. *Internuclear Ophthalmoplegia*

Multiple sclerosis may present as an extra-ocular nerve palsy, usually a sixth nerve lesion. More often diplopia occurs without weakness of any individual eye movement. This is due to disruption of the conjugate eye movement mechanism and is fully discussed in Chapter 8.

General Approach to Diplopia

Whenever a patient presents with the symptom of diplopia the following sequence of questions will usually establish the site of the lesion and provide a strong clue to the cause.

1. *Was the Onset Acute or Gradual?*

Clearly one either has or has not got diplopia, but a relentless worsening suggests infiltration of the nerves or a mechanical displacement of the globe.

2. *Is there any Variability or Remission?*

Extra-ocular nerve lesions of any cause are usually "all or none". If the symptom varies from time to time a latent strabismus or myasthenia gravis must be considered.

3. *Is there any Associated Ptosis of the Eyelid?*

An acute third nerve palsy invariably includes complete ptosis of the eyelid. Lesser degrees of ptosis or variable ptosis should suggest myasthenia gravis or a progressive ocular myopathy. Occasionally, patients with allergic swelling of the eyelid are incorrectly diagnosed as suffering from recurrent partial third nerve lesions; oedema of the eyelid during an attack establishes the diagnosis.

4. *Was there any Pain?*

A painful onset usually indicates aneurysmal dilatation of a blood vessel, either a berry aneurysm causing a third nerve palsy or an aneurysmal dilatation of the intracavernous part of carotid artery causing a third or sixth nerve palsy. Incomplete loss of eye movements and severe congestion of the eye should also raise the possibility of a granulomatous lesion in the orbit, i.e. pseudo-tumour of the orbit or Tolosa–Hunt syndrome. Herpes Zoster Opthalmicus with a nerve palsy should also be considered as the vesicular rash may take several days to appear during which time there is severe pain in the distribution of the first division of the fifth nerve.

Migraine headache may occasionally be complicated by an extra-ocular nerve palsy. A full personal and family history of headaches usually provides a clue to this possibility.

5. *Is there any Exophthalmos or Proptosis?*

Protrusion of the globe suggests the presence of either an aneurysm in the cavernous sinus, thrombosis of the cavernous sinus with vascular congestion or a tumour in the orbit.

The rapidity of onset and presence of pain usually enables the distinction to be made but the inflammatory conditions of the orbit which respond to steroids should also be considered. the fact that thyrotoxicosis is the commonest cause of exophthalmos should always be remembered.

Chapter 6

THE CEREBELLO-PONTINE ANGLE AND JUGULAR FORAMEN

The second major grouping of cranial nerves is found in the region known as the cerebello-pontine angle. This consists of a shallow triangle lying between the cerebellum, the lateral pons, and the inner third of the petrous ridge (see Figure 6.1). The vertical extent of the angle is from the fifth

Figure 6.1. The Skull Base

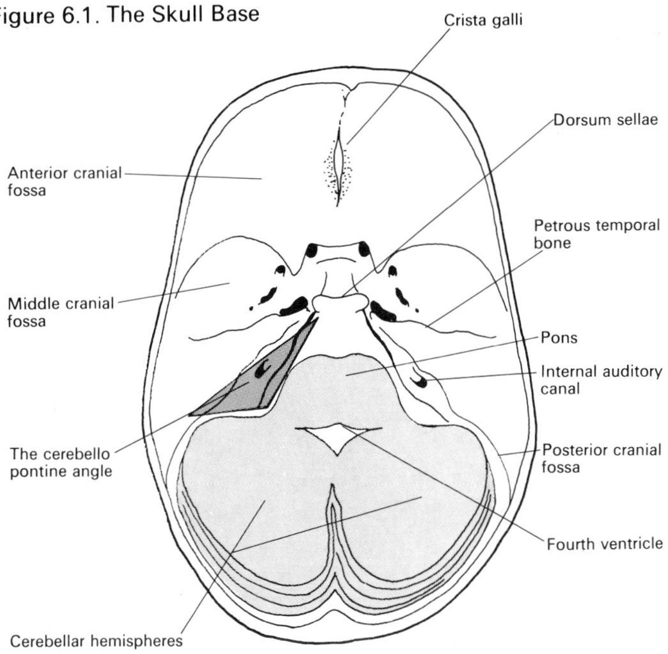

Crista galli

Dorsum sellae

Anterior cranial fossa

Petrous temporal bone

Middle cranial fossa

Pons

Internal auditory canal

The cerebello pontine angle

Posterior cranial fossa

Fourth ventricle

Cerebellar hemispheres

nerve above, on its course from the pons to the petrous apex, and the ninth nerve below, passing from the lateral medulla to the jugular foramen. The abducens nerve runs upwards and forwards on the medial edge of the area and the seventh and eighth cranial nerves traverse the angle to enter the internal auditory canal (Figure 6.5).

The hallmark of a lesion in this region is clinical evidence of damage to the seventh and eighth cranial nerves, so that a wide range of vestibular, auditory and motor abnormalities may occur. Several simple and benign conditions such as Bell's palsy enter into the differential diagnosis of more serious conditions such as acoustic nerve tumours.

It is essential to be able to evaluate the nerves in the area at the bedside, and have at least an understanding of the methods and aims of eighth nerve tests, such as auditory

function tests and the caloric test. These are described and discussed at the end of this chapter.

CLINICAL EVALUATION OF THE AFFECTED CRANIAL NERVES

1. The Trigeminal Nerve (V)

The trigeminal nerve conveys sensation from the face and provides the motor supply to the muscles of mastication, The cutaneous distribution is of great clinical importance.

Figure 6.2. The Cutaneous Distribution of the V Nerve

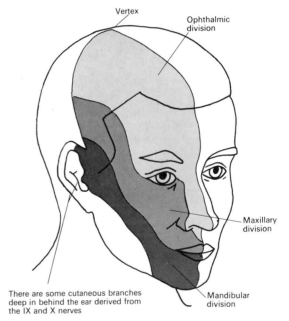

Vertex

Ophthalmic division

Maxillary division

There are some cutaneous branches deep in behind the ear derived from the IX and X nerves

Mandibular division

The sensory supply of the face is shown in Figure 6.2. Notice that the area supplied by the first division extends back to the vertex; not to the hairline and includes the nose and part of the upper lip (embryologically this is the nerve supply of the fronto-nasal process). The third division has a relatively small area of supply and it is important to remember that there is a large area over the angle of the jaw supplied by nerve roots C2 and C3. Patients with non-organic sensory loss over the face usually claim anaesthesia extending to the jawline.

The motor supply of the temporalis muscle, masseter and pterygoids is conveyed to the muscles in the mandibular division of the nerve.

The symptoms of fifth nerve damage include spontaneous pain in the face, which may be indistinguishable at times from true tic douloureux (fully discussed in Chapter 21). Conversely, patients occasionally present with a patch of painless numbness over the face, usually in the distribution of one of the branches. This is an extremely ominous sign, often indicating malignant infiltration of the nerve.

Damage to the motor supply leads to weakness of the muscles of mastication, and yet if the damage is unilateral this rarely causes significant disability and it is extremely unusual for the patient to be aware of the deficit.

Clinical Evaluation of the Fifth Nerve

The most sensitive part of the nerve appears to be those fibres subserving the corneal reflex. The earliest sign of fifth nerve damage is often an impaired or absent corneal response. If numbness of the entire face is found with an intact corneal response there are considerable grounds for doubting the organicity of the claimed sensory loss. In patients with non-organic sensory loss, the numbness often extends from the hairline to the angle of the jaw. This is an important point as anaesthesia of the face is a fairly common manifestation in non-organic disease. In the case of organic damage subsequent blunting of sensation to pin prick and finally anaesthesia may occur, but loss of the corneal reflex is an important early sign.

The masseter is the most powerful muscle in the body and even in the presence of obvious wasting of both the temporalis and masseter muscles on one side it is difficult to detect unilateral weakness of jaw closure. Jaw closure should not be tested with a finger in the patient's mouth. A human bite can be very unpleasant. Downward pressure with the thumb on the bony ledge of the patient's chin is sufficient.

Jaw opening is a much weaker movement (a fact well known to alligator and crocodile handlers) and although wasting in the pterygoids is not detectable, weakness is readily discernible. This is tested by putting a finger or fist under the patient's chin in the mid-line and asking him to open his mouth against moderate resistance. The examiner must allow the mouth to slowly open. If the muscle on the right is weak the jaw will be pushed across to the right side. This is because the action of the two obliquely arranged pterygoid muscles is to tip the jaw open and simultaneously pull it forward. It is the failure to move forward on the weak

side that causes the jaw to deviate *towards* the affected muscles.

The fifth nerve does *not* supply any of the muscles of facial expression.

The Corneal Reflex (Figure 6.3)

A wisp of cotton wool, twisted to a point, should be prepared. The examiner should hold the patient's lower lid down and ask him to look up and to the side. The area shown is stroked gently. The cotton wool should not be allowed to cross in front of the pupil or the patient will see it and blink. The less sensitive bulbar conjunctiva around the edge of the iris should not be stroked. Both eyes should shut simultaneously if the corneal reflex is present.

Figure 6.3. The correct way to elicit the corneal reflex

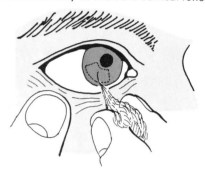

2. The Abducens Nerve (VI)

The anatomy and clinical evaluation of the sixth nerve is fully detailed in Chapter 5.

3. The Facial Nerve (VII) (Figure 6.4)

Many incorrectly think that the fifth nerve has a motor supply to the muscles of facial expression, and there are others who mistakenly think that the seventh nerve conveys sensory fibres to the face. For practical purposes the seventh nerve is purely motor, although it also carries the chorda tympani, conveying taste sensation from the anterior two-thirds of the tongue. As this nerve joins the seventh nerve in the middle ear, theoretically the presence or absence of impaired taste sensation ought to be of great localising value but in practice it is not particularly useful.

The nerve supplies the frontalis muscle and all the muscles of facial expression including platysma. It also supplies tensor tympani and a complete lesion affects auditory acuity on the affected side. The seventh nerve does *not* contribute to the innervation of the upper eyelid and ptosis is *not* a feature of a seventh nerve palsy. There *is* weakness of eye *closure* as the bottom lid is paralysed and cannot wrinkle to

Figure 6.4. Schematic Diagram of the Course and Connections of the Facial Nerve

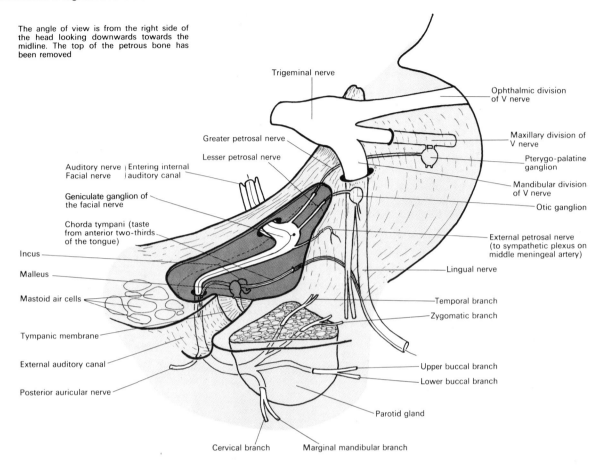

The angle of view is from the right side of the head looking downwards towards the midline. The top of the petrous bone has been removed

Trigeminal nerve

Ophthalmic division of V nerve

Greater petrosal nerve

Maxillary division of V nerve

Lesser petrosal nerve

Pterygo-palatine ganglion

Auditory nerve | Entering internal
Facial nerve | auditory canal

Mandibular division of V nerve

Geniculate ganglion of the facial nerve

Otic ganglion

Chorda tympani (taste from anterior two-thirds of the tongue)

External petrosal nerve (to sympathetic plexus on middle meningeal artery)

Incus

Malleus

Lingual nerve

Mastoid air cells

Temporal branch

Zygomatic branch

Tympanic membrane

External auditory canal

Upper buccal branch

Lower buccal branch

Posterior auricular nerve

Parotid gland

Cervical branch   Marginal mandibular branch

meet the upper lid nor can the upper lid be wrinkled. It can only passively cover the cornea which it protects. Several textbooks incorrectly include ptosis amongst the manifestations of a seventh nerve lesion. Finally, the nerve supplies the platysma muscle over the front of the neck. In some people the voluntary control of this muscle is highly developed and they can 'web' their neck by forced contraction of this muscle. It is best demonstrated when the patient tries to evert his lower lip.

Clinical Evaluation of the Seventh Nerve

One of the problems most often discussed and yet frequently misunderstood is the difference between an upper motor neurone lesion and a lower motor neurone lesion of the seventh nerve.

The difference is based on the supranuclear innervation of the seventh cranial nerve nucleus. This is fully discussed in Chapter 8. Basically, the cerebral hemisphere exerts much more control over the opposite lower face; the part most

concerned with facial expression. The forehead and eye closure mechanisms are mainly concerned with reflex eye closure and have a dual consensual type of innervation (i.e. both eyes shut simultaneously if either eye is threatened).

The simple result is that a unilateral lesion of the fibres from say the left hemisphere, as occurs in a typical C.V.A., will lead to readily detectable weakness in the lower face while eye closure and forehead movement remains intact because the other hemisphere pathways provide adequate cross innervation.

In a lower motor neurone lesion of either the nucleus or the main seventh nerve trunk, *all* muscles innervated by the seventh nerve will be affected, leading to complete loss of control of the face on that side.

The difficulty seems to stem from the terminology—an upper motor neurone lesion affects only the *lower* face, whereas a lower motor neurone lesion affects the entire face.

In evaluating a patient with facial weakness a systematic examination should be made.

1. The patient's ability to wrinkle the forehead is tested, (frontalis muscle). This is impaired in a lower motor neurone lesion.

2. The patient's ability to shut the eyes tightly is tested. In the presence of a lower motor neurone lesion the eye rolls up exposing the conjunctiva. In an upper motor neurone lesion very slight weakness of eye closure is usually detectable.

3. The patient's ability to flare the nostrils, smile and forcibly show the teeth is tested. In a lower motor neurone lesion profound asymmetry is obvious. In an upper motor neurone lesion slow and incomplete movement of the mouth on the side opposite the lesion may be noted. The weakness in an upper motor neurone lesion is rarely complete. A further problem results when the weakness is more apparent on emotional movement (a spontaneous smile) than on volitional movement (showing the teeth). This is discussed further in Chapter 8.

4. The platysma muscle is tested. The best way to do this is to ask the patient to try and evert the lower lip, while observing the neck muscles.

If it were as simple as this, there would be little problem, but there are three other considerations.

1. Everyone has some degree of facial asymmetry. In many cases it is easy to speculate that the patient has facial weakness. Often a comment such as "facial asymmetry, ? weakness" is made. If there is any doubt it is best to assume that the face is normal. The very slight but obvious weakness of eye closure that is typical of an upper motor neurone lesion is the best check. If eye closure is quite normal and symmetrical, there is probably no facial weakness.

2. In a patient with an incomplete lower motor neurone seventh nerve lesion or a recovering Bell's palsy there is often relative preservation or early recovery of the muscles of the forehead and around the eye, the residual weakness of the lower face mimicking a rather severe upper motor neurone lesion.

3. Occasionally, in patients with a greater degree of upper motor neurone control of the opposite seventh nerve than is usual, an upper motor neurone lesion can produce profound weakness of the mouth and moderately severe weakness of the eye and forehead muscles, thus mimicking a recovering or incomplete lower motor neurone lesion.

In both the latter instances one may have to rely on other symptoms and signs to establish the type of seventh nerve lesion. It is always worth obtaining old photographs of the patient and asking relatives' advice. If a close relative can see no change in the patient's expression then there is almost certainly nothing wrong.

Taste Sensation

Taste sensation should always be tested in a patient who has a lower motor neurone lesion of the seventh nerve. The tongue should be pulled out and the surface dried. A drop of sweet, salt or sour flavour is placed on a cotton wool stick and stroked along each side of the tip of the tongue. The patient should then put his tongue back in his mouth but should not swallow until he has established whether the taste was appreciated on both sides.

Taste may be completely lost, or may be delayed often with a slightly metallic flavour in incomplete lesions of the chorda tympani. Unimpaired taste sensation is *not* a reliable indication that the nerve lesion is proximal to the middle ear as these fibres are often spared.

Testing the Corneal Response when Eyelid Closure is Paralysed

When a patient has a lower motor neurone lesion of the seventh nerve eyelid closure is affected so that a normal corneal reponse cannot be seen. It is vital to be certain that the corneal reflex is intact in this situation. If it is impaired the patient clearly has more than a simple Bell's palsy and from a management point of view the eye is at considerable risk from foreign bodies if it is both anaesthetic *and* unprotected.

In this situation testing should be performed as follows:

1. The patient is asked to compare the sensation on both sides when the cornea is stroked with cotton wool as described earlier.
2. The examiner should observe whether the eyeball rolls upwards and away from the stimulus.
3. He should also observe whether the other eye shuts—as noted above, the corneal response is a consensual reflex, like the pupillary response to light.

4. The Auditory and Vestibular Nerve (VIII)

The clinical physiology of the eighth nerve is a subject in itself and is dealt with in greater detail at the end of this chapter.

CEREBELLO-PONTINE ANGLE LESIONS
(Figures 6.5, 6.6)

The terms cerebello-pontine angle tumour and acoustic neuroma are not interchangeable. There are several other less common lesions that may occur at this site.

Acoustic Nerve Tumours

When an acoustic nerve tumour develops in the cerebello-pontine angle, the following sequence of events occurs. The

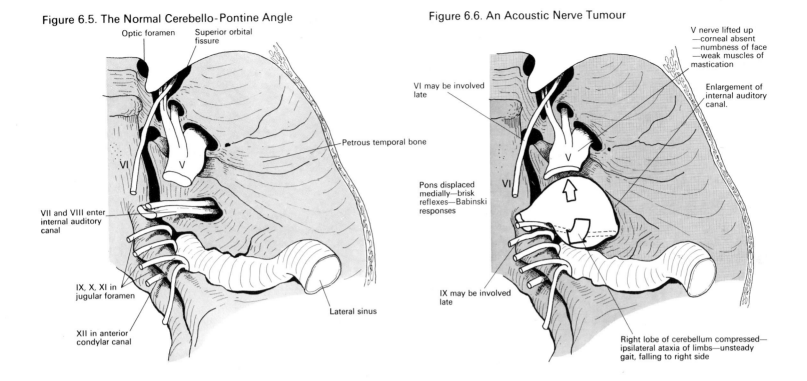

Figure 6.5. The Normal Cerebello-Pontine Angle

Optic foramen
Superior orbital fissure
Petrous temporal bone
VII and VIII enter internal auditory canal
IX, X, XI in jugular foramen
XII in anterior condylar canal
Lateral sinus

Figure 6.6. An Acoustic Nerve Tumour

V nerve lifted up
—corneal absent
—numbness of face
—weak muscles of mastication
VI may be involved late
Enlargement of internal auditory canal.
Pons displaced medially—brisk reflexes—Babinski responses
IX may be involved late
Right lobe of cerebellum compressed—ipsilateral ataxia of limbs—unsteady gait, falling to right side

tumour usually arises on the vestibular division of the nerve, but the earliest symptoms are auditory. Tinnitis (a high pitched ringing noise) is followed by slowly progressive and often unrecognised loss of hearing. Episodes of vertigo are an unusual feature in the early stages of an acoustic nerve tumour, although such tumours are usually accorded an unwarranted high position in the differential diagnosis of vertigo.

Although on anatomical grounds early damage to the seventh nerve would be anticipated, a facial nerve palsy is usually a late manifestation of an acoustic nerve lesion. However, some twitching of the facial musculature (a condition known as hemifacial spasm) may occasionally be a presenting symptom. If the seventh nerve *is* involved the chances of finding a lesion *other than* an acoustic nerve tumour are greatly increased.

The most consistent early physical sign is depression or absence of the corneal reflex. The fifth nerve is lifted up by the tumour and the afferent fibres for the corneal reflex seem to be very sensitive to distortion. Later, numbness over the face may appear but a complete fifth nerve lesion with sensory loss (other than loss of the corneal reflex) or motor weakness is very unusual. Occasionally face pain, similar to tic douloureux may occur, but again this is decidedly unusual.

The ability of the cranial nerves in the vicinity to be stretched and distorted without clinical evidence of damage, is a striking feature of the natural history and clinical findings in a patient with an acoustic nerve tumour.

When the tumour extends medially and starts to distort the brain-stem and cerebellum, more dramatic symptoms are produced. Attacks of vertigo, ataxia of gait or of the upper limbs and a mild spastic paraparesis may occur. The ataxia is usually most marked in the limbs on the side of the tumour. At this stage, brisk reflexes, extensor plantar responses and ataxia may be found, with few local signs except for deafness and a depressed corneal response. If the patient is left untreated further distortion of the brain stem may block the cerebral aqueduct leading to hydrocephalus, headache and papilloedema.

The natural history of an acoustic nerve tumour can range from two to ten years or even longer. Bilateral acoustic neuromas may occur, usually in patients with neurofibromatosis.

Other Causes of Cerebello-Pontine Angle Lesions

Meningiomas, cholesteatomas, haemangioblastomas and aneurysms of the basilar artery may all occur in the cerebello-pontine angle. Neuromas may also occur on the fifth, seventh and ninth nerves and can produce similar clinical pictures. In all the cases the sequence of events may provide the clue to the alternative pathology. An early seventh nerve palsy is an important clue being very rare in acoustic neuromas. On occasions it is not until the lesion is exposed at surgery that its nature is revealed.

A pontine glioma, a rare tumour of the brain stem, primarily occurring in small boys, typically expands the pons and produces a series of projecting knobs of tumour on the surface of the brain stem. One of these knobs may project into the cerebello-pontine angle and produce the clinical picture of an extrinsic tumour in the area. The fact that the patient is a child should always raise the possibility of this diagnosis. Pontine gliomas may also occur in the older patients and particularly in those with neurofibromatosis.

Medulloblastomas and astrocytomas of the cerebellum may push forward into the angle but the inevitable ataxia and the later development of headache, papilloedema and vomiting, usually with a total history of a few months at the most should point to this diagnosis. Again these tumours are more likely to be found in young patients.

Carcinoma of the nasopharynx may invade the skull base between the clivus and the petrous bone where the sixth nerve is especially vulnerable. Malignant infiltration of the fifth nerve usually causes either spontaneous pain or patches of numbness in the fifth nerve distribution. Neither event occurs as an early feature of an acoustic nerve tumour. Carcinoma from distant sites may reach this area and the writer has seen two patients with *acute* cerebello-pontine angle lesions caused by metastatic Hodgkins Disease.

Local meningeal involvement by syphilis or tuberculosis were important causes of the syndrome in the past.

In general whenever the possibility of a lesion in the cerebello-pontine angle is raised the clinical history and the evaluation of the physical signs should be very carefully documented and compared with the typical clinical picture of an acoustic nerve tumour. Any unusual feature should indicate the possibility of another cause.

Investigation of Patients with Suspected Cerebello-Pontine Angle Lesions

Careful history taking and examination may provide all the necessary information for a reasoned guess at the pathology of the lesion.

Routine screening tests should be made for disease elsewhere (syphilis, nasopharyngeal neoplasms etc.).

Plain skull films may be helpful and reveal erosion of the internal auditory foramen. This change is not invariably present and a normal skull film does not exclude an acoustic

nerve tumour. A meningioma can cause hyperostosis (thickening of bone) of the skull base and neuromas in other areas may cause bone erosion.

Full studies are indicated to demonstrate the degree and type of deafness and the impairment of the caloric responses. Interpretation of the caloric tests may become extremely complicated when the brain stem has also been distorted. If the intracranial pressure is not raised either air or contrast medium via the lumbar route will allow good visualisation of the cerebello-pontine angles and will demonstrate the extent of the lesion, although not the pathology.

Vertebral angiography is increasingly used in investigation and helps in both excluding an aneurysm as the causative lesion, and demonstrating the blood supply of the tumour. The high mortality rate of operations on these tumours (15–20 per cent) is due to the difficulty caused when the vessels supplying the tumour also supply the brain stem. Information as to the vascularity of the tumour is of great help to the neurosurgeon.

A raised C.S.F. protein is typical of an acoustic nerve tumour but a normal C.S.F. does not constitute an adequate screening or exclusory investigation.

OTHER CAUSES OF DAMAGE TO CRANIAL NERVES IN THE REGION

Fifth Nerve Lesions

There are four other conditions to be mentioned briefly.

1. *Trigeminal Sensory neuropathy*

This is a rare condition in which progressive numbness of the face occurs in the distribution of the fifth nerve. It may have its onset at any age and the differential diagnosis must include a continued search for a neoplasm in the nasopharynx. A period of up to two years may elapse before a neoplasm can be demonstrated so that the diagnosis of trigeminal sensory neuropathy should not be made too readily and should be kept under continuous review.

2. *Tic Doulouroux*

This condition is discussed in the chapter on face pain (Chapter 21). The features of interest in this chapter are that the pain is not exclusively confined to one division of the nerve, but usually runs along the line between the third and second, and the second and first divisions respectively. Contrary to popular misconception if sensation is tested immediately after a burst of pain, some impairment may be demonstrated. The general rule that there should be *no* sensory loss other than under this circumstance is valid, and a permanent area of numbness excludes the diagnosis (unless previous nerve section has been performed). The diagnosis is only tenable if there are no physical signs of fifth nerve damage.

3. Herpes Zoster Ophthalmicus

This condition is also briefly considered in Chapter 5 and Chapter 21. Although Herpes Zoster theoretically can affect any nerve root in the body, thoracic roots are usually affected, particularly in the younger age group. In the elderly the virus has a predeliction for the first division of the fifth nerve. The typical history is one of two to three days' excruciating pain in the forehead on one or other side. Between the third and fifth days small vesicles appear, usually in the eyebrow. At its height the rash may cover the entire cutaneous distribution of the nerve. Extra-ocular nerve palsies may occur and usually recover over six to eight weeks. The severe pain lessens with the onset of the rash in most cases but if it does not do so urgent treatment in an attempt to prevent the development of "post-herpetic neuralgia" is necessary.

4. Multiple Sclerosis

An attack of numbness of one side of the face in a young person; occasionally following local anaesthesia for dental work is quite a common symptom of multiple sclerosis.

Sixth Nerve Lesions

The causes of sixth nerve lesions have been fully documented previously, see Chapter 5.

Seventh Nerve Lesions

1. Bell's Palsy

One of the most common neurological disorders seen is Bell's Palsy. This consists of an acute seventh nerve paralysis often preceded by a history of aching pain in and around the ear on the day of onset. Otherwise the paralysis is quite painless, although the face is often described as feeling "stiff" or "numb". It is essential to be certain that there is no actual sensory loss as this is quite incompatible with the diagnosis. The palsy is usually complete at the onset, but recovery may be so rapid that the palsy appears incomplete by the time the patient is first seen. The prognosis is excellent, some eighty per cent of the patients making a complete uncomplicated recovery in two to six weeks.

The outlook may be improved by the use of steroids over a ten-day course. The main indication for the use of steroids is a complete palsy particularly if taste is also affected, suggesting severe damage to the nerve. The aetiology is thought to be a viral infection with damage to the swollen nerve caused by entrapment in the facial canal. The only important underlying diseases are diabetes and hypertension, both of which may present as Bell's palsy. Rare causes include sarcoidosis and Melkersson's syndrome, the latter associated with oedema of the face and a fissured tongue. In both conditions recurrent attacks may occur.

The most frequent and tragic mistake is for the patient to be told that Bell's palsy represents a "small stroke"—it does not! This term with all its implications should never be used in discussing this benign condition.

2. Ramsay–Hunt Syndrome (Herpes Zoster of the Seventh Nerve)

In this condition the seventh nerve is damaged by the Herpes virus. This causes certain distinct differences in the clinical picture. Very severe pain in the ear may precede the facial weakness by twenty-four to thirty-six hours, with the later eruption of vesicles in or around the external auditory meatus or over the mastoid process. Other cranial nerves may be involved, notably the fifth nerve with sensory loss over the face or numbness of the palate due to a ninth nerve lesion. The majority of patients recover to some extent but only fifty per cent of patients make a full recovery.

3. Hemifacial Spasm

This condition has many pathological similarities to trigeminal neuralgia and in fact the conditions may co-exist. Both are often caused by minor anatomical variations of blood vessels overlying the nerve inside the skull and presumably causing irritation of the nerve. Hemifacial spasm consists of continual twitching movements usually maximal around the eye and mouth. The condition is annoying and embarrassing rather than unpleasant. Consideration should always be given to the possibility of an underlying lesion although like "tic douloureux" the number of cases in which a lesion is found is small. It may occur in either sex at any age but is more commonly found in older age groups. Tumours in the cerebello-pontine angle, basilar artery aneurysms and basal meningeal lesions may all be responsible for this condition but in the majority of cases no definite cause is found.

THE EIGHTH NERVE

The eighth cranial nerve carries information from two highly specialised end organs; the vestibular apparatus and the organ of Corti. Both lie deep in the temporal bone. They are suspended in the bone in perilymph which is basically C.S.F.

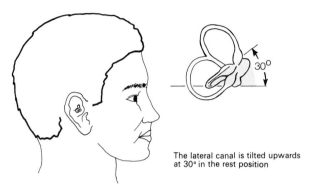

Figure 6.7. Figure to show the Position of the Semicircular Canals in the normal position

The lateral canal is tilted upwards at 30° in the rest position

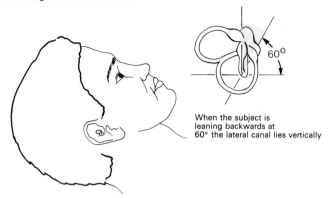

Figure to show the Position of the Semicircular Canals during *The Caloric Test*

When the subject is leaning backwards at 60° the lateral canal lies vertically

and is in continuity with the subarachnoid space. A highly specialised fluid with a high protein content, known as endolymph fills the semicircular canals and the scala media of the cochlear.

The Vestibular Apparatus (Figure 6.7 and 6.8)

1. *The Semi-Circular Canals*

The semi-circular canals are three fine tubes arranged as shown in Figure 6.7. Note that the lateral canal is tilted up 30° at the front; it is *not* horizontal. The six canals work as three matched pairs in three planes as indicated in the figure. At the end of the canal that joins the utricle is a swelling called the ampulla. This contains the cupola and the hair cells. The cells are polarised to respond to movement in one direction only by the position of the single kinocilium on each cell. In the lateral canal movement towards the utricle stimulates the cupola. The vertical canals are stimulated by movement *away* from the utricle.

Activity in the canals is transmitted to the vestibular nucleus on the same side of the brain stem and then to the eye muscle nuclei as discussed in Chapter 7. The desired end result is that whatever the position of the head the eyes look straight ahead.

2. *The Otolith Organs*

The Utricular Mechanism

The otolith organ in the utricle senses tilting of the head. It is shaped like a flat plate tilted up at the anterior end. It is covered with hairs polarised towards the bend. Head tilt is sensed by the variation in pressure of the calcium carbonate crystals on the hairs produced by gravity.

The Saccular Mechanism

The organ in the saccule senses angular acceleration of the head. It is shaped like a shield with a central ridge facing forwards. Forward movement forces the crystals to attempt to slide down the slope on either side proportional to the speed and angle of the movement.

Vestibular Function Tests

1. *Gait and Stance*

Patients with a unilateral disorder of vestibular function tend to veer or fall to that side. The same is true of cerebellar disease so that any distinction between the two has to be made on other grounds. The Romberg test is *not* a specific test of vestibular function.

2. *Nystagmus*

Nystagmus is discussed in detail in Chapter 8.

3. *The Caloric Test*

This is the most useful test of vestibular function. Ideally a standardised test using thermostatically controlled water temperature should be used. The test is based on the fact that the cupola can be deflected by convection currents set up in the semi-circular canals if they are heated or cooled. The lateral canals can be easily stimulated by hot or cold fluid running through the external auditory canal. A further advantage is that the patient's head can be held still so that the resulting nystagmus is easily observed.

a. The patient sits on a couch with his head back at 60° to bring the lateral canals to the vertical position. This is because it is easier to produce convection currents in a vertical column of fluid. The test should not be performed if the ear drum is perforated.

b. Water at 30°C and 44°C is run into each ear in turn. A thermostat is used to keep the temperature steady and 250 mls. of water are allowed to flow over 40 seconds in the standardised test.

Figure 6.8. Schematic Diagram of Right Vestibular Apparatus

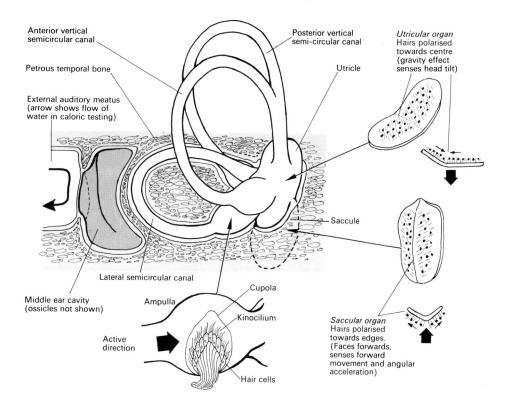

c. While the water is running the patient looks at a point straight ahead. This produces vertigo and easily observed nystagmus as the canals are stimulated or inhibited and the eyes are pushed or pulled to either side. The duration of the nystagmus is timed. The normal duration is 2 minutes ±15 seconds.

Explanation of results (Figure 6.9)

a. Cold water cools the apex of the canal and fluid flows towards the cool area *away* from the utricle. The cupola is inhibited.

b. Hot water heats the apex of the canal setting up a convection current towards the utricle. This stimulates the cupola.

c. With the knowledge that an active semicircular canal moves the eyes to the opposite side it follows that cold water upsets the balance and the normal canal pushes the eyes towards the cold stimulus. Conversely, the hot water activates the canal and pushes the eyes away from the stimulated ear.

The two abnormalities that may be detected are called canal paresis and directional preponderance.

Canal Paresis

If the semicircular canals or the VIIIth nerve are damaged an incomplete or defective response to both hot or cold water in the *affected* ear will be found.

Directional Preponderance

The central connections of the vestibular nerve are such that cold water in one ear has the same effect as hot water in the other. If it is found that nystagmus cannot be induced to one side it indicates that the vestibular nucleus of the appropriate side is defective. This is known as directional preponderance.

There are some situations in which both canal paresis and directional preponderance may be combined. This is often encountered when an acoustic nerve tumour or other posterior fossa lesion is displacing the brain stem.

4. Positional Nystagmus

When a patient's main symptom is vertigo occurring only when the head is in a certain position, positional testing is essential.

Figure 6.9. Diagram to Illustrate the Mechanism of the Caloric Test

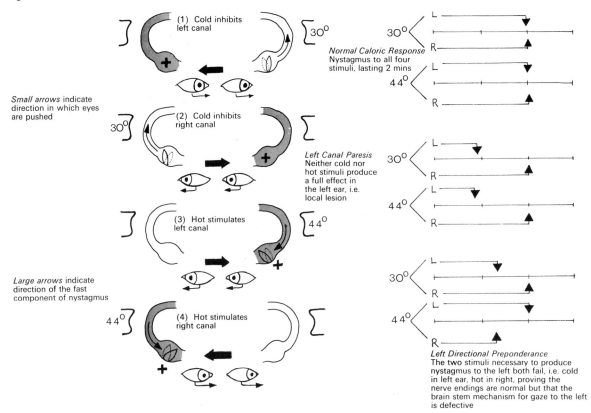

(1) Cold inhibits left canal

Small arrows indicate direction in which eyes are pushed

(2) Cold inhibits right canal

(3) Hot stimulates left canal

Large arrows indicate direction of the fast component of nystagmus

(4) Hot stimulates right canal

Normal Caloric Response
Nystagmus to all four stimuli, lasting 2 mins

Left Canal Paresis
Neither cold nor hot stimuli produce a full effect in the left ear, i.e. local lesion

Left Directional Preponderance
The two stimuli necessary to produce nystagmus to the left both fail, i.e. cold in left ear, hot in right, proving the nerve endings are normal but that the brain stem mechanism for gaze to the left is defective

The patient's head is held by the examiner with the patient sitting with his back towards the end of a couch. The patient is then quickly lowered with his head turned to the right or left until the head is off the end of the couch and below the horizontal position. Acute vertigo with brisk nystagmus occurs when the affected vestibular apparatus is in the underneath position. There are two types of response.

a. Nystagmus starts after a ten to fifteen second delay, lasts some fifty seconds and is directed towards the underneath ear. If the test is repeated the response is less dramatic or absent. This is the benign type.

b. If the nystagmus comes on immediately, persists as long as the position is maintained or is in the opposite direction, it is of the central type. Repeated testing will produce repeated responses. There is a high likelihood that the patient has a tumour in the posterior fossa.

More complex vestibular tests including electro-nystagmography will not be discussed in detail. Their main advantage lies in the fact, that using electrical recording with the eyes closed, the optic fixation reflexes are abolished. These reflexes are strong enough to suppress peripheral vestibular nystagmus but have no effect on nystagmus due to central pathway, cerebellar nystagmus. This allows a distinction to be made that may be impossible on clinical examination.

The Auditory Apparatus (Figure 6.10)

The organ of Corti has a similar basic structure and consists of receptor hair cells arranged in a spiral tube. The cavity of the tube is divided into three compartments by two membranes stretched across its centre, a roof membrane (of Reissner) and a tightly stretched basilar membrane. The closed cavity between them is filled with endolymph and the cavities on either side with perilymph. The receptor cells lie on supporting tissue arising from the basilar membrane. The hair processes are embedded in a thin membrane that bridges across the organ of Corti, known as the tectorial membrane. When the basilar membrane vibrates in response to a sound wave the tectorial membrane has a shearing effect on the hairs. At the apex of the cochlear the membrane has a diameter of 0·5 mm. and at the base 0·04 mm., responding to low tones and high tones respectively. The pressure wave is transmitted through the perilymph by the pump-like effect of

Figure 6.10. Section of part of the Cochlear Spiral

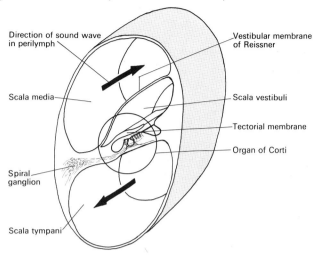

The Anatomy of the Organ of Corti

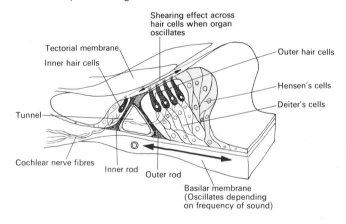

the stapes in the oval window and the shock wave passes to the round window where the energy is dissipated.

Hearing can be tested at the bedside in the following ways.

a. A simple test can be performed with a watch and quantitated by measuring the distance from the ear at which the watch can still just be heard.

b. If a watch cannot be heard at all a whispered voice at about eighteen inches should be tried, gradually raising the voice until it becomes audible. It is essential to occlude the opposite ear with a finger while performing this test.

c. The tuning fork tests help distinguish between hearing loss due to middle ear disease (conductive deafness) and that due to eighth nerve damage (perceptive deafness).

The Rinne Test

A 512 cycle tuning fork is held on the mastoid until it is no longer audible. If it is then held by the external auditory canal it will still be audible to the normal ear. This is documented as AC>BC. In perceptive deafness this situation persists, but in conductive deafness BC>AC as air conducted sound depends on intact auditory ossicles for its transmission.

The Weber Test

If the tuning fork is then placed on the vertex it should be heard equally in both ears if hearing is normal. In perceptive deafness the fork will not be heard in the affected ear. In conductive deafness, the fork will be heard equally well in both ears as the auditory ossicles are circumvented.

Electrophysiological Tests of Hearing

Classical audiometric testing includes pure tone audiometry, speech audiometry and the measurement of tone decay. These tests require considerable expertise and patient co-operation and are not easily used in young children. This is a subject in itself and can only really be appreciated by seeing the tests performed. Basically pure sounds of known frequency and intensity or a series of words are presented to the patient via earphones. The positive or correct response is plotted on standard graphs and the distinction between conductive and perceptive deafness can be made.

Recent advances in electrophysiological testing allow not only hearing to be tested but also neural activity in the cochlear, auditory nerve and brain stem pathways can be studied.

Acoustic or stapedius reflex testing is performed using an airtight probe in the external auditory meatus. The probe injects the sound, permits the pressure in the canal to be controlled and detects movement of the tympanic membrane. The stiffening of the membrane when a noise is presented to the ear is detected, requiring no co-operation from the patient.

Electrocochleography (ECog) is performed by inserting a long needle electrode through the tympanic membrane. Small potentials generated in the cochlear itself and in the auditory nerve and brain stem can be detected and studied using averaging techniques. Of special interest to neurologists, is the recording of a stream of potentials in the brain stem set up by an auditory stimulus. A series of five potentials are detected by an electrode over the mastoid process and information about brain stem function can be obtained. This promises to be of value in diseases affecting the brain stem, such as multiple sclerosis.

CLINICAL DISORDERS OF THE EIGHTH NERVE AND ITS CONNECTIONS

The insidious development of deafness and the late symptom of vertigo in cerebello-pontine angle lesions has been stressed. Only acute disorders of the eighth nerve produce dramatic symptoms such as tinnitus, acute deafness or vertigo. The most frequent cause of tinnitus is probably the rushing noise, synchronous with the pulse, that occurs in elderly arteriopathic patients and occasionally drives them to suicide. Vertigo, however, is a very frequent and distressing symptom. The most important point is to establish that the patient really has vertigo. Patients invariably use the expressions "dizzy" or "giddy" and too often these terms are uncritically accepted as vertigo. Closer questioning may reveal that the patient feels "lightheaded", "woozy" or "faint" but does *not* have the characteristic spinning sensation of vertigo. Once these "non-vertiginous" patients have been excluded relatively few disorders need be considered and most have a very characteristic history. The majority of patients in the "non-vertigo" group are suffering from an anxiety state or hyperventilation syndrome; these conditions are fully discussed in Chapter 22.

History is all important in patients with vertigo and the type of sensation, the circumstances under which it occurs, the associated symptoms, duration and frequency of attacks must all be established.

The major causes of vertigo are:

1. Benign positional vertigo
2. Vestibular neuronitis
3. Ménières Disease
4. Migraine
5. Multiple sclerosis
6. Drugs, including alcohol
7. Brain stem ischaemic attacks
8. Temporal lobe epilepsy

Benign Positional Vertigo

This condition occurs mainly in middle age. It may follow upper respiratory tract infections or quite mild head trauma. In most cases no cause can be found. This history is very striking. The patient complains of sudden attacks of vertigo while putting his head back on to the pillow to go to sleep or while getting up in the morning. Attacks during the day are unusual, and once an attack has occurred and ended, usually within fifty seconds, the patient can move about without a recurrence. The condition usually remits spontaneously over a period of weeks to months. Positional testing as described previously should be carried out and a careful distinction made between the benign form and the type indicating a tumour in the posterior fossa.

Vestibular Neuronitis

This is a common disorder that occasionally occurs in epidemic form and is thought to be due to a viral infection of Scarpa's ganglion, or of the brainstem vestibular system. The onset is abrupt with very severe ataxia and vertigo, often with severe vomiting. No position is completely comfortable and preferentially the patient lies quite still on his back. The recovery period may take several weeks with decreasing but disabling vertigo persisting during this period.

Ménière's Disease

Although this diagnosis is often suspected it is quite a rare disease of the elderly. Attacks are usually of sudden onset preceded by a full or bursting sensation in the head and followed by a roaring or hissing noise in the ear, which disappears as the ear becomes deaf later in the attack. Intense vertigo is present from the onset, but the disturbance of the otoliths is the main problem and the patient may be unable to stand or may feel as though he is somersaulting over backwards. Attacks may last up to 24 hours and leave the patient exhausted. It is the associated auditory symptoms that are the key factor in this history.

Migraine

Nausea and vertigo are common components of the migraine syndrome and many patients feel these symptoms are worse than the headache! The onset of a characteristic headache (see Chapter 20) should leave little doubt as to the diagnosis. Problems may arise when the headaches are completely replaced by the vestibular symptoms. It is essential to explore fully the previous headache history of any patient with unexplained attacks of vertigo and vomiting.

Multiple Sclerosis

Although multiple sclerosis may cause an episode of acute vertigo the majority of patients also have symptoms such as diplopia, numbness of the face, weakness or ataxia of a limb or dysarthria to indicate a more widespread brainstem lesion. None of these additional symptoms can occur with a simple disorder of the vestibular apparatus. Furthermore, in multiple sclerosis the cochlear fibres entering the brainstem may also be damaged, leading to deafness in one ear. This combination of signs may lead to diagnostic errors and Meniere's Disease may be suspected. The persistence of an attack over a two to three week period—and the patient's age—usually excludes Ménière's Disease.

Drugs

Many drugs and alcohol cause vertigo as a side effect. The drugs include all anti-convulsants, many sedatives, carbamezepine (Tegretol), some antibiotics, chloroquine, methysergide maleate (Deseril), and aspirin, which may also cause tinnitus. A careful history of drug ingestion and dosage should be regarded as part of the routine questioning in any patient who complains of vertigo.

Brain stem Vascular Disease

Although vertigo is the single most common symptom of brain stem vascular disease it does not follow that vertigo in an elderly patient is invariably due to vertebral-basilar ischaemia. As in the case of multiple sclerosis, a careful enquiry for *other* symptoms of brain stem disease should be made. It is unwise to accept this diagnosis uncritically. Brain stem vascular disease is very much overdiagnosed in elderly patients who have brief attacks of vertigo on hot days, in bathrooms and when standing up suddenly.

Temporal Lobe Epilepsy

An occasional patient with temporal lobe epilepsy will report vertigo as a symptom, often as a component of the prodromal phase of the attack. Subsequent events should leave little doubt that vertigo was part of an epileptic event. Discharges from the posterior temporal lobe are usually responsible (see also Chapters 10 and 22).

JUGULAR FORAMEN SYNDROMES

The jugular foramen is an extremely difficult area to illustrate and understand. The ninth, tenth and eleventh cranial nerves enter the internal part of the foramen lying on the medial side of the sigmoid sinus. The foramen itself angles forwards and laterally under the petrous bone which is excavated by the slight ballooning of the sigmoid sinus as it bends downwards to become the jugular bulb. The three cranial nerves emerge in front of the jugular bulb lying between it and the carotid artery which enters the carotid canal just anteriorly. There are two other structures to be considered; (a) The twelfth (hyoglossal) nerve which exits through the anterior condylar canal and comes into close relationship with the three other nerves outside the skull. (b) The cervical sympathetic which ascends into the area on the carotid artery; it does not exit from the skull via the foramen. It follows that if the cervical sympathetic is involved in a jugular foramen syndrome the lesion is certain to be outside the skull (this point is amplified later). (See Figures 6.11, 6.12)

CLINICAL EVALUATION OF THE LAST FOUR CRANIAL NERVES

1. The Glosso-Pharyngeal Nerve (IX)

A frequent error is the use of the expression "ninth nerve palsy". There is no such thing. From a practical point of view the nerve is purely sensory. The only muscle supplied by the nerve is the stylo-pharyngeus, which cannot be tested clinically. The error is made because of an almost universal misconception that the ninth nerve is motor to the palate. When the gag reflex is tested the stimulus is relayed in the ninth nerve but the resulting palatal movement is mediated by the *tenth* nerve. This reflex is too gross for accurate clinical diagnosis.

Sensation should be tested by touching the palate gently with an orange stick on each side, and then with the patient saying "Aah" touching the posterior pharyngeal wall on both sides. The patient should be asked to compare these gentle stimuli.

If there is any doubt, pain sensation should be tested in the same areas using a long hat pin. It is vital to test for such sensory loss in all the clinical situations discussed in this chapter.

Taste sensation over the posterior third of the tongue has no value in clinical diagnosis.

2. The Vagus Nerve (X)

The vagus is the motor nerve to the palate and the vocal cords. Weakness of the palate may cause nasal regurgitation of food, and nasal speech. The paralysed side of the palate does not move and is pulled across to the intact side when the patient says "Aah".

Paralysis of one vocal cord will allow that cord to lie permanently and limply in the midline. This leads to hoarseness, loss of volume of the voice and an inability to cough explosively—the so called "bovine" cough.

Examination of the tenth nerve should include examination of palatal movements, the patient's voice, and the patient's ability to cough.

3. Spinal Accessory Nerve (XI)

The spinal accessory nerve is motor to the sternomastoid and the upper part of the trapezius muscle. The complex central control of this nerve is discussed in Chapter 11. From a practical point of view, damage to the nerve itself results in wasting and weakness of the sternomastoid and upper trapezius. Like so many things in neurology these signs are very easily overlooked unless one is specifically alerted to the possibility of an abnormality.

Figure 6.11. The Jugular Foramen—Diagrammatic Sagittal Section

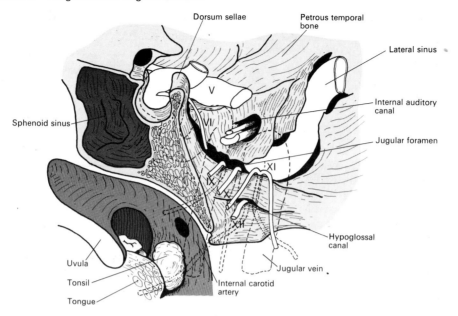

Figure 6.12. The Jugular Foramen —seen diagrammatically from below

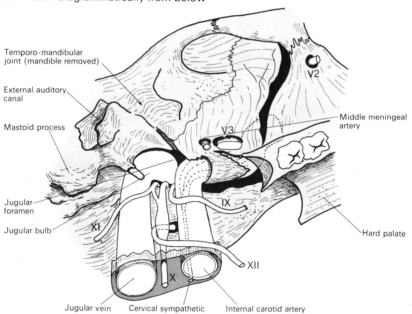

4. The Hypoglossal Nerve (XII)

The twelfth nerve is the motor nerve to the tongue. The tongue muscle in addition to moving the tongue from side to side, also moves it up and down. In fact the tongue is a piece of muscle pulling against itself.

Unilateral damage to the nerve supply leads to wasting, weakness and fasciculation of that side of the tongue. The wasting and fasciculation are best seen with the tongue lying in the floor of the mouth. Normal tongues show flickering movements when held out for more than a few seconds—a source of considerable anxiety to generations of medical students! On attempted tongue protrusion the muscle on the weak side cannot balance the forward push of the muscle on the intact side, and as a result the tongue deviates *towards* the weak side.

5. The Cervical Sympathetic

Horner's syndrome has been discussed in detail in Chapter 2.

6. The Anatomy of Swallowing

Several cranial nerves are involved simultaneously in chewing, bolus formation and swallowing. The whole sequence of events is fully detailed in Figure 6.13.

CLINICAL PRESENTATIONS

Due to the proximity of the last four cranial nerves several combinations of nerve lesions are possible, depending on the site of the causative lesion.

The presenting symptoms are similar whatever the diagnosis. They include loss of strength or hoarseness of the voice, nasal speech, difficulty in swallowing with nasal regurgitation of fluids or aspiration of food particles with attacks of choking.

The accidental observation of weakness and wasting of the sternomastoids and trapezii or tongue wasting noted by a dentist may also lead to referral.

Both the ninth and tenth nerves convey some sensation from the region of the external auditory canal and the area behind the ear. Deep aching pain in and around the ear may herald damage to these nerves in the region of the jugular foramen. Headache may also occur as these nerves convey pain fibres from the dura of the posterior fossa. Irritation of these nerves may cause referred pain in the occipital region.

As noted in Chapter 2, a Horner's syndrome can be easily overlooked by the patient but may occasionally be a presenting symptom.

Figure 6.13. The Anatomy and Physiology of Swallowing

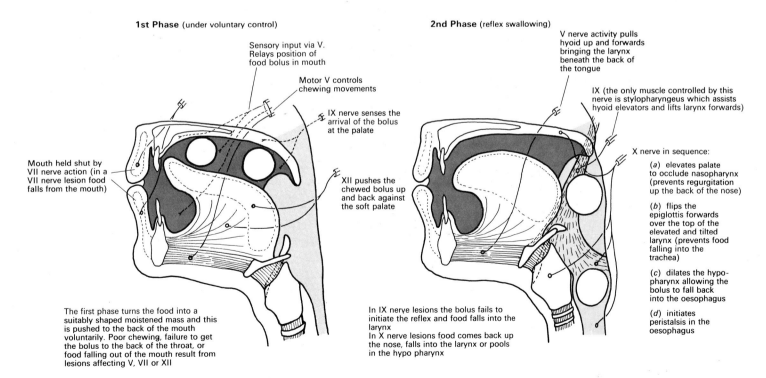

1st Phase (under voluntary control)

Sensory input via V. Relays position of food bolus in mouth

Motor V controls chewing movements

IX nerve senses the arrival of the bolus at the palate

Mouth held shut by VII nerve action (in a VII nerve lesion food falls from the mouth)

XII pushes the chewed bolus up and back against the soft palate

The first phase turns the food into a suitably shaped moistened mass and this is pushed to the back of the mouth voluntarily. Poor chewing, failure to get the bolus to the back of the throat, or food falling out of the mouth result from lesions affecting V, VII or XII

2nd Phase (reflex swallowing)

V nerve activity pulls hyoid up and forwards bringing the larynx beneath the back of the tongue

IX (the only muscle controlled by this nerve is stylopharyngeus which assists hyoid elevators and lifts larynx forwards)

X nerve in sequence:

(*a*) elevates palate to occlude nasopharynx (prevents regurgitation up the back of the nose)

(*b*) flips the epiglottis forwards over the top of the elevated and tilted larynx (prevents food falling into the trachea)

(*c*) dilates the hypopharynx allowing the bolus to fall back into the oesophagus

(*d*) initiates peristalsis in the oesophagus

In IX nerve lesions the bolus fails to initiate the reflex and food falls into the larynx
In X nerve lesions food comes back up the nose, falls into the larynx or pools in the hypo pharynx

The Syndromes

1. Vernet's Syndrome (of the Jugular Foramen)

This consists of damage to the three nerves that traverse the jugular foramen itself, i.e. cranial nerves IX, X and XI. A lesion inside the skull is more likely to cause this restricted syndrome because a lesion outside the skull is likely to affect the twelfth cranial nerve and the cervical sympathetic as well.

2. Collet—Sicard Syndrome (of the Posterior Lacero-Condylar Area)

The Collet—Sicard syndrome consists of damage to the last four cranial nerves. In Figure 6.12 it will be seen that as the foramen opens from the skull it is adjacent to the foramen lacerum, just above the condyle of the occipital bone. The last four cranial nerves lie close together in this area. This syndrome could also occur with a lesion inside the head, but an intracranial lesion extensive enough to affect all four nerves (see Figure 6.11) would usually distort the brain stem and produce signs of long tract damage.

3. Villaret's Syndrome (of the Posterior Retropharyngeal Space)

Again referring to Figure 6.12 the reader will see that in the anterior part of the area lying immediately behind the naso-pharynx, the cervical sympathetic is extremely vulnerable. Villaret's syndrome consists of damage to the IX, X, XI and XII nerves *and* a Horner's syndrome.

CAUSES OF JUGULAR-FORAMEN SYNDROMES

Lesions Inside the Skull

Any of the lesions that can cause the cerebello-pontine angle syndrome can also extend down and involve the last four cranial nerves in numerical sequence. The diagnosis is easy if the fifth and seventh nerves are also affected, as there is no lesion that could occur *outside* the skull and produce such a combination.

Tumours that specifically occur inside the skull in this region are neurinomas of the ninth, tenth or twelfth nerves. They occur most often on the twelfth nerve with a marked predilection for young females and occur on the left side in a ratio of 9:1. The reason for this is unknown. Meningiomas and epidermoid tumours (cholesteatomas) may also occur in this area and tend to cause distortion of the brain stem. This produces long tract signs and symptoms such as a mild or intermittent tetraparesis.

Lateral brain stem lesions are unusual except for vascular accidents. Although these syndromes may include a Horner's syndrome, they rarely cause diagnostic confusion because of the almost invariable spinothalamic sensory loss on the opposite side of the body which leaves no doubt that the cranial nerve damage is due to intrinsic brain stem disease (see also Chapter 11).

Lesions in the Jugular Foramen or Outside the Skull

Of the lesions discussed above both meningiomas and neurofibromas may extend out through the foramen in a dumb-bell fashion—sometimes presenting as a mass at the angle of the jaw.

A Horner's syndrome is certain evidence that the lesion is outside the skull; as the cervical sympathetic ascends *into* the area and does not pass through the foramen.

Attempts should also be made to see if a palpable mass is present at the angle of the jaw, or any cervical lymphadenopathy. It is important to realise that a bony hard mass is normally palpable in this area—it is the tip of the transverse process of the atlas!

Other Causes

1. Poly-Neuritis Cranialis

This is a somewhat dubious entity which basically consists of multiple cranial nerve palsies for which no cause can be established and which may well recover. The writer has seen several examples in elderly patients in whom intensive investigations including multiple naso-pharyngeal biopsies failed to demonstrate a cause and who recovered completely under observation. Some of the reported cases have also suffered from diabetes or syphilis, and the nerve lesions may represent a variety of transient nerve palsies similar to those that may involve the extra-ocular nerves. An important practical point is that although the suspicion of metastatic carcinoma must be high, irradiation without tissue diagnosis is not justified, unless relentless progression of the syndrome can be established. Isolated twelfth nerve palsies with recovery after a few weeks may occur and may be due to a similar pathology to Bell's palsy. In all cases follow up should be continued until full recovery has occurred.

2. Glomus or Carotid Body Tumours

These tumours arise in the chemo-ectodermal tissue that is normally present in the carotid body and may be found ectopically in the inner ear and around the ninth and tenth nerves. Neoplastic changes in this tissue produces highly vascular erosive tumours that may destroy the petrous temporal bone and present as a vascular nodule in the external auditory canal.

Depending on the exact site of the glomus tumour a cerebello-pontine angle syndrome associated with an internal and/or an external jugular foramen syndrome may result. These tumours occur in either sex with a peak incidence in the third and fourth decades.

3. *Glosso-Pharyngeal Neuralgia*

This very rare form of neuralgia consists of attacks of severe pain in the throat when fluid or food is swallowed. The pain is excruciating and similar to that of tic douloureux. Exploration to cut the nerve often reveals aberrant vessels coursing across the nerve or unsuspected neuro-fibromas, or cholesteatomas adjacent to the nerve. It is always wise to regard the syndrome as potentially symptomatic (i.e. indicating an underlying lesion) until proved otherwise by events or surgical exploration.

Investigation of the Jugular Foramen Syndrome

Having established the combination of nerve palsies, the two most important clinical signs to be excluded are a Horner's syndrome and evidence of brain stem compression (such as a spastic paraparesis). The former indicates an extracranial lesion and the latter an intracranial lesion.

If the lesion is outside the skull routine haematological studies and chest and paranasal sinus x-rays assume significance and direct examination of the nasopharynx and larynx is a part of the routine evaluation. Skull x-rays are rarely of value although a careful skull base film should be taken.

If the lesion is intracranial air encephalography or contrast studies (myelography) are necessary. If the lesion is outside the skull a carotid angiogram may demonstrate a mass displacing the upper carotid artery.

As an example of the jugular foramen syndrome—

CASE REPORT

A 76-year-old man presented with a history of weight loss, a mass at the angle of his jaw, dysphagia and a hoarse voice. On examination the following signs were present:

1. There was a hard tender mass at the angle of his jaw.
2. The left palate was insensitive to touch and pinprick.
3. The left palate was weak and he had a bovine cough.
4. There was wasting and weakness of the left sternomastoid and trapezius muscles.
5. The left side of the tongue was slightly wasted, fasciculating and deviated to the left on protrusion.
6. He had a left Horner's syndrome.

In this case the mass and the Horner's syndrome indicated that the lesion was extracranial. Biopsy revealed a squamous carcinoma, probably metastatic from the lung.

A certain amount of easily acquired skill is necessary to detect multiple lower cranial nerve palsies. The provisional diagnosis and investigative approach depend on the accurate detection of associated signs. Jugular foramen syndromes are examples of conditions where clinical findings alone provide nearly all the information necessary to diagnose and treat the patient.

Chapter 7

CONJUGATE EYE MOVEMENTS AND NYSTAGMUS

The eyes have central connections that function like the steering linkage on a car, allowing the eyes to move together, that is, the movements are "conjugate". In the absence of these controlling mechanisms the eyes rove in an aimless way. If these mechanisms fail to develop, as in the case of someone who is blind from birth, wild roving eye movements are a very obvious feature.

Three basic control mechanisms are established in the first few months of life, provided that the child has normal vision.

1. The ability to look in any desired direction, until an object of interest is found. These movements occur as little flicks of the eyes, called "saccadic movements". They essentially supply the brain with a series of still pictures until the desired object is located. They are under voluntary control and are initiated in the frontal lobes.

2. The ability to hold the object on the same point of the retina in spite of any movement it may make. These pursuit movements of the eyes are smooth to avoid jerky vision. They are controlled by the parieto-occipital area in close liaison with the visual cortex.

3. Ideally the eyes are held in the straight ahead position most of the time. This is achieved by the continual adjustment of the eye position in relation to the position of the head in space and is maintained by vestibular activity and proprioceptive information from the neck muscles integrated at brain stem level.

PATHWAYS OF CONJUGATE GAZE CONTROLLING MECHANISMS

It must be stressed that many of the pathways to be discussed are only presumed to exist. None of the descending pathways can be followed beyond the general area of the pretectal region and the lateral pontine reticular formation. The rough position of the pathways has been deduced from clinical evidence provided by lesions in the brain stem and their effects on eye movements.

Voluntary Gaze Mechanism (Figure 7.1)

The cortical areas controlling voluntary gaze lie in the premotor strip of the frontal lobe (area 8). This area has an intimate connection with the parietal control area, which it can override at any time to change the direction of gaze. The descending pathways pass in the corona radiata through the anterior limb and genu of the internal capsule, closely associated with the corticobulbar fibres to the brain stem nuclei. From the internal capsule the fibres rotate to lie medially and dorsally in the cerebral peduncle (follow the arrows on the figure). The main pathway passes to the pons and at some point decussates to the opposite side. The exact point is not established. Here it ends in a presumptive 'pontine centre for lateral gaze', which may lie in the para-abducent nucleus, or in the vestibular nucleus itself. The adjacent sixth nerve nucleus is activated from this area and so is the opposite paired medial rectus muscle, by a very important relay, back across the midline and up to the opposite third nerve nucleus. Thus, both eyes look to the left or right simultaneously. This relay pathway is the medial longitudinal fasciculus. The fundamental importance of this tract is shown by its presence in all vertebrates, and in its being the first tract to myelinate in man. A less well-documented pathway controlling vertical gaze also exists. Clinical evidence would suggest that this pathway is mediated via the basal ganglia and the area underlying the superior colliculus.

Pursuit Eye Movement Mechanism (Figure 7.2)

The object to be followed is located by voluntary effort. The eye "locks in" on the object, and the eyes then only move in response to movements of the object, which is kept focused on the macular part of the retina. Thus a direct relay from the visual cortex, forward to area 19 controls the movement. This area projects via corticotectal and corticotegmental fibres into the midbrain and pons. There is also a large forward projection that gives the frontal eye fields information as to where to direct voluntary gaze, although it is unlikely that the parietal area actively controls frontal eye field activity.

Vestibular and Cerebellar Influences on Eye Movements

These influences are best understood if we examine what happens when one lateral semicircular canal is stimulated.

Figure 7.1. Voluntary control (frontal eye fields)
Start at circle to follow complete pathway

Area 19
parieto-occipital
eye field

Pathway mediating
voluntary vertical
movements and
convergence

? Via basal
ganglia

Via anterior limb
and genu of the
internal capsule

Start here

Area 8
frontal eye field

III

VI

Medial longitudinal
fasciculus (relay
back up to opposite
III nerve)

Lateral pontine
gaze centre

Adducting eye (III)   Abducting eye (VI)

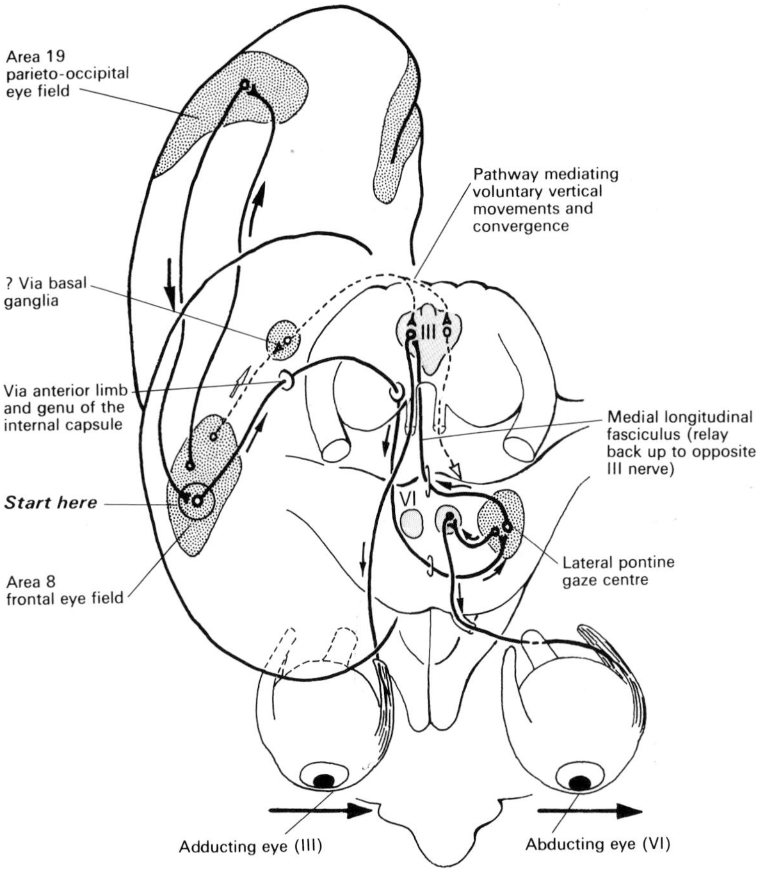

Figure 7.2. Pursuit eye movements (parieto-occipital eye fields)
Start at circle to follow complete pathway

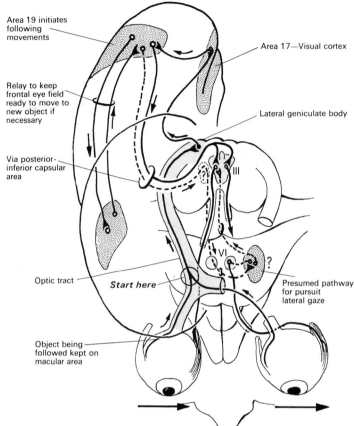

Area 19 initiates
following
movements

Area 17—Visual cortex

Relay to keep
frontal eye field
ready to move to
new object if
necessary

Lateral geniculate body

Via posterior-
inferior capsular
area

III

Optic tract

Start here

VI

Presumed pathway
for pursuit
lateral gaze

Object being
followed kept on
macular area

The lateral canal is only stimulated by forward movement of the endolymph within it (follow arrows on Figure 7.3 from the left labyrinth. See also Chapter 6).

If the head is rotated sharply to the left, the fluid in the left labyrinth moves forward and stimulates the cupola. For the eyes to keep looking straight ahead (the ultimate aim of the whole process) the eyes must deviate to the right side. This is performed by the activity in the medial vestibular nucleus, provoked by the canal stimulation relaying across to the opposite sixth nerve, and back up the medial longitudinal fasciculus to the third nerve nucleus on the same side. Thus both eyes simultaneously move to the right. The cerebellum plays some role through a facilitatory mechanism for the movement relayed through the fastigial nucleus of the cerebellar roof nuclei. Contributory information also comes from the proprioceptive organs of the neck muscles via the spinovestibular tract.

The role of the cerebellum is far from clear. In addition to the above, essentially vestibular reflex pathway that is facilitated by cerebellar activity, there is a prominent flocculo-oculomotor tract, the only direct cerebellar connection with the eye muscle nuclei. This pathway, by its connection with the *opposite* third nerve, and presumably by a relay down to the sixth nerve on its own side, would tend to move the eyes in the opposite direction. This pathway may help explain why nystagmus in cerebellar disease is in the opposite direction to that occurring in vestibular disease. Experimental studies on the role of the cerebellum in eye movements have produced complex results and clinical lesions and stimulation experiments often result in divergence of the eyes!

This difficulty is mentioned because whenever nystagmus is discussed, cerebellar disease is always prominent in discussion, although the nystagmus caused by cerebellar disease is the least understood and clinically the least certain cause of nystagmus that is encountered. We will refer to

Figure 7.3. Vestibular and Cerebellar Influence on Eye Movement
Start at circle to follow complete pathway

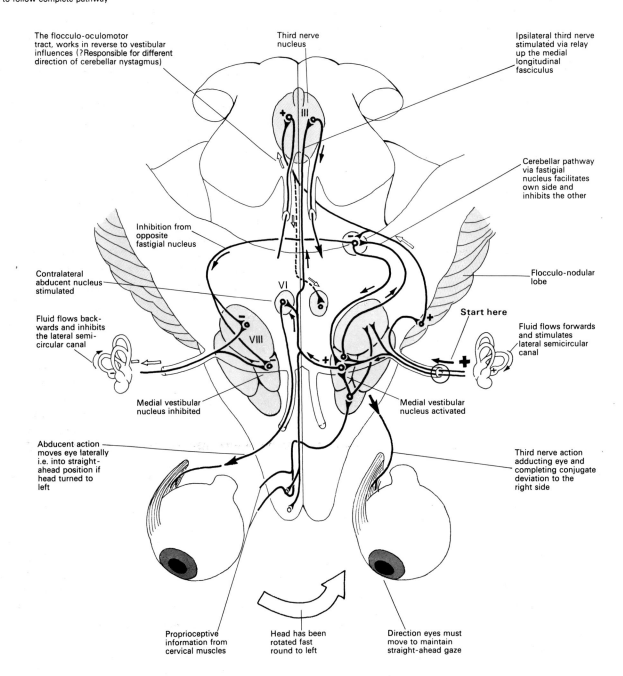

The flocculo-oculomotor tract, works in reverse to vestibular influences (?Responsible for different direction of cerebellar nystagmus)

Third nerve nucleus

Ipsilateral third nerve stimulated via relay up the medial longitudinal fasciculus

Cerebellar pathway via fastigial nucleus facilitates own side and inhibits the other

Inhibition from opposite fastigial nucleus

Contralateral abducent nucleus stimulated

Floccular-nodular lobe

Start here

Fluid flows backwards and inhibits the lateral semi-circular canal

Fluid flows forwards and stimulates lateral semicircular canal

Medial vestibular nucleus inhibited

Medial vestibular nucleus activated

Abducent action moves eye laterally i.e. into straight-ahead position if head turned to left

Third nerve action adducting eye and completing conjugate deviation to the right side

Proprioceptive information from cervical muscles

Head has been rotated fast round to left

Direction eyes must move to maintain straight-ahead gaze

these pathways again in later discussion of the clinical features of nystagmus.

Vertical Eye Movements

Vertical eye movements do not require the participation of the sixth nerve and the controlling mechanisms lie mainly in the midbrain beneath the superior and inferior colliculi. The importance of basal ganglia pathways in these movements can be deduced from some important clinical observations to be discussed later.

The ability to converge the eyes is critical to maintaining close binocular vision. This movement utilises both medial

60

rectus muscles simultaneously. To do this it was theorised that a midline "centre for convergence" existed, and this was long held to be in the nucleus of Perlia, lying between the third nerve nuclei. Experimental work has failed to confirm the validity of this view and divergent squints may result from damage anywhere from the thalamus to the lateral pons or cerebellar peduncles. It seems unlikely that a specific midline mechanism exists.

CLINICAL DISORDERS OF CONJUGATE GAZE MECHANISMS

In each of the controlling areas lesions that damage the pathways may cause inbalance between the two sides by either over-activity or under-activity of the damaged area.

Lesions in the Frontal Cortex and Anterior Internal Capsule

Over-activity of the Frontal Eye Field (see Figure 7.4)

Epileptic seizures arising in the appropriate area of the frontal cortex cause what are called "frontal adversive attacks". In these episodes the attack commences with the head and eyes being forcibly deviated away from the discharging frontal cortex. The side of the body to which the deviation has occurred may then be involved by focal motor activity and ultimately the attack may progress to a generalised seizure.

Under-activity of the Frontal Eye Field

Damage to the frontal eye field by a vascular occlusion may render the patient unable to look to the opposite side. This deficit is rarely seen as rapid compensation occurs and the eye movements appear to be normal within hours. However, residual evidence may be found in the patient having difficulty in maintaining gaze in that direction or in the development of some nystagmus caused by this weakness when attempting to do so. If the patient is subsequently anaesthetised or becomes comatose, the eyes will deviate towards the damaged side of the cortex, because of the unopposed activity of the intact opposite frontal lobe. The unconscious patient with a frontal lesion therefore looks away from his hemiplegic side (see Figure 7.5).

Bilateral damage to the frontal cortex or the appropriate pathways in the internal capsule may lead to total loss of voluntary control over eye movements. There are several relatively rare causes of this condition. A congenital variety exists called congenital oculomotor apraxia. The affected child moves his whole head around to find the desired object. An acquired form of oculomotor apraxia may occur

in arteriosclerotic patients who have suffered bilateral cerebral vascular accidents. If the lesions responsible are in the anterior internal capsule the loss of control of eye movements is often accompanied by other evidence of pseudo-bulbar palsy (see Chapter 9). The insidious development of the same type of damage to both pathways is seen in a condition called progressive supranuclear degeneration (Steele–Richardson–Olzewski syndrome), and may also occur as a component of Jakob–Creutzfeld disease (see Chapter 10). Both conditions are complicated by dementia.

Lesions in the Parieto-Occipital Cortex

Over-activity of the Parieto-Occipital Cortex

Seizures originating in the parieto-occipital area cause deviation of the eyes to the opposite side, but in this situation the movement will often be accompanied by visual hallucinations. These usually consist of flashing lights and coloured blobs. A generalised convulsion may ensue but focal motor activity, other than the eye movement is not a feature of a focal seizure arising in the occipital lobe.

Under-activity of the Parieto-Occipital Cortex

Damage to the parieto-occipital cortex is often associated with other parietal lobe difficulties which may make testing impossible. Similarly, if an homonymous hemianopia coexists (as it often does if the lesion is a vascular one), the patient may be unable to follow an object because it keeps vanishing into the hemianopic field. In these cases it is essential to keep the object to be followed just inside the midline, in the intact half of the patient's vision and to move it slowly.

The nystagmus that occurs while watching passing telegraph poles from a moving train is dependent on the integrity of this fixation mechanism. Loss of this so-called opticokinetic nystagmus to one side is important clinical evidence of a lesion in the opposite parietal lobe. It is tested by spinning a drum marked with vertical lines, in front of the patient, and asking him to watch the lines. The drum is spun in opposite directions to provoke nystagmus to both right and left. This can be voluntarily suppressed by a few people but it is also a good test for hysterical blindness. The drum is spun in front of the suspected patient's eyes; if nystagmus occurs, in the direction of rotation, vision is intact.

Lesions Affecting Basal Ganglia

Although the anatomical pathways that link the basal ganglia with eye movements are unknown, there is adequate clinical evidence of their importance. For reasons that are not

DIAGRAMS TO ILLUSTRATE EYE MOVEMENT DISORDERS ASSOCIATED WITH SEIZURES AND HEMIPLEGIA

Figure 7.4. Frontal Adversive Seizure

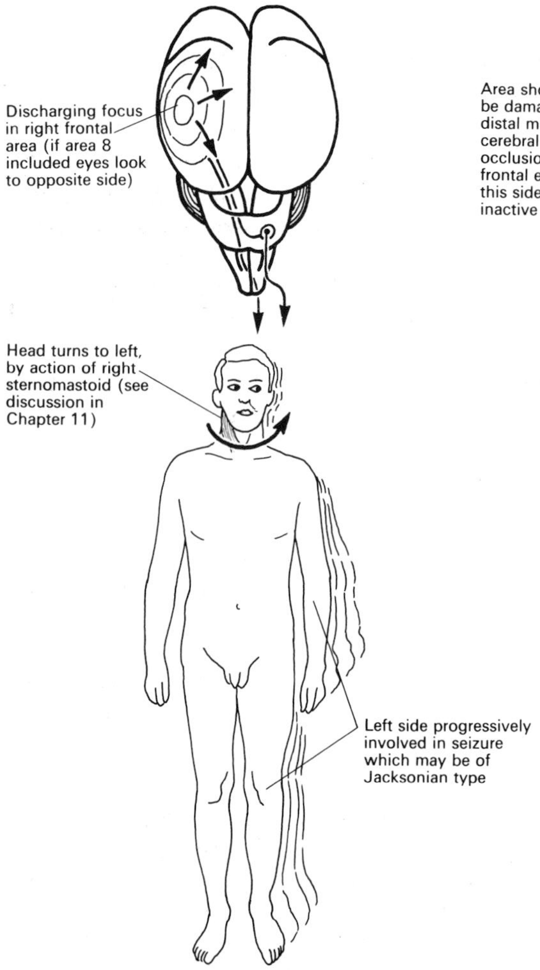

Discharging focus in right frontal area (if area 8 included eyes look to opposite side)

Head turns to left, by action of right sternomastoid (see discussion in Chapter 11)

Left side progressively involved in seizure which may be of Jacksonian type

Figure 7.5. Right Frontal Damage

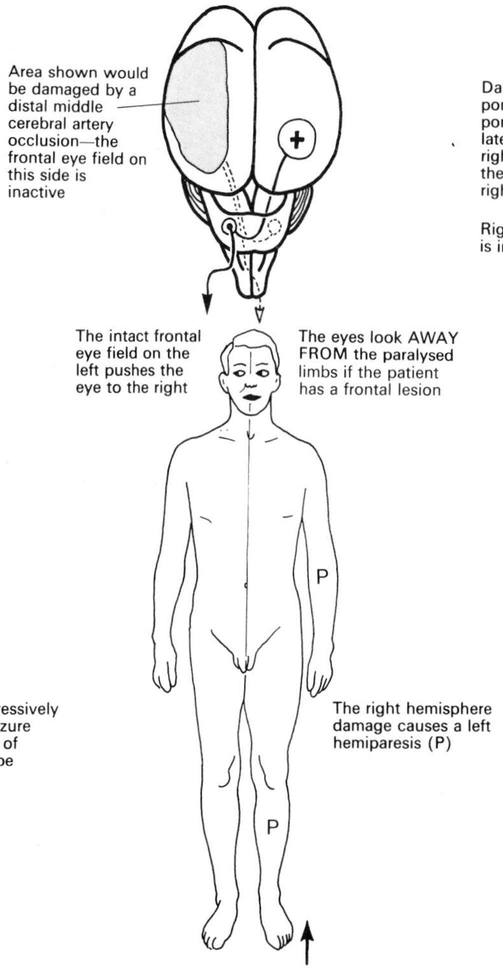

Area shown would be damaged by a distal middle cerebral artery occlusion—the frontal eye field on this side is inactive

The intact frontal eye field on the left pushes the eye to the right

The eyes look AWAY FROM the paralysed limbs if the patient has a frontal lesion

The right hemisphere damage causes a left hemiparesis (P)

Figure 7.6. Right Pontine Damage

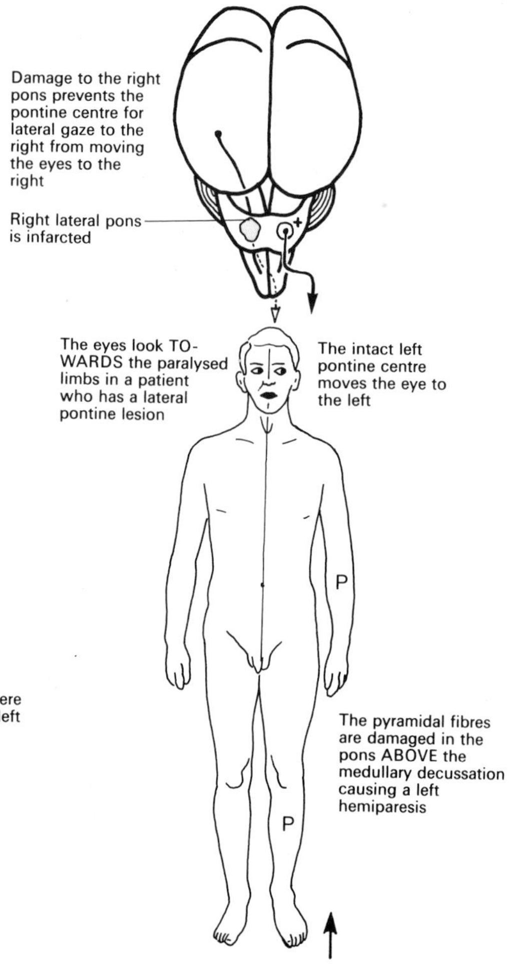

Damage to the right pons prevents the pontine centre for lateral gaze to the right from moving the eyes to the right

Right lateral pons is infarcted

The eyes look TO-WARDS the paralysed limbs in a patient who has a lateral pontine lesion

The intact left pontine centre moves the eye to the left

The pyramidal fibres are damaged in the pons ABOVE the medullary decussation causing a left hemiparesis

clear the basal ganglia mechanisms seem to be predominantly concerned with movements in the vertical plane—possibly the tendency to jolt up and down while walking is automatically compensated for by synchronised up and down eye movements.

Over-activity of Basal Ganglia

This problem is the cause of attacks of oculogyric crisis. These usually consist of a fixed deviation of the eyes in an upwards direction. Lateral deviation or downward deviation occurs less frequently. These attacks are a feature of post-encephalitic Parkinsonism. In this condition compulsive thoughts or actions and a frank confusional state may co-exist with the attack. Other causes included phenothiazine hypersensitivity, post-head injury state and neurosyphilis.

Under-activity of Basal Ganglia

Impairment of vertical gaze is quite a frequent finding in elderly persons. Impaired upward gaze is also an early and frequent sign in both parkinsonism and Huntington's chorea. In both diseases attempted upward gaze may cause jerky vertical nystagmus due to weakness of the movement.

Lesions Affecting the Collicular Area

There are several manifestations of lesions in this area. The signs are thought to be caused by pressure and distortion of underlying structures in the midbrain, and not by damage to specific pathways traversing the colliculi. The general name for the clinical picture produced is Parinaud's syndrome. Any combination of impaired upward gaze, impaired downward gaze, pupillary abnormality or loss of accommodation reflex may occur. In general, loss of upward gaze associated with dilated pupils that are fixed to light, suggests a lesion at the level of the superior colliculus. Loss of downward gaze, normal pupil reactions to light and loss of convergence suggest that the lesion is slightly lower, in the area of the inferior colliculus. Lesions of the pineal gland, ranging from pinealomas, teratomas, gliomas and undifferentiated pineal tumours may produce this clinical picture. Other causes are rare, but include encephalitis, Wernicke's encephalopathy, neurosyphilis and multiple sclerosis.

Retractory Nystagmus

This is a very rare sign of disease in the collicular area and consists of an inward and an outward movement of both eyes when the patient attempts to look upwards. Presumably it is produced by all the extra-ocular muscles acting simultaneously—jerking the globe back into the orbit on attempted upward gaze; in an attempt to overcome the inability to look upwards.

Lesions Affecting the Pontine Area

Damage to the "centre for lateral gaze' results in an inability to look to the side of the lesion. There is often a co-existent sixth nerve palsy on the same side but the failure of *either* eye to move on attempted lateral gaze indicates a gaze palsy. If hemiplegia occurs it will be on the opposite side, as the lesion is above the pyramidal decussation. Therefore, if the patient is unconscious the eyes will deviate towards the hemiplegia (see Figure 7.6). This condition may be seen with basilar artery thrombosis, multiple sclerosis, pontine gliomas and Wernicke's encephalopathy. The full clinical picture of a lateral pontine lesion is discussed in Chapter 11.

Internuclear Ophthalmoplegias (Figure 7.7)

There is considerable variation in textbook classifications of internuclear ophthalmoplegias. To avoid adding to this confusion three main varieties will be described. The basic internuclear ophthalmoplegias are due to an upset of the mechanisms that link the eyes and gaze becomes disconjugate (i.e. the eyes move independently).

1. Divergent Squints (Figure 7.7A)

Occasionally examples are seen in which, far from there being weakness of convergence, the eyes are actually divergent. Essentially, there is paralysis of both medial recti. This condition occurs in hypertensive brain stem lesions and multiple sclerosis. Divergence may be complicated by skew deviation of the eyes, in which one eye looks up and out and the other looks down and out. This is usually associated with pontine lesions in the region of the cerebellar peduncles. The abnormality may be further dramatised by the presence of see-saw nystagmus in which the eyes jerk up and down alternately.

2. Classical Internuclear Ophthalmoplegia (Figure 7.7B)

In this relatively common variety the medial longitudinal fasciculus is damaged and the medial recti fail to move synchronously with the lateral recti on attempted lateral gaze to either side. Yet when each eye is tested alone medial rectus function is evident but incomplete. (Test by covering the abducting eye and making the adducting eye follow the finger.) The majority of examples of this condition occur in multiple sclerosis and in fact the condition is almost pathognomonic of this disease. Unilateral unternuclear ophthalmoplegia is invariably caused by a vascular lesion of the paramedian area of the brain stem (see Chapter 11).

Examples of these ophthalmoplegias;

CASE REPORT

A girl, 23 years of age, presented during her third episode of multiple sclerosis with a left lower motor neurone seventh nerve palsy and complete divergence of the eyes. Three days after starting a course of ACTH the facial weakness had cleared and the eyes improved to the extent that she had a classical internuclear ophthalmoplegia. Within a week her eye movements were normal. She thus demonstrated consecutively two of the varieties of ophthalmoplegia.

CASE REPORT

A man, 56 years of age, was treated with insulin shock therapy in the Middle East, during a toxic confusional state. On recovery he had diplopia on looking to the left side. When seen a year later he had a unilateral internuclear ophthalmoplegia. This presumably resulted from a vascular lesion during a variety of metabolic insults caused by fever, dehydration and hypoglycaemia.

Other causes include pontine glioma, encephalitis, Wernicke's encephalopathy and anticonvulsant drug intoxication.

3. Internuclear Ophthalmoplegia (Figure 7.7C)

The third variety of internuclear ophthalmoplegia also encountered quite frequently in multiple sclerosis is the reverse of the classical variety. Neither eye abducts completely while adduction is complete. The medial longitudinal fasciculus therefore seems to be intact, but the relay to the sixth nerve on both sides is impaired. If not due to a bilateral sixth nerve palsy (test by covering each eye) the mechanism may be as suggested in Figure 7.7C.

In both the latter varieties of internuclear ophthalmoplegia, nystagmus of the laterally moving eye is a feature

Figure 7.7. Internuclear Ophthalmoplegias

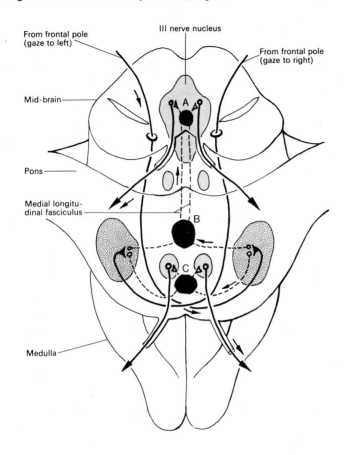

From frontal pole (gaze to left)

III nerve nucleus

From frontal pole (gaze to right)

Mid-brain

Pons

Medial longitudinal fasciculus

Medulla

Figure 7.7A. Lesion at A

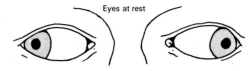

Eyes at rest

Divergent squint due to bilateral involvement of medial recti and loss of the convergence mechanism

Figure 7.7B. Lesion at B

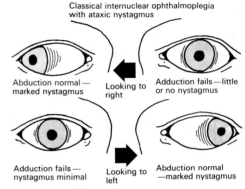

Classical internuclear ophthalmoplegia with ataxic nystagmus

Abduction normal — marked nystagmus

Looking to right

Adduction fails — little or no nystagmus

Adduction fails — nystagmus minimal

Looking to left

Abduction normal — marked nystagmus

Figure 7.7C. Lesion at C

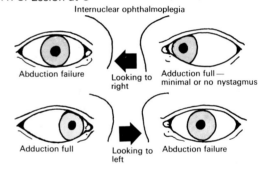

Internuclear ophthalmoplegia

Abduction failure

Looking to right

Adduction full — minimal or no nystagmus

Adduction full

Looking to left

Abduction failure

and the classical variety is sometimes referred to as "internuclear ophthalmoplegia with ataxic nystagmus". The disconjugate movements plus the asymmetrical nystagmus cause frank diplopia or blurring of vision, often severe enough to prevent reading.

Neither symptom occurs in conjugate gaze palsies as the eyes maintain their relative positions at all times, but as noted previously, whenever there is weakness of conjugate movement nystagmoid movements in the direction of weak gaze are a common feature.

NYSTAGMUS

The basic pathological feature common to all causes of nystagmus is that there is weakness in maintaining the conjugate deviation of the eyes or an inbalance in the postural control of the eye movements. In either case there is

a tendency for the laterally deviated eyes to drift slowly back to the central position (this is the pathological component), and to regain the original position by a fast flick (this is the movement that is recorded as the direction of the nystagmus). One of the major problems for the student arises from the fact that nystagmus is defined in the direction of the *fast* movement which is *not* the abnormal part of the process. It is the slow drift that is pathological—*not* the more easily observed fast flick. It follows that minor degrees of nystagmus will only be manifest on full lateral gaze to the weak side. If more severe, it may appear on the slightest deviation to the weak side. If very marked, it may also be apparent at rest as fine jerky movements of the eye from side to side. Qualitatively, it may be defined as fine or coarse (based on the amplitude of movement), horizontal, vertical or rotatory. The other quality, usually described as pendular, is a specific feature of ocular nystagmus and is discussed separately below. Although at first sight the quick movement would appear to be a deliberate attempt by the occipito-parietal motor area to restore fixation, the movement persists even following transcollicular section of the brain stem. The activity is therefore thought to be generated in the pons. However, the occipito-parietal motor area does have significance in the physiological phenomenon of opticokinetic nystagmus mentioned before. It is *absence* of opticokinetic nystagmus that is pathological, and this finding points to a lesion in the pursuit gaze pathway or the opposite parieto-occipito-temporal cortex. Conversely, in cerebellar nystagmus the optic fixation reflexes may be strong enough to inhibit the slow drift and prevent nystagmus from occurring. Thus cerebellar nystagmus may only be manifest in the dark or with the eyes closed. This can be shown by electronystagmography, which is performed in the dark with the eyes closed and the eye movements are recorded electrically from electrodes placed over the eyelids.

Varieties of Nystagmus

Nystagmoid Jerks

Coarse jerking movements of the eyes occur if the patient is made to follow a moving object too far or too fast. The examiner should aim to take the edge of the iris of the adducting eye to the caruncle and no further. Similarly, if the examiner holds the object closer than two feet from the patient's eye it will cause convergence and this in turn will provoke nystagmoid jerking on minimal lateral eye movements. Nystagmoid jerks have no pathological significance; they do not represent minimal nystagmus.

Congenital Nystagmus

This condition, which is often familial, occasionally causes unnecessary concern, as it produces very dramatic nystagmus. It is present from birth. The movements are non-stop and pendular, i.e. there is no fast and slow phase, just a steady "wobble" of the eyes. The head may nod in the opposite direction, which serves to stabilise the retinal image. The movements become even more dramatic when the patient directs his gaze in any direction, but invariably the eyes oscillate from side to side—the movements do not become vertical on upward gaze. One of the features that indicates that nystagmus is of the congenital variety is that in spite of the very gross jerking the patient has no sensation of the movement of his eyes and no subjective nausea or vertigo. Recently acquired nystagmus of this severity is usually associated with nausea and vertigo on attempted lateral gaze.

An important differential diagnosis of congenital nystagmus in the first few years of life is the condition known as spasmus mutans. In this situation the child develops fast, fine but variable movements of the eyes. The head also nods, but not in a compensatory direction, usually up and down, and often the head nodding precedes the onset of the eye movements. The condition is benign but may last weeks to months. It is essential to exclude any ocular abnormality as similar eye movements occur in children with impaired vision (but not total blindness) caused by congenital macular disease, congenital cataracts, total colour blindness and albinism.

Nystagmus Caused by Vestibular Disease

Any lesion affecting the semicircular canals, the eighth nerve or the vestibular nuclei will seriously upset the push-pull effect of the vestibular control of eye movements. Let us assume that the left-sided vestibular elements have been damaged in Figure 7.3. Activity in this pathway normally pushes the eyes to the right, therefore reduced activity will lead to weakness of eye movements to the right side. On attempting gaze to this side the intact vestibular mechanism on the right, coupled with the weakness of the damaged left side will force the eyes to drift back to the midline. The quick jerk to restore the gaze will be to the right side, i.e. the nystagmus is away from the side of the vestibular lesion.

There are several distinguishing features in lesions affecting the different parts of the vestibular pathway. With destruction of the labyrinth by Ménière's Disease, nystagmus does not occur, because of central compensation for the absence of any input. A similar situation exists after acute labyrinthine destruction when the initial imbalance settles. Similarly in slowly occurring damage to the eighth nerve (an acoustic nerve tumour) compensation often prevents development of nystagmus. When it does occur in this situation it often reflects brain stem or cerebellar damage from the extension of the tumour into the cerebello-pontine angle. With central lesions of the vestibular apparatus (multiple sclerosis, cerebral vascular accidents, gliomas, syringomyelia) compensation cannot occur and the nystagmus and associated symptoms of vestibular damage tend to persist. Although nystagmus from a peripheral lesion is horizontal or rotatory, that arising from a central lesion may also be vertical. The eyes move up and down, usually doing so on attempted upward gaze. Horizontal nystagmus on looking upward is *not* vertical nystagmus. Although widely held to be pathognomonic of intrinisc brain stem disease, vertical nystagmus can result from distortion of the brain stem by an extrinsic lesion, and is quite often seen in patients with drug toxicity, especially that caused by diphenylhydantoin (Epanutin) and other anticonvulsants.

The most clearcut examples of vestibular nuclear nystagmus are seen in vascular lesions of the brain stem which are usually strictly unilateral. In multiple sclerosis, bilateral damage, and involvement of other pathways produces very complex nystagmus, such as that found in association with internuclear ophthalmoplegia as discussed above.

Nystagmus Caused by Cerebellar Lesions (see also Chapter 12)

As already mentioned the exact mechanism of cerebellar nystagmus is not known. Although nystagmus is a feature of unilateral cerebellar disease, in some cerebellar degenerations and midline cerebellar disease, nystagmus may be absent even though the patient may be so ataxic as to be unable to sit without support. Many hold that cerebellar disease only causes nystagmus when vestibular pathways are damaged, and yet this view has to explain why when nystagmus is found it is in the reverse direction to vestibular disease affecting the same side. If we consider the flocculo-occulomotor pathway in Figure 7.3, which normally tends to move the eyes *towards* the active side of the cerebellum, weakness of this activity could lead to difficulty in looking at the damaged half of the cerebellum, and the fast jerk to restore gaze would be *towards* the damaged cerebellar hemisphere. This explanation certainly fits the clinical situation as nystagmus in cerebellar disease is maximal towards the side of the lesion.

Other Causes

There are a multitude of rare varieties of nystagmus beyond the scope of this text. However, there are several common causes of nystagmus that cannot be based on anatomical features. All sedative drugs, especially barbiturates and glutethimide, and anticonvulsants, especially diphenylhydantoin (Epanutin), primidone (Mysoline) and carbamezepine (Tegretol) can cause severe vertigo and dramatic nystagmus following deliberate or accidental intoxication. Alcohol and one of its complications—Wernicke's encephalopathy—are also associated with nystagmus. Following head injuries with loss of consciousness, transient nystagmus following recovery of consciousness is quite common and does not seem to carry any serious prognostic significance. Persistent nystagmus may occur in the event of a fracture though the petrous bone damaging the labyrinth or eighth nerve (see Chapter 23).

A comprehensive list of causes of nystagmus without an understanding of the underlying pathophysiology is of little use.

The importance of testing for nystagmus correctly, and recording in detail the quality, direction and other features is not sufficiently appreciated. The almost universal finding recorded in the neurological examination of patients—"a few nystagmoid jerks" does not indicate great clinical acumen. On the contrary it demonstrates poor clinical technique and a failure to recognise that this is not a physical sign.

DISEASES AFFECTING THE CEREBRAL HEMISPHERES

There are three basic ways in which cerebral hemisphere functioning can be compromised:

1. Infiltrative or compressive neoplasms either primary or secondary.
2. Vascular lesions including vascular occlusions, haemorrhages, emboli, subdural and extradural blood clots.
3. Diffuse neuronal dysfunction either due to degenerative processes or metabolic disorders.

Neoplastic lesions tend to occur in the lobes of the brain whereas vascular lesions occur in specific vascular territories which fortunately for the diagnostician are not anatomically the same as the lobes of the brain. Finally, extremely diffuse damage to the hemispheres is usually readily recognisable although the cause can rarely be established.

Chapter 8

THE CEREBRAL HEMISPHERES: 1. THE LOBES OF THE BRAIN

GENERAL FEATURES OF DISEASE IN THE CEREBRAL HEMISPHERES

Intellectual and Behavioural Disorders

For the highest levels of intellectual functioning the entire brain must be intact. Yet quite extensive lesions in some areas may produce little or no identifiable deficit, whereas a small lesion in the dominant hemisphere may have a devastating effect on speech function and comprehension. In the presence of a cerebral neoplasm additional features such as raised intra-cranial pressure, cerebral oedema and brain displacement may add non-specific generalised intellectual or behavioural changes to the focal signs of the underlying lesion. For this reason any statement by a patient's relative to the effect that a recent intellectual decline or change in personality has occurred should be taken very seriously, even if no definite abnormality is detectable on simple testing. So often the patient himself is unaware of, or denies such a change and it is always vital to get reports from employers and workmates to supplement the history given by the patient and his family.

Memory impairment, loss of concentration, irritability, loss of motor skills or inappropriate behaviour may all mark the onset of symptoms of a cerebral lesion. As examples the following cases may be cited:

CASE REPORT

A middle-aged industrial chemist, always an extrovert, became more expansive in his behaviour and one day while driving with his wife suggested that she should drive for a while. As soon as she stepped from the car to go round to the driving seat, he drove off and left her stranded. He had no explanation for this behaviour. The only physical sign was a right Babinski response. Investigation demonstrated a large meningioma over-lying the left parietal area. No satisfactory explanation can be advanced for the behavioural upset but his behaviour was normal following the removal of the meningioma.

CASE REPORT

The doorman at a large London hotel started greeting eminent guests at the door in a familiar manner. By lunchtime numerous complaints had been received by the manager who found the doorman entertaining the occupants of the entrance hall to a selection of army songs. On examination he had bilateral extensor plantars and mild papilloedema. His behaviour until that day had been exemplary. A chest x-ray revealed a large carcinoma of the lung and subsequently multiple cerebral metastases were demonstrated by a cerebral scan.

More specific disabilities may provide clues as to the localisation of the underlying lesions.

1. Frontal lobe lesions cause striking memory impairment to the point of dementia, often coupled with marked physical inertia (see later explanation). A frequently associated feature is a deterioration in the social behaviour especially in respect of micturition. This is probably related to the location of the cortical centre for micturition in the second frontal gyrus. Urinary incontinence occurring in the early stages of the history in a patient with intellectual decline should always be regarded as indicating a frontal lesion until proven otherwise. The unusual use of bad language in inappropriate circumstances is another feature.

2. Temporal lobe disorders may also cause personality changes with memory impairment. The slow deterioration may be punctuated by episodic bizarre personality change with sudden onset and cessation. These often turn out to be complex psychomotor seizures and may last for days at a time with residual confusion between the more obvious attacks. The possibility of a temporal lobe disorder should be considered in any patient with sudden attacks of altered behaviour.

3. Parietal lobe lesions produce manifestations that vary depending on the patient's cerebral dominance. The majority of patients (including the majority of left-handed patients) are left hemisphere dominant.

Dominant hemisphere parietal lesions produce dysphasia with either inability to understand commands, inability to speak or a combination of both.

The evaluation of patients who are unable to communicate requires some degree of skill and time. A very common error and dangerous assumption is that poor communication is synonymous with confusion.

CASE REPORT

A middle-aged alcoholic female became irrational and "confused". This was attributed to an amnestic syndrome and she was transferred to a mental hospital where it was discovered that she was "dysphasic". Subsequent investigation and operation disclosed a glioma in the temporal lobe of the dominant hemisphere.

CASE REPORT

An elderly coloured male was taken to hospital and left by his relatives, who departed before giving any history. He was "confused" and could give no account of himself. The neurological service was asked to see him at their leisure with a diagnosis of "chronic brain syndrome". Examination revealed both receptive and motor dysphasia, a mild right hemiparesis and a slightly dilated left pupil in an extremely drowsy man. Immediate investigation revealed a massive subdural haematoma which was successfully evacuated.

The methods available for screening patients for dysphasia will be detailed later, but the main point must be reiterated; speech difficulties can easily be mistaken for confusion by the unwary examiner.

Lesions affecting the non-dominant parietal lobe do not affect speech function but cause unusual deficits in acquired skills such as cutting up food, dressing, getting out of the bath, and geographic orientation. The complete preservation of speech function which allows the patient to discuss, while not understanding these disabilities is a feature of the condition which is known dyspraxia.

CASE REPORT

A man came home to find his 70-year-old wife sitting in an empty bath making repeated but ineffectual efforts to get out. She could not understand why she was having such difficulty and may have been stuck in the bath for four hours. After her husband had helped her from the bath she needed help to dress. There was evidence of a right hemisphere lesion on physical examination, which proved to be due to a cerebro-vascular accident.

CASE REPORT

A 56-year-old man suffered a series of attacks of paraesthesiae in the left arm during an influenzal illness. There were no definite sequelae. On the day he returned to work he took two and a half hours to travel the half mile to work and was seen wandering in the wrong direction by neighbours. When he arrived at work he was unable to find his way to his bench. He was sent home and his wife found that he had great difficulty putting on his pyjamas. No abnormality was found on angiography but a vascular lesion of the non-dominant parietal lobe was probably the cause.

Combinations of peculiar behaviour, wearing clothes back to front, inability to dress, getting lost around the house or in the street, or sudden inability to perform skilled tasks such as carpentry are all suggestive of a lesion in the non-dominant parietal lobe.

Bedside Evaluation of Intellectual Function

An assessment of the patient's mental state, intelligence and specific evaluation for dysphasia should be made. Considerable information in all these spheres can be obtained while passing the time of day with the patient and during the actual history taking.

His mood, attitude towards his disability, attitude towards the examiner and third parties are readily detectable without specific testing.

1. Mental State

Formal testing of the mental state is often confined to asking the patient the date and day of the week. Anyone who has spent more than a few days in a hospital bed will know how difficult this becomes! The monotony of routine, the irrelevance of the date, and the isolation from the outside world readily produces some degree of confusion about time and date in the most alert patient. General questions on the content of the day's newspaper, or the news on the radio, are usually much more useful although they are at first sight less specific than the date. Nursing reports of the patient's behaviour and manner are also extremely useful in making this general evaluation. An assessment of the patient's memory for remote, recent and immediate events should be made and wherever possible checked with a relative.

2. Intellectual Function

Testing can be performed at the bedside but subtle alterations are very unlikely to be detected by the occasional examiner. Formal psychometric testing is essential especially where no immediately obvious abnormalities are apparent. For clinical notes the "100 minus 7" test is traditionally used although for full interpretation both accuracy and the time taken are important. This is so badly affected by anxiety and fright that to base the whole assessment on this test would be entirely inappropriate. The ability to learn a lengthy sentence, such as the typical Babcock sentence, is useful however. A perseveration of errors as well as the time taken to complete the sentence gives useful information. The test sentence (which the examiner must also know by heart!) is, "There is one thing that a nation must have to be rich and great, and that is a large, secure supply of wood". Most patients can learn this sentence accurately in three to five attempts. However, the test is subject to all the problems of anxiety, speech difficulty and memory disturbance. The results are not specific for any condition. Another test of memory and concentration consists of asking the patient to learn a series of numbers forwards and backwards. Normally patients can learn seven numbers forwards and five backwards. Explaining the meaning of proverbs and general knowledge tests, the names of public figures, capitals of countries etc. can be very difficult as the general interests of the patient will influence their performance.

One dysphasic patient unable to name any simple objects or describe the meaning of simple words such as brunette was asked the meaning of "piscatorial", his face lit up and he answered in a flash "appertaining to a fish". Needless to say he was a keen fisherman. The writer experienced considerable difficulty while working in the U.S.A. when attempting dysphasia and intelligence testing as he had little common ground with the patients in public affairs or sport.

Finally, the patient's ability to repeat, paraphrase or explain a simple story can be tested. Many patients who are slightly confused regard the examiner with incredulity when the story is related and it requires a certain amount of self-control and preliminary explanations to perform this test without calling your own sanity into question.

Cowboy Story:

A cowboy went to San Francisco with his dog, which he left at a friend's house while he went to buy a new suit of clothes. Dressed in his grand new suit he came back to the dog, whistled at it, called it by name and patted it. The dog would have nothing to do with him in his new coat and hat and gave a mournful howl. Coaxing the dog was of no avail, so the cowboy went away and put his old suit on again and the dog immediately showed its wild joy on seeing its master as it thought he ought to look.

3. *Dysphasia and Dyspraxia*

Dysphasia testing is best left until one has a clear idea as to how confused or disorientated a patient is, yet as already mentioned it is important to be certain that the patient has full comprehension of the spoken word and is capable of making a well-informed, appropriate answer to a question before taking the case history. It is essential that the patient is not distressed by testing and it is best not to pursue any difficulty for too long.

a. Establish that the patient can understand the spoken word by his ability to close his eyes, stick out his tongue and show either his right or his left hand to command. A severely confused demented or dysphasic patient may stick out his tongue at the first command and may continue to stick it out on every subsequent command. This may represent perseveration or may be the only motor act that the patient can be persuaded to perform.

b. If the patient cannot understand spoken commands he may be able to read them. The same simple responses should be asked for in writing, i.e. "put out your tongue" etc. showing the command to the patient on a card.

c. The patient's spoken answers, if any, should be recorded. In patients with nominal aphasia (difficulty in naming objects) a remarkably good command of language is possible but the sentences may lack nouns. To avoid the problem he may use an alternative to the noun. A patient who was asked to name his wedding ring, pointed to his wife and said, "I've been with her a long time."

d. The patient may be able to express himself better in writing and should be asked to write his name and address and write a simple sentence to dictation.

e. Object-naming is a very simple test and is perhaps the most useful at the bedside. It can also be most distressing for the patients and casual bystanders should not be allowed to listen to or laugh at the patient's disabilities. Naming simple objects such as a pen and its nib, or a watch and its hands will usually detect nominal aphasia.

f. The patient should read and discuss a passage from a book or newspaper to test his ability to both read *and understand* what he is reading.

Abnormalities in the performance of these tests indicates impairment of understanding the written or spoken word and imply dysphasia and therefore damage to the dominant parietal lobe. Once one dysphasic difficulty has been detected the site of damage is localised and no further localising information can be added by more exhaustive testing.

Dyspraxia is the equivalent of "dysphasia" in the non-dominant parietal lobe. The presenting history usually includes examples of lost skills such as difficulty in feeding or getting out of the bath. Simple tasks such as removing the dressing gown, lighting a cigarette or folding a piece of paper are readily observed. Allowances for any motor deficits or ataxia should obviously be made but in many cases these functions are normal, making the considerable difficulty that the patient has with apparently simple tasks even more dramatic. Constructional tests using either matches to copy simple figures and shapes or drawing things from memory fall into the same category. As with dysphasia the demonstration of difficulty in one sphere of activity provides sufficient localising information. At a higher level of testing the patient's ability to draw a plan of the ward or of an area of his home can be tested. A taxi driver performed well on all tests until asked to sketch a plan of Trafalgar Square—explaining his main complaint of difficulty in doing his job!

In summary patients may appear to be confused because of general depression of intellectual function which may vary with the conscious level, or because of dysphasic difficulties causing them difficulty in both understanding and communicating verbally, or they may have problems in the performance of simple tasks due to dyspraxia. Distinction between these possibilities is vital. Dysphasia or dyspraxia indicate a focal abnormality in the dominant and non-dominant hemispheres respectively, whereas confusion may indicate an altered level of consciousness or a metabolic disorder affecting the whole brain. This would require an entirely different approach to further investigation and treatment.

Motor Disorders in Hemisphere Disease

For normal motor function the patient must have intact sensory feedback and cerebellar control of his limbs. Patients often say that they are "unsteady" or "numb" when they mean "weak". If these descriptive terms are taken at face value an entirely incorrect view of their disability will be obtained. It is essential to ask the patient to elaborate on these terms in the same way as he should be asked to elaborate on the term "blackout". In a severe parietal lobe lesion the limbs on the opposite side may lie useless and completely ignored by the patient although they may not be weak. At a less severe level the outstretched arm, held out normally when the eyes are open, may fall away when the eyes are closed; this is not due to weakness but due to deficient appreciation of its position. In cerebellar disease the outstretched arm may show wild oscillations and even rise when the eyes are shut. This outstretched arms test is a very useful one for screening a patient and should be evaluated systematically.

1. Observe the outstretched hands. Are there any abnormalities of the hands themselves, such as finger clubbing? Do they shake? Does one arm have difficulty in maintaining its position?

2. Can the patient play the piano in mid air quickly and rhythmically? If not, the less efficient hand may be affected by a mild pyramidal lesion (in a right-handed patient the movements are often normally slightly better performed with the right hand).

3. When the eyes are closed, do the hands remain level? Does one rise up or oscillate (indicates cerebellar disease)? Does one fall away (indicates defective sensation or weakness)?

If the patient is drowsy or will not move his limbs to command because of dysphasia, the spontaneous movements of the suspect limb should be observed. If the examiner pinches the skin of the patient's anterior chest wall, the patient will invariably use his best arm to pull the examiner's hand away. If the good arm is then held down while the test is repeated the affected limb will move if it is able to do so. The legs may be tested by painful stimuli to each leg in turn, and at the same time the gross sensory function of the two sides can be assessed.

Full Evaluation of Motor Function in the Presence of a Hemisphere Lesion

We have considered gross defects of motor function in the semi-conscious patient above. In many instances one is looking for a very subtle deficit and the secret of evaluation lies in knowing how to look for minor motor disability.

1. The Face

We have previously mentioned the problem of the asymmetrical face and the frequent assertion that this represents a mild upper motor neurone lesion. We can now elaborate on upper motor neurone facial weakness as encountered in patients with hemisphere lesions.

There are two types of facial movement, voluntary facial grimacing and smiling, and involuntary grimacing and smiling as a true emotional response. The former function is probably mediated through classical motor pathways from the motor strip and the emotional responses through supplementary motor areas lying deep in the insula and temporal lobes. Therefore, the facial movements should be carefully observed during history taking and spontaneous smiles provoked and carefully observed. Then a forced smile should be tested and the patient's ability to show the teeth (with the almost inevitable patient response "they are false").

Quite obvious facial weakness on one test may be coupled with normality on the other. The type of weakness may have localising significance, emotional weakness usually indicating a lesion affecting the temporal lobe.

2. The Limbs

When testing the limbs we are looking for pyramidal weakness. This concept is vital to accurate diagnosis and yet is surprisingly neglected in most textbooks and teaching, as indicated by the number of doctors who test limb power by assessing the hand grips and the strength of the quadriceps muscles. These are the two movements *least* likely to be affected in cerebral disease!

The distribution of weakness is best remembered by recalling the typical posture and gait of a patient recovering from a stroke. The arm is flexed (the flexor group of muscles being strong), and the leg extended (the extensors being strong). Functionally this is ideal; if the situation were reversed few patients would ever regain the ability to walk after a stroke.

In the arm the weak groups are those controlling shoulder abduction elbow extension, wrist extension and finger abduction. The intact spastic groups adduct the arm to the side of the body, and flex the arm at the elbow and wrist.

In the leg, the weak groups are the hip flexors, the hamstrings and the dorsiflexors of the foot. The strong spastic muscles are the glutei and quadriceps which hold the hip and knee stiff and the plantar flexors which keep the foot slightly flexed—causing it to scrape along the ground as the patient walks.

This pattern of weakness indicates damage to pyramidal pathways and is typical of a deep hemisphere lesion, or damage to the main motor pathways (the cortico-spinal tracts in the brainstem or spinal cord).

If the whole area of cortex supplying a limb is damaged the extra-pyramidal pathways are unable to take over and *global, flaccid* weakness of the limb occurs associated with brisk reflexes and an extensor plantar response. This also explains how a patient with a small infarction in the internal capsule has a good prognosis for recovery whereas if the left middle cerebral artery is occluded the prognosis for recovery is poor and the patient has the added problem of dysphasia due to the damage to the speech cortex. This is discussed further in the next chapter.

Motor Evaluation Should Answer the Following Questions

1. Is there any facial weakness, either voluntary or emotional?
2. Is there any fall away of the outstretched hands?
3. Is there any disparity between piano-playing movements of the hands or toe wiggling (the equivalent test in the feet)?
4. Is there any tone increase on the affected side?
5. Is there any reflex asymmetry (brisker on the affected side) or an extensor plantar response?
6. Is there weakness in the pyramidal distribution, bearing in mind that proximal movements (shoulder abduction and hip flexion) may be demonstrably weak when the only peripheral signs are impaired fine movements?

SENSORY DISORDERS IN HEMISPHERE DISEASE

The main symptom of damage to the sensory cortex is sensory epilepsy. This usually consists of episodes of tingling parasthesiae progressing to numbness. It is very unusual for focal pain to be produced although it can happen. Due to considerable motor representation in the sensory cortical area the sensory symptoms are often associated with some twitching of the same limb or limbs. The sensory symptoms are usually strictly unilateral.

CASE REPORT

A 70-year-old man complained of severe low back pain and pain radiating down the entire right leg. On examination an orthopaedic surgeon found brisk reflexes and an extensory plantar response. When seen the next day he was densely hemiplegic and semiconscious. A large metastatic deposit in the leg area of the sensory strip was found. It is thought that his early symptoms were a form of sensory epilepsy.

CASE REPORT

A 42-year-old engineer had suffered from attacks of tingling and numbness of the left hand, extending to the left side of the chest and head since the age of nineteen. As these episodes often occurred at meal times they had long been ascribed to "indigestion"! Three weeks before admission he suffered two major epileptic fits each beginning with these sensory symptoms but progressing to focal jerking of the arm and face and then loss of consciousness.

A loud bruit was heard over the entire right side of the head and angiography revealed an angioma occupying the bulk of the right hemisphere.

The sensory loss caused by a superficial lesion is rarely complete. In fact, *total* loss of *all* sensory modalities on one side is extremely unusual, and should raise doubts as to the organicity of the findings. Due to bilateral cortical projections and some sensory appreciation of poorly localised touch, pain and vibration at thalamic level these sensations may be relatively spared. The modalities that are specifically affected by a cortical lesion are accurate localisation of touch, two point discrimination, joint position sense and temperature appreciation. Other "popular" modalities such as the recognition of numbers scratched on the skin and stereognosis (recognition of an object placed in the hand) are really composite sensory functions requiring all modalities to be intact, and are not specific forms of sensation. They do depend on the sensations particularly appreciated at cortical level and will therefore often be very severely impaired by a cortical lesion. Asking the patient to compare the textures of bed coverings is a useful screening test, but is subject to the same objection of relative non-specificity. Abnormalities in these tests suggest diffuse damage to the sensory cortex.

To detect very minimal dysfunction the test for sensory extinction is used. The theoretical basis of the test is probably the same as that for extinction hemianopia, illustrated in figure 3.3. The patient is lightly touched on either limb and occasionally simultaneously on both limbs. The ability to recognise a light touch on one limb, but failure to detect the same touch when both limbs are touched at the same moment is called sensory extinction and has the same significance as cortical sensory loss.

If the lesion lies deep in the hemisphere at thalamic level or in the subthalmic area more dramatic sensory loss will be found. In the early stages of a progressive lesion, or in the recovering stages of a vascular lesion damaging the sensory pathways at thalamic level, extremely unpleasant deep poorly localised pain down the opposite side of the body may occur. These sensations may occur spontaneously or be provoked by any stimulus to the affected side of the body. This is called the Dejerine—Roussy syndrome and is discussed further in the next chapter.

CASE REPORT

A 52-year-old woman presented with a two-month history of difficulties affecting the right side. This had started as a tingling in the right hand and simultaneous numbness of the right big toe. At the same time she became aware that the right leg was clumsy. Over the following six weeks the entire right side became numb and yet hypersensitive to touch. For four weeks she had noticed increasing weakness of the right arm and right leg. She had had a slight left-sided headache throughout. She had had a left mastectomy seven years previously for carcinoma of the breast. Examination revealed a hemiplegic gait with minimal weakness on formal testing and flexor plantar responses. There was severe impairment of *all* sensory modalities on the entire right side of the body. Investigation and craniotomy revealed a large necrotic metastasis in the posterior part of the left thalamus.

This is a typical example of the history of a thalamic lesion and a good example of the type of sensory deficit found in such cases.

Testing Techniques in Sensory Evaluation

Traditionally a wisp of cotton wool is used to test light touch sensation. A mere touch with a finger tip is just as effective and can be very accurately repeated from side to side.

When testing pain sensation, the examiner should use a slightly blunted pin. One must deplore the increasing use of an intravenous needle carried in the lapel. This punctures the skin and may even draw blood with the attendant risk of infection. There is no need to draw blood to cause pain. It is essential to be sure that it is the *painful* sensation that is appreciated and not just the touch.

Two-point discrimination can only be used as a test when the patient has already been able to appreciate and localise a single light touch. Clearly there is no point in performing the test if the patient is unable to sense a light touch. The test is only reliable at the finger tips, the average female being able to detect 2–3 mm. separation and males (especially manual workers) up to 5 mm. separation. Although it is stated that appreciation of greater than 4 cm. separation on the legs is abnormal the figure varies so widely that the test must be regarded as unreliable in the lower limbs.

Joint position sense can be tested in the hands and feet. The distal interphalangeal joint should be steadied by holding each side of the joint, and the distal phalanx moved up and down by holding the side of the finger or toe. If the pulp and nail are held the "push-pull" stimulus will affect the results. Always start with the patient watching the toe or finger so that he understands what is required. He may then close his eyes for formal testing (Figure 8.1).

Vibration sense, tested with a 128 cps. tuning-fork, is another test of dubious clinical value. It is not a specific modality carried in a specific pathway. The sensation probably travels in both dorsal columns and spinothalamic pathways and is appreciated bilaterally at thalamic level. In hemisphere lesions vibration will only be lost in association with dense loss of other modalities due to a lesion in the region of the thalamus. The value of vibration sense in the diagnosis of peripheral nerve and spinal cord lesions will be discussed in a later chapter.

Figure 8.1. The Correct Way to Test Joint Position Sense

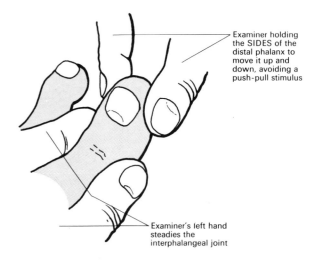

Examiner holding the SIDES of the distal phalanx to move it up and down, avoiding a push-pull stimulus

Examiner's left hand steadies the interphalangeal joint

Temperature sensation need rarely be tested routinely. With cortical lesions the loss is usually identical to the pain sensation loss. Temperature sense loss is never found in isolation.

Sensory testing in routine screening for a hemisphere lesion should include the following:

1. Light touch is tested on both sides and extinction testing performed as discussed above.
2. Joint position sense is tested on both sides.
3. Pain appreciation is evaluated on both sides—short of actual pain loss altered appreciation of pain has the same significance.

If these simple tests reveal no abnormality further testing is unnecessary.

Figure 8.2. The Frontal Lobes (shown pulled apart)

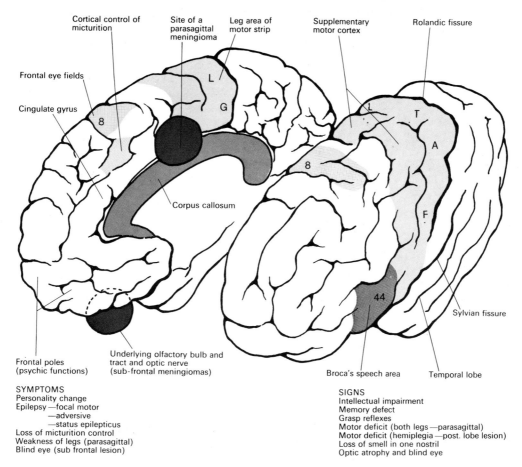

Cortical control of micturition
Site of a parasagittal meningioma
Leg area of motor strip
Supplementary motor cortex
Rolandic fissure
Frontal eye fields
Cingulate gyrus
Corpus callosum
Frontal poles (psychic functions)
Underlying olfactory bulb and tract and optic nerve (sub-frontal meningiomas)
Broca's speech area
Temporal lobe
Sylvian fissure

SYMPTOMS
Personality change
Epilepsy —focal motor
      —adversive
      —status epilepticus
Loss of micturition control
Weakness of legs (parasagittal)
Blind eye (sub frontal lesion)

SIGNS
Intellectual impairment
Memory defect
Grasp reflexes
Motor deficit (both legs—parasagittal)
Motor deficit (hemiplegia—post. lobe lesion)
Loss of smell in one nostril
Optic atrophy and blind eye

CLINICAL DISORDERS OF THE LOBES OF THE BRAIN

1. The Frontal Lobes (Figure 8.2)

The frontal lobes include all the hemisphere anterior to the Rolandic fissure. They extend much further posteriorly than is generally appreciated. The two lobes are interconnected in the midline by the corpus callosum which unfortunately allows for easy spread of frontal lobe tumours across the midline in a "butterfly" distribution. The areas of clinical importance are the motor strip (Area 4), the supplementary motor area (Area 6), the frontal eye fields (Area 8), the cortical centre for micturition (the medial surface of the frontal lobe) and the important connections with the temporal lobe, parietal lobe, basal ganglia, hypothalamus and cerebellum. In addition in the dominant hemisphere there is Broca's speech area. This area controls the motor mechanisms concerned with articulation. The olfactory bulb and tract, and the optic nerve lie immediately under the lobe.

Clinical Features of Frontal Lobe Damage

The frontal lobes play a major role in personality, particularly in respect of acquired social behaviour. Patients with frontal lobe lesions will often present with personality disorders. Loss of drive, apathy, decreasing concern about personal appearance, personal hygiene, family affairs or business all occur. An apathetic dementia results. In some cases increasing disinhibition causes trouble. Urinating in public, inappropriate bad language and anti-social behaviour without concern for the effect on others occurs. Severe decline in intellect is coupled with memory impairment until obvious dementia occurs. In any demented patient where there is a history of personality change or micturition problems *before* the dementia becomes established, urgent consideration should be given to the possibility of a frontal lobe tumour. Patients with parasaggital lesions are particularly likely to present in this way.

CASE REPORT

A 60-year-old woman had been behaving somewhat peculiarly for nearly five years. The earliest symptom was apparent while driving when passengers noticed that she always drove in and out of bus bays to the alarm of the people waiting at the bus stop. Her business acumen declined and she was unable to cope with the introduction of V.A.T. Finally, her air letters to her son in Canada arrived written only in the margins so that when the letter was opened the message was destroyed. She was extremely peculiar in affect and slightly hypomanic but there were no definite neurological signs. Investigation demonstrated a large right subfrontal meningioma.

The particular type of micturition disturbance associated with a frontal lobe lesion is an abrupt awareness that the bladder is full coupled with the inability to prevent the bladder from emptying immediately. The patient loses the ability to inhibit the micturition reflex. As personality changes ensue, this causes less and less concern (to the patient)!

CASE REPORT

A 56-year-old female became increasingly disinterested in her household duties and incontinent of urine. However, it was not until she voided on her husband's prize roses that he sought advice on her account. An enormous parasaggital meningioma was removed with full recovery.

Epileptiform attacks are a frequent feature of frontal lobe lesions. There are three types of seizure that point to a frontal lobe disturbance.

1. *Adversive Fits*

Due to the presence of the frontal eye fields in area 8, a discharge in this region often causes the head and eyes to turn away from the discharging cortex. these are called "adversive seizures" and are typical of a frontal lesion.

2. *Focal Motor Epilepsy*

Focal Jacksonian fits and unilateral motor convulsions are usually due to a lesion in or near the main motor cortex in the precentral gyrus of the frontal lobe. However, surprisingly frequently the lesion is actually found in the parietal area. The discharge in these cases probably arises in the motor cells in the sensory strip. The simultaneous onset of tingling parasthesiae with the focal fit should indicate this possibility.

3. *Status Epilepticus*

It has recently been recognised that as many as fifty per cent of patients who suffer an attack of status epilepticus *early* in the course of their illness are eventually shown to have a frontal tumour.

Patients with lesions in the orbital part of the frontal lobe or subfrontal lesions such as olfactory groove or sphenoidal ridge meningiomas may develop intellectual deficits due to frontal lobe damage. These lesions may also cause blindness in one eye or loss of sense of smell in one or other nostril, and these problems may not be noticed by the dementing patient. For this reason it is essential to examine vision and sense of smell extremely carefully in demented patients.

Because the motor strip is so far back, compared with the size of the frontal lobe, intellectual deterioration, micturition disturbance or focal epileptic attacks are often the earliest symptoms of a frontal lobe tumour, long before definite physical signs appear. The possibility of a frontal tumour should always be pursued as far as possible on suspicion alone, even if there are no physical signs.

CASE HISTORY

A 64-year-old bus driver complained of a variety of unexplained symptoms and was eventually dismissed on medical grounds. About a year later he began to become morose and uncommunicative and complained of headaches. He rapidly deteriorated and memory difficulties were noted. The picture was thought to be due to a severe retarded depression and he was admitted to a mental hospital for electroconvulsive therapy. After three treatments he became drowsy and developed a mild left hemiparesis. Neurological examination revealed gross papilloedema and a mild left hemiparesis. A very large oedematous Grade 3 astrocytoma was resected from the right frontal lobe. Following surgery the patient had no motor deficit and no recollection of events for several weeks prior to his admission.

Physical Signs of Frontal Lobe Lesions

As indicated above, physical signs may be a late feature of a frontal lobe lesion. The need to look for optic atrophy, check for normal vision in both eyes and careful testing of the sense of smell has already been mentioned.

One of the most useful tests is the grasp reflex. It is also difficult to elicit. In the fully conscious patient stroking the palm is liable to serious misinterpretation! It is easier if the examiner holds the patient's hand with two or three fingers in the palm while gently rotating and flexing the arm as tone is assessed. Then as he lets go gentle pressure is exerted against the base of the patient's fingers. An involuntary increase in the grasp which traps the examiner's fingers is a positive response. In the unconscious or drowsy patient the test is useful and performed by gently pulling against the patient's fingers. A bilateral grasp response has no localising value but a unilateral grasp reflex provides strong evidence of a disturbance in the opposite frontal lobe.

If the lesion is situated posteriorly in the lobe damage to the motor strip may cause increased reflexes and a Babinski response on the opposite side of the body. If the dominant hemisphere is affected the patient may also have motor aphasia (inability to speak but with full understanding of instructions). This is almost invariably coupled with detectable weakness of the right face and right arm.

Parasaggital lesions are particularly likely to cause micturition disturbances and intellectual upset. As the area of cortex supplying the leg lies either side of the midline at this point, increased reflexes in both legs and *bilateral* extensor plantar responses may be found. Direct disruption of frontal lobe influences over the basal ganglia and cerebellum may cause "pseudo-Parkinsonism" or "pseudo-cerebellar" signs in addition to the apathy due to dementia. It is easy in such a case to make the mistaken diagnosis of arteriosclerotic dementia and Parkinsonism. For this reason the majority of neurologists insist on full investigation before a patient is allowed to be labelled as demented with the hopeless prognosis that this diagnosis carries.

2. The Parietal Lobes (Figure 8.3)

The parietal lobes are quite small extending from the Rolandic fissure anteriorly to the parieto-occipital fissure posteriorly and the temporal lobe below. The functional overlap between parietal, occipital and temporal lobe function in this area, and the physical continuity of the lobes makes anatomical boundaries of little practical significance.

The sensory cortex is organised in the same way as the motor strip with a large representation for information from the face and arm on the lateral surface and the trunk and leg areas on the top and in the parasaggital area.

Speech function is concentrated in the supramarginal and angular gyri, and in the upper part of the adjacent temporal lobe. The visual association areas (Area 19) are adjacent to the occipital lobe (see extinction hemianopia, Chapter 3). The same region is also responsible for the phenomenon of optico-kinetic nystagmus discussed in Chapter 7.

Clinical Features of Parietal Lobe Damage

The clinical features of dominant and non-dominant parietal lobe dysfunction have been discussed earlier in this chapter. To summarise, the following physical signs should be sought in patients with a suspected parietal lobe disorder.

1. Evidence of cortical sensory loss or sensory inattention.
2. Evidence of dysphasia if a dominant hemisphere lesion is suspected.
3. Evidence of dyspraxia if a non-dominant hemisphere lesion is suspected.

Figure 8.3. Parietal and Occipital Lobes (from behind and above)

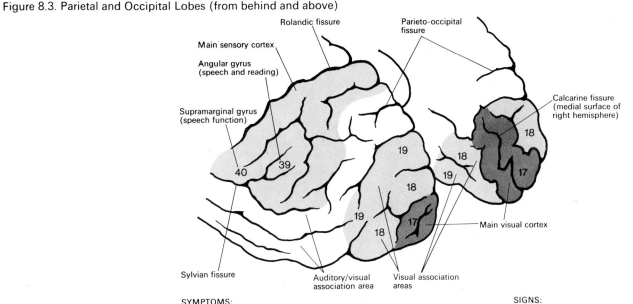

SYMPTOMS:
Parietal lobe:
Sensory seizures
Dysphasia (dominant hemisphere)
Dressing apraxia   \ (non-dominant
Geographical confusion / hemisphere)
Occipital lobe:
Seizures with flashing light aura
Visual field defects
Dyslexia and visual agnosia (if area
   19 and forward involved)

SIGNS:
Parietal lobe:
Cortical sensory loss
Sensory inattention
Attention hemianopia
Dysphasia/dyspraxia
Optico-kinetic nystagmus lost
Occipital lobe:
Homonymous field defects
Dyslexia or alexia

4. Evidence of an attention hemianopia or a frank hemi-anopia if a parieto-temporal lesion is present.
5. Loss of optico-kinetic nystagmus (Chapter 8).
6. "Soft" motor signs such as increased reflexes, mild facial weakness, and an extensor plantar response on the side opposite the suspected lesion.

3. The Occipital Lobes (Figure 8.3)

The occipital cortex has already been described in Chapter 3. Tumours in the occipital pole have epileptic potential but are relatively rare. Seizures preceded by visual hallucinations, consisting of unformed flashes of light and colours should be regarded as arising in the occipital lobe. Any field defect that is produced by a tumour in the lobe will not spare the macular cortex (a feature of vascular lesions, see next chapter and Chapter 3). Damage to areas 18, 19 and 37 in the adjacent parietal lobe responsible for visual association may cause varying degrees of psychic blindness such as visual agnosia (inability to recognise objects) or alexia (inability to read).

CASE REPORT

A middle-aged architect suffered from attacks of flashing lights in the right field of vision for ten years. Following one attack, vision did not recover and the hemianopia did not spare the macular. He also had great difficulty reading, writing and spelling indicating damage to the adjacent parietal area. This was not consistent with a simple vascular lesion and further investigation and operation revealed an occipito-parietal astrocytoma.

4. The Temporal Lobes (Figures 8.4, 8.5)

The anatomy of the temporal lobe is extremely difficult to grasp due to the way the lobe is folded in on itself under the overhanging frontal and parietal lobes and the extensive and important areas that are rolled in under the hemisphere. Furthermore, the connections of the lobe to the hippocampal area, the cingulate gyrus and the insula make the "functional" temporal lobe much more extensive than its physical boundaries. The "limbic system" which includes many of these functions is discussed in Chapter 12.

One can only summarise some of the many functions of the temporal lobe that find expression in clinical disorders. These include:

1. The central representation of auditory and vestibular information.
2. Memory function in the hippocampal gyrus.
3. Visual association areas.
4. Central representation of taste and smell.
5. The upper homonymous visual field pathways (Chapter 3).

Figure 8.4. The Temporal Lobe

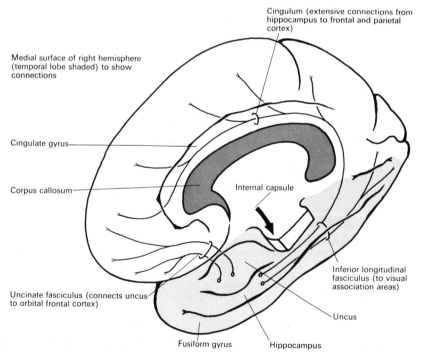

Cingulum (extensive connections from hippocampus to frontal and parietal cortex)

Medial surface of right hemisphere (temporal lobe shaded) to show connections

Cingulate gyrus

Corpus callosum

Internal capsule

Inferior longitudinal fasciculus (to visual association areas)

Uncinate fasciculus (connects uncus to orbital frontal cortex)

Uncus

Fusiform gyrus   Hippocampus

Figure 8.5. Lateral Surface of Left Temporal Lobe (anterior part shown cut off, Sylvian fissure pulled open)

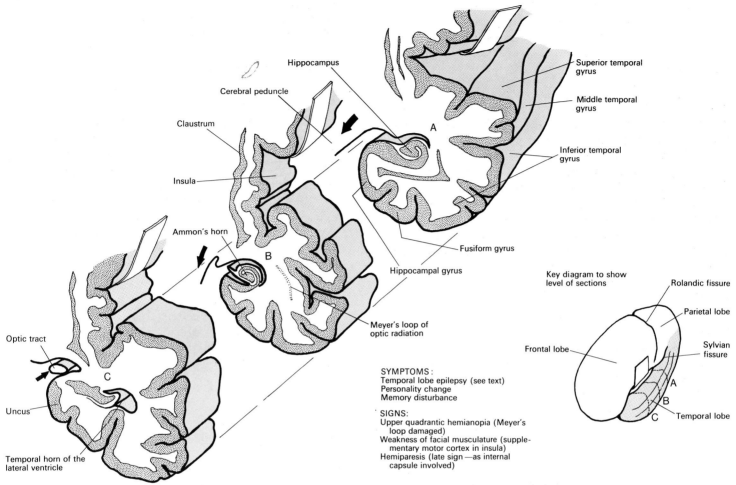

SYMPTOMS :
Temporal lobe epilepsy (see text)
Personality change
Memory disturbance

SIGNS:
Upper quadrantic hemianopia (Meyer's loop damaged)
Weakness of facial musculature (supplementary motor cortex in insula)
Hemiparesis (late sign —as internal capsule involved)

6. The entire visual radiation at the parieto-occipital-temporal junction.
7. Supplementary motor areas concerned with facial expression, eating, emotional responses to pain and pleasure.
8. Many aspects of behaviour via frontal lobe connections.
9. Central control of visceral motility, sexual and respiratory function.

Clinical Features of Temporal Lobe Disease

The clinical symptoms of temporal lobe disease can be of bewildering complexity. Fortunately the great frequency with which the disordered function is "epileptic" in nature makes recognition of the lesion possible. The important clinical pointer is that however bizarre and whatever the nature of the upset, the sudden onset and offset of the disturbance points to a paroxysmal disturbance in the temporal lobe, generally known as a "psychomotor" seizure. This term emphasises the behavioural upset that is a feature of such attacks, which is unlike any other form of epilepsy. Consciousness is not necessarily lost and motor dexterity is often maintained. These disorders are discussed in greater detail in Chapters 12 and 22.

Patients may relate a variety of typical prodromal events closely related to temporal lobe functions. They may describe vertigo, auditory or visual hallucinations, smell or taste hallucinations, unpleasant visceral symptoms, déjà-vu sensations, uncontrollable deep breathing, sexual fantasies or just a peculiar feeling "as if something awful was going to happen".

Motor accompaniments vary and peculiar grimacing, chewing, sucking or kissing mouth movements, repeated fiddling with clothing and sometimes removal of clothing may occur. Patients may drive many miles during an attack and become lost.

Focal motor seizures affecting the face and arm in particular (by activation of supplementary motor areas in the insula) may occur and the seizure may progress to loss of consciousness and a major convulsion.

Following a temporal lobe attack the patient is often very confused and in this state may physically attack over-helpful bystanders. Contrary to popular opinion, aggressive behaviour *during* the attack is very unusual.

Physical Signs of Temporal Lobe Lesions

Lesions in the temporal lobe almost invariably cause temporal lobe epilepsy unless they are extremely acute lesions such as haematomas or highly malignant gliomas. It is important to remember that only ten per cent of patients with temporal lobe seizures are harbouring a tumour, so that exclusory investigation is not indicated *unless* there are other reasons to suspect a neoplasm. The main reasons are physical signs and these are as follows.

Subtle personality change may occur. These are less dramatic than in frontal lobe lesions and may mimic depressive or psychotic disorders more often than dementia. There is a high incidence of impotence in males with temporal lobe tumours so that this symptom combined with personality change should arouse suspicion. Unilateral lesions rarely cause significant memory impairment.

A careful search for an upper quadrantic homonymous hemianopia is very important. This would provide evidence of damage to Meyer's loop (Chapter 3). If a complete hemianopia is present the lesion has spread into the adjacent parietal lobe, and appropriate parietal lobe problems may be found including dysphasia.

As the face area of the motor cortex is that most likely to be affected by a temporal lobe mass, a mild facial weakness should also be sought. Otherwise physical signs occur extremely late in the course of the disease and the picture then becomes one of a rapidly developing hemiparesis with confusion, headache, dysphasia (if on the dominant side) and personality change indicating a rapidly expanding lesion.

THE DIAGNOSIS AND INVESTIGATION OF CEREBRAL TUMOURS

The cardinal symptoms and signs of a cerebral tumour are said to be headache, vomiting and papilloedema. In fact these are very rarely the presenting symptoms unless the tumour is in the posterior fossa or has blocked the flow of C.S.F. This means that the majority of tumours produce more subtle symptoms and signs as already described in this chapter.

Headaches are discussed in detail in Chapter 20. In relation to cerebral tumours the following features are worth considering:

a. Headache is *not* an inevitable symptom of a cerebral tumour and is often so mild that the patient only mentions it in response to a direct question.
b. Less than one per cent of patients referred to hospital with headaches have a cerebral tumour.
c. Tumour headache is *not* particularly severe, it has a dull relentless quality. An association with vomiting certainly increases the chances of finding a serious cause but as a broad generalisation the more severe the headache the *less* likely it is to be due to a tumour.

Epileptic seizures in relation to tumours at different sites have already been discussed. As in the case of headache it is essential to have a sense of proportion about epilepsy and cerebral tumours:

a. In patients under twenty years of age the incidence of cerebral tumours causing epilepsy is 0·02 per cent.
b. Even in patients in the age group 45–55, the decade with the highest incidence of cerebral tumours, only ten per cent of patients with recent-onset epilepsy prove to have a cerebral tumour.
c. Epileptic seizures are more likely to occur when the underlying tumour is an infiltrating glioma than a surface lesion such as a meningioma. As gliomas occur twice as frequently as meningiomas the patient who has a fit due to a tumour usually proves to have a malignant glioma or astrocytoma.

From this it follows that a first seizure occurring in a patient aged twenty-one or more does *not* automatically mean that the patient has a cerebral tumour. Extensive investigation is only indicated if there are features discussed earlier in this chapter. In patients who have physical signs the tumour incidence rises to fifty per cent. In all patients with epilepsy a long-term follow-up is essential and the onset of physical signs should prompt investigation. A complete set of negative investigations early in the course of the illness does *not* exclude a neoplasm. Occasionally five to ten years elapse before other evidence of a slow growing tumour becomes apparent. Epilepsy due to a tumour is *not* particularly difficult to control and difficulty in controlling epilepsy is not evidence of an underlying tumour. However, if the epilepsy *starts* as an episode of status epilepticus there is a fifty per cent risk that the patient has a frontal tumour and full investigation *is* indicated in this instance.

In childhood the majority of cerebral tumours occur in the cerebellum (medulloblastomas or cystic astrocytomas), the pons and the optic nerve or chiasm. Supratentorial tumours are rare. Therefore early headache, vomiting ataxia or visual disturbance *are* common features of a tumour in the child and conversely epilepsy is very unusual. (Clinical details of posterior fossa tumours in childhood are to be found in Chapters 3, 6, 11 and 12.)

In the adult supratentorial tumours account for ninety per cent of cerebral neoplasms increasing the likelihood of an epileptic presentation and decreasing the incidence of headache as there is more space available for tumour expansion. Only cerebellar tumours (in the adult haemangioblastomas and metastases) and tumours that block C.S.F. flow (pinealomas, ependymomas of the fourth ventricle and intraventricular tumours) cause headache and vomiting as early features.

Pathological Features and Clinical Management

Childhood

In childhood cerebellar tumours are the main problem and pre-operative pathological diagnosis is difficult. Half the tumours consist of a small astrocytoma associated with a large cystic cavity. Complete removal with a low risk of recurrence is often possible. The other half consist of highly malignant medulloblastomas; tumours of disputed tissue origin usually arising in the vermis and extending down the superior medullary velum or peduncles into the brainstem with less possibility of complete resection. They also tend to seed the C.S.F. and secondary deposits in the lumbar theca are found. They are usually radiosensitive and combined surgery and radiotherapy (including the whole spinal canal) may achieve impressive cure rates. Pontine gliomas are discussed in Chapter 11 and optic nerve gliomas in Chapter 3. Neither are really resectable but often are moderately radiosensitive and significant symptomatic improvement and survival can be achieved. In the adult these particular gliomas occur with greatest frequency in patients with neurofibromatosis.

Adulthood

In the adult the first difference is the twenty to thirty per cent chance that *any* cerebral tumour is a metastasis. In the male carcinoma of the bronchus is the usual cause and in the female carcinoma of the breast. Therefore a chest x-ray and careful breast examination are the first and most important investigations in any patient of the appropriate sex with a cerebral tumour. Almost any other tumour may metastasise

to the brain but renal carcinoma, large bowel tumours and malignant melanomas are those most likely to do so. Large bowel tumours show a particular tendency to metastasise to the cerebellum, and in general metastases occur more frequently in both the parietal lobe and cerebellum than would be anticipated if spread were on a random basis.

Primary cerebral tumours occur in the lobes in a frequency roughly proportional to the size of the lobe, i.e. frontal/temporal/parietal and occipital. The primary cerebellar tumour that specifically occurs in the adult is the haemangioblastoma. This consists of a small highly vascular nodule of tumour often in association with a large haemorrhagic cyst. Complete resection is often possible and the prognosis is probably the best for any cerebral tumour. Occasionally these tumours produce erythropoeitin and cause polycythaemia. They may also be associated with vascular tumours in the retina (Hippel–von Lindau disease).

In the cerebral hemispheres half the tumours are malignant gliomas or astrocytomas with four grades of malignancy, I–IV, in order of increasing malignancy. An important subvariant is the oligodendroglioma, which occurs mainly in the frontal lobe and shows the greatest tendency to calcify. Many patients survive fifteen to twenty-five years with this type of tumour due to its exceedingly slow growth. The general prognosis of gliomas and astrocytomas is related to both the site and histological grading. Seventy-five per cent of patients with Grade IV tumours are dead within nine months, and even with Grade I and II tumours seventy-five per cent of patients are dead within three years.

There is little to be gained by early diagnosis of these infiltrating malignant tumours for the following reasons. Those tumours arising in silent areas (i.e. in regions not associated with specific symptoms or signs) tend to remain asymptomatic until very large and even then may carry a good prognosis because they are accessible and resectable by virtue of their site. Whereas tumours arising in vital areas cause early symptoms and signs but are often inoperable because the deficit produced by surgery would be unacceptable. The chance of operation depends on the site of the tumour and survival on the histological grading. Paradoxically it is better to have a highly malignant glioma in the frontal pole than a low grade glioma in the parieto-temporal region!

The relative incidence of tumours in different sites are indicated in Figure 8.6.

Tumours outside the substance of the brain include meningiomas, intraventricular lesions, pinealomas and neurofibromas. They produce either local signs if strategically sited or non-specific signs and raised intracranial pressure if they interfere with the circulation of the C.S.F. (Figure 8.7).

Figure 8.6. Tumour Frequency in Different Sites in the Adult

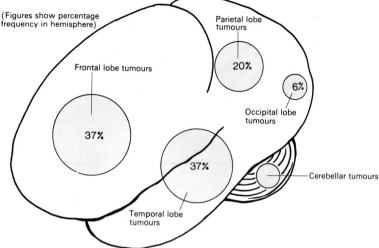

(Figures show percentage frequency in hemisphere)

Frontal lobe tumours — 37%

Parietal lobe tumours — 20%

Occipital lobe tumours — 6%

Temporal lobe tumours — 37%

Cerebellar tumours

Figure 8.7. Main Tumour Sites (other than in hemispheres)

Note. The shaded areas are intended to represent the site and not the relative frequency of occurrence

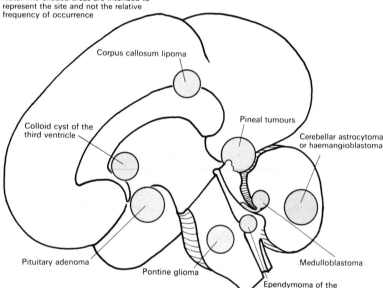

Corpus callosum lipoma

Colloid cyst of the third ventricle

Pineal tumours

Cerebellar astrocytoma or haemangioblastoma

Pituitary adenoma

Pontine glioma

Medulloblastoma

Ependymoma of the fourth ventricle

Meningiomas account for twenty per cent of intracranial tumours; and arise from the dura particularly in areas where it is densely adherent to bone. The sites and relative frequencies are indicated in Figure 8.8. Lesions along the falx Ⓐ are known as parasagittal tumours and typically produce frontal syndromes and cause technical complications by their tendency to invade the sagittal sinus. Surface meningiomas Ⓑ at first sight are highly favourable but often present formidable technical problems and successful removal may be marred by considerable neurological deficit.

Figure 8.8. The Common Sites of Meningiomas and Neurofibromas

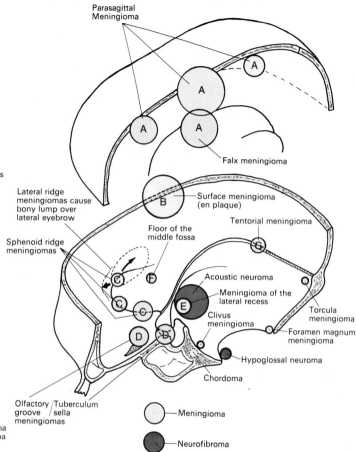

Parasagittal Meningioma

Falx meningioma

Surface meningioma (en plaque)

Tentorial meningioma

Lateral ridge meningiomas cause bony lump over lateral eyebrow

Floor of the middle fossa

Sphenoid ridge meningiomas

Acoustic neuroma

Meningioma of the lateral recess

Torcula meningioma

Clivus meningioma

Foramen magnum meningioma

Hypoglossal neuroma

Chordoma

Olfactory groove / Tuberculum sella meningiomas

○ — Meningioma

● — Neurofibroma

Tumours along the sphenoid ridge Ⓒ tend to produce extraocular nerve palsies at the inner end and middle third, and marked hyperostosis if in the lateral third producing a bony boss over the pteryion. Complete surgical removal is usually technically impossible and relentless progression of signs and frequent recurrences are the rule. Lesions at Ⓓ the olfactory groove or tuberculum sellae cause anosmia, visual failure and dementia. Meningiomas in the lateral recess Ⓔ are a rare cause of the cerebello-pontine angle syndrome (Chapter 6). Those on the free edge of the tentorium Ⓖ or at the confluence of the great veins Ⓗ tend to obstruct C.S.F. flow and produce the symptoms and signs of obstructive hydrocephalus (headache, vomiting and papilloedema). Rarely meningiomas arise on the front of the brainstem and in the foramen magnum. Their clinical features will be found in Chapters 11 and 15 respectively.

Neuromas account for seven per cent of intracranial tumours and nearly all arise on the acoustic nerve (Chapter 6).

They may also occur on the 5th, 9th, 10th and 12th cranial nerves (see also Chapter 7). It is worth restating that even in the best hands the surgical mortality of an acoustic nerve tumour approaches twenty per cent. This underlines the fact that the terms benign and malignant are almost meaningless in relation to cerebral tumours; it is the technical aspects that determine the prognosis.

Pituitary adenomas account for ten per cent of all primary intracranial tumours and are discussed in detail in Chapter 3.

Other extracerebral tumours are rare and each account for one per cent or less of cerebral tumours. Intraventricular tumours include pedunculated meningiomas, ependymomas (particularly in the floor of the fourth ventricle), gliomas extending into the ventricle and benign colloid cysts of the lining of the third ventricle or the septum pellucidum. Lipomas of the corpus callosum are rare and may achieve considerable size. Pinealomas tend to infiltrate the midbrain (see Chapters 2 and 8) and cause early obstruction of the aqueduct. Tumours in the ventricle can often be resected via the ventricle, but pinealomas are usually treated by irradiation, the obstructed aqueduct being bypassed by a shunt (a polythene cannula from the lateral ventricle into the cisterna magna).

CEREBRAL ABSCESS AND INFECTIVE GRANULOMAS

One of the most important differential diagnoses of cerebral tumour is cerebral abscess. The diagnosis may be extremely difficult to make to the extent that it is not until pus is encountered during needle aspiration of a cerebral mass that the diagnosis becomes apparent. This is particularly true in those situations in which a chronic low-grade abscess has developed in the absence of overt underlying disease.

In a classical case of cerebral abscess the presentation is acute with a toxic "meningitic" onset with fever quickly followed by confusion and focal neurological signs over a matter of days.

This typical course usually occurs in patients in whom the risk is recognisable. This includes patients with pneumococcal pneumonia; patients with rheumatic heart disease; and patients with cyanotic heart disease (venous blood bypasses the filtering effect of the lungs). In the pre-antibiotic era patients with chronic osteomyelitis, septic foci in the sinuses and chronic ear disease were also at great risk. Although this risk has been reduced so has awareness of the possibility of cerebral abscess and this is felt by many to account for the delay in diagnosis that is so often fatal. The prognosis for patients with cerebral abscess has *not* improved in the last twenty years. Finally cerebral abscess may complicate head injuries particularly those involving the paranasal sinuses and the middle ear. This is discussed further in Chapter 23.

A clue to the possible source of infection can sometimes be found in the site of the abscess. Blood-borne infections from the lungs or heart, like cerebral metastases and emboli, tend to lodge in the parietal lobes. Frontal abscesses are usually secondary to disease in the paranasal sinuses and temporal lobe and cerebellar abscesses from disease in the middle ear.

The infecting organism, particularly from local lesions in the sinuses and ears is usually the pneumococcus, although in some instances no definite organism can be cultured. For this reason, penicillin in adequate doseage (up to twenty-four mega units per twenty-four hours) is the most reliable treatment unless cultures and sensitivities suggest otherwise.

Too often, inadequate treatment with newer antibiotics in the mistaken belief that the abscess is due to an unusual or resistant organism is responsible for therapeutic failure. Blood cultures, C.S.F. cultures (if the fluid can be safely obtained—see below) and aspirated pus from the abscess should be obtained before antibiotics are given.

Suspected cerebral abscess is probably the most dangerous situation in which to perform a lumbar puncture. With the rapid onset and considerable oedema that usually occurs the risk of coning is high. Papilloedema rarely has time to develop and its absence cannot be taken as evidence that there is no risk.

As examples of the different types of presentation of cerebral abscess the following cases may be cited.

CASE REPORT

A 60-year-old man with known compensated cyanotic heart disease presented with a seven-day history of headache, drowsiness and increasing dysphasia. He had been running an intermittent fever. A lumbar puncture at the referring hospital revealed a pressure of 260 mm and the fluid contained fifty-six cells, fifty per cent polymorphs and fifty per cent lymphocytes. The protein was 100 mgm. per cent and the C.S.F. sugar normal. Further investigation revealed an abscess in the left temporal lobe which was successfully drained.

The history, presentation and underlying disease made the diagnosis obvious in this patient but he was fortunate to survive the ill-advised lumbar puncture.

CASE REPORT

A 32-year-old female who had had a normal pregnancy and delivery two years previously presented with a two-month history of headache and focal epileptic seizures involving the left face and left arm. In retrospect it was possible that an isolated focal fit occurred a year previously. Prior to admission an attack left her with permanent weakness of the left face and arm and a peculiar affect. Right carotid angiography revealed an avascular mass in the right frontal lobe. At craniotomy for glioma pus was encountered and a β-haemolytic streptococcus was cultured. She made a full recovery following surgery.

This history is typical of the sub-acute "space-occupying lesion" type of presentation, in a clinical setting in which the original source of infection is not certain.

Other infective diseases causing cerebral masses are relatively rare in Great Britain. The syphilitic intracerebral gumma has become a museum disease and intracranial tuberculoma has become an extremely rare disease although in India tuberculosis accounts for twenty per cent of all intracranial masses. Hydatid cysts are rare in Europe but account for thirty per cent of intracranial tumours in several South American countries. Clearly these disorders must be considered in immigrants and those who have served overseas in these areas.

(Other infectious diseases of the nervous system are discussed in Chapter 26.)

INVESTIGATION OF A SUSPECTED CEREBRAL MASS

Details of special investigations and interpretation are to be found in Chapter 25. Only details directly applicable to the diagnosis of cerebral tumours will be considered in this section.

1. The history and physical examination should be reviewed for any evidence to suggest an underlying primary neoplasm. Negative chest x-rays and a normal breast examination will exclude the majority of primary neoplasms. All previous surgical procedures should be reviewed. Very often patients have not been told or have forgotten the removal of a malignant tumour many years previously.

2. Plain skull films are almost always normal. Gross sella erosion is usually found only in the presence of obvious raised intracranial pressure and pineal shift usually parallels very obvious clinical evidence of a large mass in one hemisphere. Abnormal intracranial clacification may occasionally provide a diagnostic clue and the x-rays are usually abnormal in patients with a pituitary tumour. It is unusual for x-rays to do anything other than confirm clinical findings. Apparently abnormal skull films in the absence of symptoms and signs should always be interpreted with caution. This often happens when skull films are taken after a minor head injury and some unrelated abnormality is suspected.

3. An E.E.G. is more likely to be abnormal with an intrinsic tumour although it may be misleadingly normal in some cases. However, as a general rule an E.E.G. is more likely to raise false diagnostic possibilities, and when grossly abnormal often does no more than confirm very obvious physical signs. Interpretation by the clinician in charge of the case is more likely to avoid unnecessary investigation of dubious abnormalities.

4. Ultrasound investigation although finding its place at first in cerebral disease diagnosis no longer holds a significant place in investigation. The problem of reflection of sound waves from the skull have not yet been overcome and usually the shift of the midline is only certain when the clinical situation is already obvious.

The investigations discussed so far, although often showing abnormalities usually do so only when the situation is already clinically obvious. They do *not* advance the diagnosis but merely add supportive evidence and can occasionally be misleadingly normal in the most difficult clinical situations.

5. Radioisotope scanning is the first of the investigations providing accurate and occasionally pathologically useful information. The highest accuracy is achieved in meningiomas, cerebral abscesses and metastases (provided the latter are over 2 cm. in diameter). This is probably due to the combination of increased vascularity and oedema in these lesions. The diagnostic accuracy rapidly falls off in the case of gliomas and astrocytomas. Even in the most malignant tumours a false negative rate of thirty to forty per cent is possible and in low grade tumours the success rate is as low as twenty per cent. A negative scan may practically exclude meningiomas, abscesses and metastases but does *not* exclude other tumours. Furthermore acute vascular accidents cause positive scans and cannot be distinguished from a tumour unless the scan uptake decreases with time. Unfortunately the clinical situation may not allow the luxury of waiting and repeating the scan six weeks later.

6. The recent advent of computerised axial tomography (EMI scanning)—a form of computerised x-ray densitometry holds great promise for the future and although enormous advantages are already apparent the technique is still under evaluation and only available in a few centres in Great Britain.

7. Angiography was introduced in 1936 and remains an indispensable aid to tumour diagnosis. (Its role in vascular disease is discussed in the next chapter.) However, even angiography may fail to detect tumours in certain areas where shift of known vessels is not produced or lesions that do not develop a pathological circulation. However if the patient is suspected of having a tumour on one side a

carotid angiogram on the appropriate side is the investigation of choice, and the investigation most likely to indicate the site, and often the nature of the lesion.

8. Lumbar air encephalography is contraindicated in patients with suspected cerebral tumours as is lumbar puncture. There are occasional exceptions to this rule but only under close neurosurgical supervision (the whole problem is amplified in Chapter 25). In patients with tumours and particularly those with obstruction of C.S.F. pathways ventriculography is the procedure of choice unless angiography has already indicated the site and nature of the lesion. Air or sodium iophendylate (myodil) is put into the lateral ventricle via a burr hole and allowed to pass through the foramen of Munro into the third ventricle and down the aqueduct to the 4th ventricle until the site of the obstruction is seen. The shape and direction of the obstructive deformity often indicates the probable diagnosis.

The diagnosis of cerebral tumours is in the first instance based on the history and physical signs. Subsequent investigation is based on a sequence of investigations as seems appropriate to the clinical diagnosis. At all stages a continual review of the situation and the evidence provided by the tests already performed is evaluated and the need to continue the investigations considered. It is quite possible to fail to demonstrate a tumour at the first attempt and it should always be remembered that there is no absolutely exclusory test.

The need to continue to follow patients once suspected of having a tumour is evident. The expense, and risk of unnecessary investigation on the mere "suspicion" of a tumour should be apparent. Full tumour exclusion should only be considered when the clinical suspicion backed up by signs and screening investigation indicate a *real* possibility of detecting a tumour.

Chapter 9

THE CEREBRAL HEMISPHERES: 2. VASCULAR DISEASES

In the previous chapter the anatomy of the hemispheres was described and this knowledge applied to the detection of dysfunction in various areas. This has special application in the detection of cerebral tumours.

When we consider the blood supply of the cerebral hemisphere the single most important point to remember is that each lobe does not have an individual blood supply so that vascular disease usually produces an entirely different set of syndromes although on occasions some overlap with lobe disease can occur.

At the simplest level a hemiparesis means no more and no less than that there is an abnormality in the opposite hemisphere. A very common error is to assume that "hemiparesis" is synonymous with a "stroke", an assumption that may have disastrous consequences.

To make the differentiation between a neoplastic or other space occupying lesion and a stroke one must rely very substantially on the history and yet the abruptness of onset that characterises a vascular lesion *may* occur with a cerebral tumour, and conversely but much less frequently a stroke may have a sub-acute onset that mimics a tumour. Therefore, a very accurately plotted anatomical extent of the lesion can be critical in making the differential diagnosis and distinguishing those patients who should be considered for further investigation.

THE ARTERIAL BLOOD SUPPLY OF THE CEREBRAL HEMISPHERES

The hemispheres are supplied by the terminal branches of the carotid and basilar arteries. There are anastomoses between the various branches over the cortex and the efficiency of these is often critical in determining the final outcome of major vessel occlusions (Figure 9.1).

1. The Anterior Cerebral Artery (Figure 9.2)

The anterior cerebral artery sweeps forward and over the genu of the corpus callosum and then backwards as two vessels, the pericallosal and callosomarginal arteries, supplying the parasaggital cortex including the entire motor and sensory cortex controlling the leg.

Shortly after its origin the anterior cerebral artery gives off an inconstant branch known as the recurrent artery of Huebner. If present, this vessel contributes to the blood supply of the nerve fibres in the internal capsule destined to supply the cranial nerve nuclei and the arm on the opposite side.

The two anterior cerebral arteries are joined by a short anterior communicating artery which allows collateral flow to the opposite hemisphere if the carotid artery is occluded on either side. Whenever carotid ligation is contemplated in the treatment of an aneurysm the patency of this vessel has to be demonstrated angiographically before ligation is performed.

2. The Middle Cerebral Artery (Figure 9.4)

This artery originates at the bifurcation of the internal carotid artery just above the cavernous sinus. The vessel then passes laterally between the upper surface of the temporal lobe and the inferior surface of the frontal lobe to reach a position deep in the Sylvian fissure. Here it divides into three main vessels which pass upwards and backwards in the fissure giving off branches that exit along the length of the fissure to supply the surface of the hemisphere. These are the precentral, central, posterior parietal and posterior temporal arteries.

As the middle cerebral artery passes laterally it gives off a series of six to twelve long thin penetrating vessels that enter the anterior perforated substance to supply the basal ganglia and part of the internal capsule. These are the Lenticulostriate arteries. Terminal branches of the main vessel reach the occipital pole (see below) and probably provide an independent blood supply to the macular cortex at the tip of the lobe.

3. The Posterior Cerebral Artery

The posterior cerebral arteries are formed by the bifurcation of the basilar artery in the interpeduncular space (Figure 9.2 and Figure 9.4). Each vessel passes round the cerebral peduncles lying between the medial surface of the temporal lobe and the upper brain stem. Along its length each gives off vessels supplying the inferior medial surface and hippocampal area of the temporal lobe. A series of

Figure 9.1. Diagram to Show the Course of the Carotid and Vertebral Arteries in the Thorax and Neck

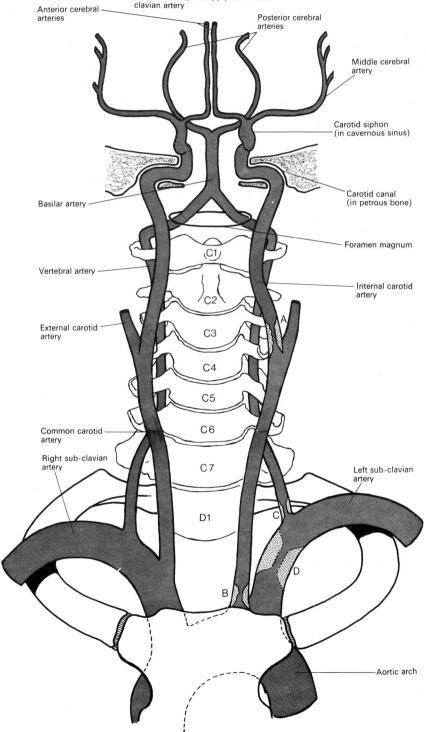

A, B, C are common atheroma sites
Lesions at A & B produce transient hemiparetic schaemic attacks
Lesions at C produce brainstem ischaemic episodes
Lesions at D produce the "subclavian steal syndrome"—blood passes up the left carotid artery and back down the left vertebral artery to supply the left sub-clavian artery

Anterior cerebral arteries

Posterior cerebral arteries

Middle cerebral artery

Carotid siphon (in cavernous sinus)

Basilar artery

Carotid canal (in petrous bone)

Foramen magnum

C1

Vertebral artery

Internal carotid artery

C2

External carotid artery

A

C3

C4

C5

Common carotid artery

C6

Right sub-clavian artery

C7

Left sub-clavian artery

D1

C

D

B

Aortic arch

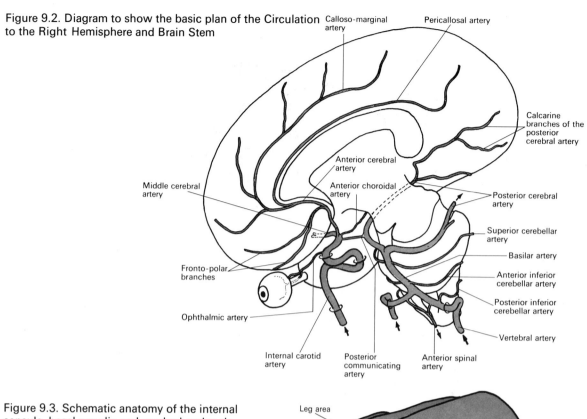

Figure 9.2. Diagram to show the basic plan of the Circulation to the Right Hemisphere and Brain Stem

Calloso-marginal artery

Pericallosal artery

Calcarine branches of the posterior cerebral artery

Anterior cerebral artery

Anterior choroidal artery

Middle cerebral artery

Posterior cerebral artery

Superior cerebellar artery

Basilar artery

Anterior inferior cerebellar artery

Posterior inferior cerebellar artery

Fronto-polar branches

Ophthalmic artery

Vertebral artery

Internal carotid artery

Posterior communicating artery

Anterior spinal artery

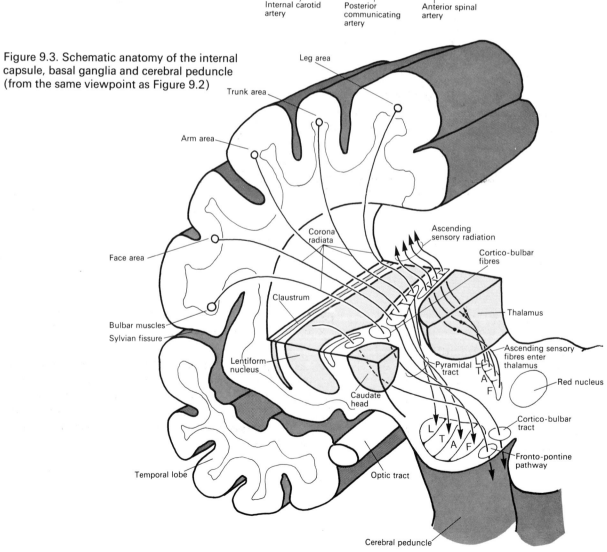

Figure 9.3. Schematic anatomy of the internal capsule, basal ganglia and cerebral peduncle (from the same viewpoint as Figure 9.2)

Leg area

Trunk area

Arm area

Corona radiata

Ascending sensory radiation

Cortico-bulbar fibres

Face area

Thalamus

Claustrum

Ascending sensory fibres enter thalamus

Bulbar muscles

Sylvian fissure

Pyramidal tract

Red nucleus

Lentiform nucleus

Caudate head

Cortico-bulbar tract

Temporal lobe

Optic tract

Fronto-pontine pathway

Cerebral peduncle

Figure 9.4. The Blood Supply of the Deep Structures of the Hemisphere

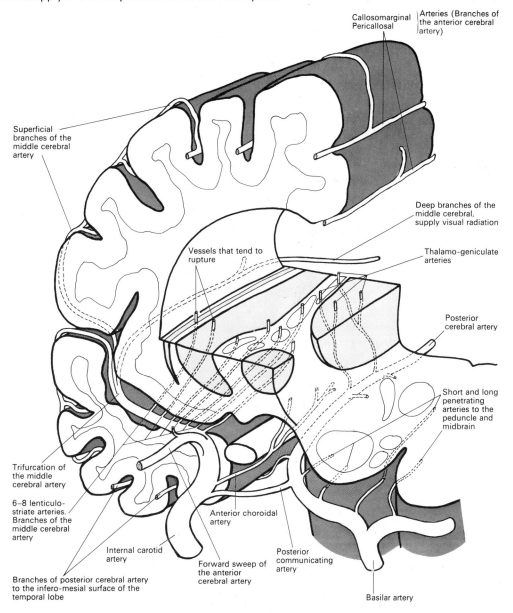

Callosomarginal
Pericallosal
Arteries (Branches of the anterior cerebral artery)

Superficial branches of the middle cerebral artery

Vessels that tend to rupture

Deep branches of the middle cerebral, supply visual radiation

Thalamo-geniculate arteries

Posterior cerebral artery

Short and long penetrating arteries to the peduncle and midbrain

Trifurcation of the middle cerebral artery

6–8 lenticulo-striate arteries. Branches of the middle cerebral artery

Anterior choroidal artery

Posterior communicating artery

Internal carotid artery

Forward sweep of the anterior cerebral artery

Branches of posterior cerebral artery to the infero-mesial surface of the temporal lobe

Basilar artery

penetrating vessels supply the dorsolateral brain stem, the thalamus, posterior internal capsule and sublenticular and retrolenticular visual radiations. These are the thalamogeniculate and thalamo-perforating arteries.

The main vessel terminates as the calcarine artery, supplying the visual cortex with the exception of the macular cortex at the tip of the pole. This has a dual or independent blood supply from the middle cerebral artery (see macular sparing hemianopia, Chapter 3).

THE CLINICAL PICTURES PRODUCED BY CEREBRAL BLOOD VESSEL OCCLUSIONS

The term occlusion is used reservedly. Following a C.V.A. it is unusual to find a vessel actually occluded. This is because most occlusions are probably due to embolic blockage with rapid subsequent recanalisation. However, a few minutes obstruction of flow in any vessel leads to irreversible damage to the territory supplied.

There are three main patterns of damage that can occur:

1. Occlusion of the main trunk of the parent vessel.
2. Occlusion of one of the important penetrating arteries.
3. Occlusion of one of the terminal branches.

We will consider these three possibilities for each vessel in turn.

Figure 9.5. Anterior Cerebral Artery Occlusion

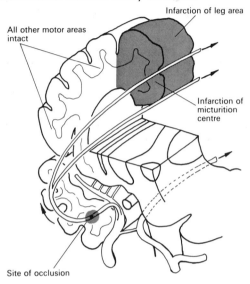

Anterior Cerebral Artery Occlusion (Figure 9.5)

1. *Main Trunk Occlusions*

Anterior cerebral artery occlusions are quite rare. The picture depends to some extent on whether the recurrent artery of Heubner is present.

   a. If there is *no* recurrent artery the face and arm will not be affected, but the entire leg area of the cortex is destroyed. This causes flaccid paralysis of the leg, with cortical sensory loss.

   b. If there *is* a recurrent artery and the block occurs proximal to its origin, the anterior internal capsule will also be infarcted giving rise to a typical upper motor neurone facial weakness and a spastic arm with considerable potential for recovery (because the overlying arm cortex is intact) but a useless flaccid leg (because all cortical control of the limb is lost).

Because the paracentral lobules are also damaged, voluntary control of micturition is often impaired. Incontinence of urine is the almost invariable consequence. In some instances this combination of incontinence and flaccid weakness of the leg may lead to an ineffectual search for a cauda equina lesion. The clinical evidence against this is that in spite of the flaccidity of the leg the reflexes rapidly return and become *brisk* and the plantar response is *extensor*. These findings would be very unusual with a cauda equina lesion which usually cause areflexia and absent plantar responses (see Chapter 15).

Furthermore considerable intellectual deficit and memory disturbance may occur due to damage to fronto-parietal and fronto-temporal fibres in the cingulate gyrus.

In all cases if there is any evidence that the other leg is also affected (i.e. the lesion is not strictly unilateral) a para-saggital tumour must be excluded. Vascular occlusions affecting the hemisphere should *not* produce *bilateral* signs.

2. *Perforating Artery Occlusion*

If the recurrent artery of Heubner is present and is occluded, weakness of the face and arm will occur; this will be of pyramidal type. Even if the dominant hemisphere is involved dysphasia does not occur because the cortex is unaffected. This is a very rare syndrome.

3. *Terminal Branch Occlusion*

The terminal vessels primarily supply the cortex controlling the leg and infarction affects both motor and sensory function. Flaccid weakness of the leg with brisk reflexes and an extensor plantar response is found. The sensory loss affects accurate touch perception and joint position sense, i.e. is of the cortical type. This makes it almost impossible to mobilise the patient as even with splints to stiffen the leg the patient has lost awareness of its position. With distal lesions intellectual disturbances and bladder dysfunction may be less severe than that caused by a main trunk occlusion.

Middle Cerebral Artery Occlusions

1. *Main Trunk Occlusions* (Figure 9.6)

Middle cerebral occlusion causes massive infarction of the bulk of the hemisphere. There is often considerable cerebral oedema which may cause coma. There are also important differences between the hemispheres with global dysphasia if the dominant hemisphere is affected, and severe dyspraxia or even denial of the existence of the whole left side if the non-dominant hemisphere is affected.

From a motor point of view the lesion destroys both pyramidal and extrapyramidal mechanisms, hence a flaccid type of weakness of the face and arm, with little or no potential for recovery is found. The leg cortex is spared but is so extensively "undercut" by the lesion that even the leg rarely improves significantly.

This is quite the most devastating type of C.V.A. with very minimal improvement to be anticipated and a real chance

Figure 9.6. Distal Middle Cerebral Artery Occlusion

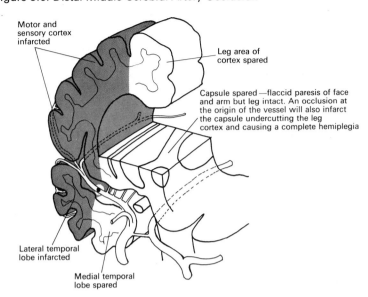

Motor and sensory cortex infarcted

Leg area of cortex spared

Capsule spared—flaccid paresis of face and arm but leg intact. An occlusion at the origin of the vessel will also infarct the capsule undercutting the leg cortex and causing a complete hemiplegia

Lateral temporal lobe infarcted

Medial temporal lobe spared

that the patient may die from the acute swelling of the infarcted hemisphere. Hemianaesthesia and a complete hemianopia are usually associated with the hemiparesis. The clinical picture can be identical with that produced by total occlusion of the carotid artery in the neck, with cross circulation via the anterior communicating artery keeping the anterior cerebral area perfused and the posterior cerebral circulation functioning normally. These anastomoses may be so efficient that patients are sometimes seen who have complete carotid artery occlusion and no neurological deficit.

2. *Perforating Artery Occlusions* (Capsular C.V.A.) (Figure 9.7)

A cerebral vascular accident due to occlusion of one of the lenticulostriate vessels is both the most frequent and the most favourable that occurs. Several of these vessels may be occluded without demonstrable effect. The evidence for this statement takes two forms. First, extrapyramidal syndromes are extremely rare in vascular disease of the brain and yet a substantial part of the basal ganglia is supplied by these vessels. Secondly, there is the evidence provided by "pseudo-bulbar palsy". The explanation of this condition is rarely understood by physicians. The mechanism is as follows; a vessel supplying the cortico-bulbar fibres to the brain stem nuclei becomes occluded. Because most of these nuclei have 50:50 innervation from each hemisphere, little or no deficit occurs and the episode may pass unnoticed. If some time later, the cortico-bulbar fibres on the *other* side are damaged the cranial nerve nuclei are abruptly deprived of

all control. Speech, chewing and swallowing become impossible. Significant recovery is unusual. The syndrome is most often seen in diabetic or hypertensive patients, as both groups are prone to develop widespread small vessel disease.

When the vessel supplying the main motor pathways of the capsule is occluded, a typical "capsular C.V.A." occurs. The only evidence of cortico-bulbar fibre damage is a mild upper motor neurone facial weakness. Both limbs on the opposite side are affected, resulting in a flaccid hemiparesis. In the acute stage no reflexes or plantar responses can be elicited. Within hours, tone starts to return, the reflexes become brisk and an extensor plantar response will be found. As the tone increases power returns in a pyramidal distribution. The flexor groups in the arm and the extensor groups in the leg become strong. The functional importance of this distribution of power results in the majority of patients leaving hospital with the typical hemiplegic gait. Physiotherapy capitalises on this functional distribution and helps the patient to learn to use the compromised limbs, but recovery would have occurred in any case.

There is rarely any sensory deficit or field defect, as both these pathways lie in the vascular territory of the posterior cerebral artery. A combination of hemiplegia, hemianaesthesia and hemianopia is not typical of capsular infarction and the prognosis in such cases is poor. These patients have either had a middle cerebral artery occlusion

Figure 9.7. Capsular Infarction (lenticulo-striate artery occlusion)

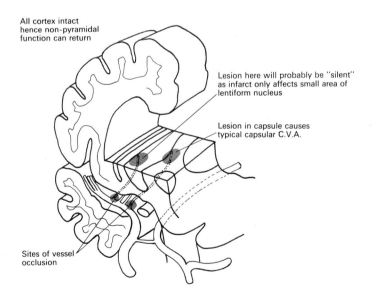

All cortex intact hence non-pyramidal function can return

Lesion here will probably be "silent" as infarct only affects small area of lentiform nucleus

Lesion in capsule causes typical capsular C.V.A.

Sites of vessel occlusion

(see above), an anterior choroidal artery occlusion (see later), or a haemorrhage into the internal capsule.

A capsular lesion is not accompanied by dysphasia because the parietal cortex is unaffected.

A distinction must be made between dysphasia and dysarthria. Dysarthria refers to poor phonation. With a capsular lesion in the acute stages, severe weakness of the face may lead to slurring of speech but the patient understands the spoken word, and uses words correctly. There is really no reason at all for there to be any confusion about the use of these terms.

3. Terminal Branch Occlusions

There are four major peripheral branches on each side.

a. The Dominant Hemisphere

The precentral artery supplies the motor areas for the face and arm and Broca's speech area. Occlusion of this vessel causes flaccid paralysis of the face and arm and total inability to speak, but with full comprehension. As the patient is also unable to write his anguish and frustration is considerable. Recovery is minimal although speech therapy may occasionally have a modest success in helping these patients to say a few key words.

If the central artery is occluded weakness of the face and arm occurs with mild dysphasic difficulties.

Occlusion of the posterior parietal artery produces *complete* aphasia with loss of comprehension and loss of speech, even though the patient may well be able to phonate and even say single irrelevant words, or new words of his own making (neologisms), or incoherent sentences of otherwise normal words (word salads). There may be a mild hemiparesis and cortical sensory loss but this is usually impossible to ascertain due to the lack of communication.

Occlusion of the superior temporal artery tends to cause receptive aphasia. The patient may be able to speak but the sentences are irrelevant and inappropriate to the examiner's question.

b. The Non-dominant Hemisphere

Superficial branch occlusions in the non-dominant hemisphere produce similar findings although the dysphasic difficulties are replaced by dyspraxia. Precentral and central branch occlusions cause a flaccid monoplegia of the arm and face. Occlusions of the posterior parietal and superior temporal arteries may cause mild sensory difficulties in the left face and arm and more generalised difficulties such as dressing apraxia or geographical disorientation and difficulty with skilled tasks.

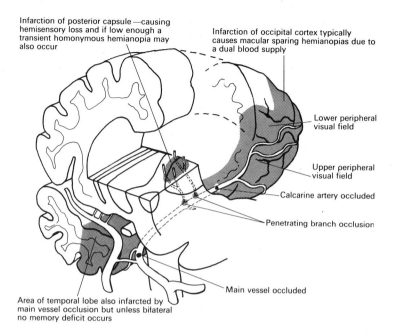

Figure 9.8. Posterior Cerebral Artery Occlusions

Infarction of posterior capsule—causing hemisensory loss and if low enough a transient homonymous hemianopia may also occur

Infarction of occipital cortex typically causes macular sparing hemianopias due to a dual blood supply

Lower peripheral visual field

Upper peripheral visual field

Calcarine artery occluded

Penetrating branch occlusion

Main vessel occluded

Area of temporal lobe also infarcted by main vessel occlusion but unless bilateral no memory deficit occurs

Posterior Cerebral Artery Occlusions

1. Main Vessel Occlusions

The effects of a complete posterior cerebral artery occlusion can be very variable as there are anastomoses between the vessel and the middle cerebral arteries. Variable degrees of confusion and memory deficit can occur but these are more suggestive of *bilateral* damage due to occlusion of the basilar artery than occlusion of a single posterior cerebral artery. There may also be some sensory deficit and a field defect due to thalamo-geniculate artery occlusion.

2. Perforating Vessel Occlusion

Occlusion of one of the thalamo-geniculate vessels produces a more readily recognisable clinical picture. The posterior limb of the internal capsule, part of the thalamus and the visual radiation, are affected, resulting in hemi-anaesthesia with loss of all sensory modalities, and complete hemianopia (the visual radiation is damaged in its entirety). Often a good recovery is achieved but the main risk is the subsequent development of the Dejerine–Roussy syndrome which follows this type of C.V.A. When this happens the initial numbness is replaced by paraesthesia, or a painful sensation which becomes excruciating in severity when the affected limb is touched, or even continual pain without provocation. This thalamic pain may drive the patient to suicide and is rarely responsive to drugs or surgical procedures. Occasionally control may be achieved with Diphenylhydantoin (Epanutin) or Carbamezepine (Tegretol) combined with Imipramine (Tofranil).

If the branches to the upper brain stem are affected Hemiballismus may occur. This is the *only* extra-pyramidal syndrome typically produced by vascular disease. It consists of the abrupt onset of wild flinging movements of the limbs on one side of the body. It may subside spontaneously but can usually be arrested dramatically by 50 mgms. Chlorpromazine I.M.I.

CASE REPORT

A middle-aged woman with severe aortic stenosis was an inpatient awaiting surgery. Early one morning she acutely developed severe flinging movements of the left limbs, fracturing the left humerus against the cot side. Within minutes she had severe angina and the violent movements continued; with serious effects on the damaged limb. Within minutes of giving 50 mgs. of Chloropromazine intramuscularly all movement ceased. It did not recur. A cerebral embolus into the region of the sub-thalamic nucleus was thought to be responsible (see also Chapter 12).

3. *Terminal Branch Occlusion*

Occlusion of the calcarine artery causes a macular sparing hemianopia (see Chapter 3). This quite frequently occurs in otherwise fit young persons during the course of a migraine attack. There is no need to embark on full investigation of a patient who presents with a macular sparing hemianopia unless other physical signs are present. Incomplete lesions can cause a variety of incomplete hemianopias but in all cases the deficit will be absolutely congruous and will spare the macula, making identification easy.

Anterior Choroidal Artery Occlusions

The anterior choroidal artery arises directly from the carotid artery and runs backwards along the optic tract to the area under the internal capsule and eventually supplies the choroid plexus of the lateral ventricle. It has a variable distribution that includes the optic tract, and the basal ganglia. At one stage surgical ligation was attempted as a possible treatment for parkinsonism, but this occasionally produced devastating disabilities including hemiparesis, and was quickly abandoned.

It seems likely that some patients who develop hemiparesis, hemisensory loss and hemianopia and who clearly have not had a middle cerebral artery occlusion (i.e. no flaccidity, no drowsiness, no dysphasia or dyspraxia), have suffered an occlusion of the anterior choroidal artery and have infarcted the subcapsular area and the optic tract.

THE DEVELOPMENT OF SYMPTOMS AND SIGNS OF A VASCULAR ACCIDENT

The various clinical pictures produced by infarction of various areas of the central nervous system have been outlined. If the damage is clearly in one of these territories, the chance that the lesion is a vascular one is high. However, the majority of diagnoses of "stroke" are based on historical features. We will examine some of these features critically to show how valuable an accurate topographical diagnosis can be in substantiating a clinical impression.

The Abrupt Onset of Symptoms

The term a "stroke" emphasises the single characteristic feature of a vascular accident—the very abrupt onset. Yet so often the patient, often elderly and living alone, is found drowsy, confused and dysphasic and the mode of onset cannot be established. In such instances it is safest to pursue other diagnostic possibilities.

Drowsiness or increasing neurological deficit over a period of hours can occur following a middle cerebral occlusion but if the onset was not very abrupt, metabolic disorders, subdural or extradural haematomas, or meningeal infection must be excluded. In the elderly patient meningitis may present as a stroke-like illness, with confusion, minimal pyrexia and little neck stiffness.

A further cause of acute hemiparesis with or without confusion that should always be considered is hypoglycaemia. There is clinical and experimental evidence that poor perfusion of one hemisphere may lead to focal symptoms such as hemiparesis when the blood sugar reaches dangerously low levels.

Conversely the extremely abrupt onset of disability can occur with a cerebral tumour.

CASE REPORT

A 28-year-old pregnant woman collapsed and became deeply unconscious while preparing a meal. She had a complete right hemiparesis and fixed dilated pupils. A skull x-ray revealed half an inch of pineal shift to the left side. She died while further investigations were being arranged. She was found to have an extensive infiltrating glioma of the left thalamus. She had been asymptomatic until she collapsed.

A Stuttering Onset of Symptoms

Whenever a neurological event has occurred it is always important to establish whether there were any premonitory symptoms. For example, however abrupt the onset of the hemiparesis, if there was a prior history of several weeks' headache, personality change or ill health the diagnosis of a stroke would clearly be in doubt.

Repeated identical brief episodes of hemiparesis with full recovery quite often occur and such episodes are called transient ischaemic attacks. These are widely regarded as a sign of an impending stroke and in general angiography is indicated in an attempt to locate an operable athero-sclerotic lesion in the appropriate carotid artery. Even this assumption is not always reliable.

CASE REPORT

A 56-year-old man gave a history of several brief attacks of left-sided weakness over a six-week period. There were no residual signs and he was extremely hypertensive. Hypotensive therapy was begun and angiography was not performed in view of the very high blood pressure. A few weeks later a similar episode occurred without recovery. An angiogram performed elsewhere revealed a glioblastoma multiforme in the right hemisphere.

This is a good example of the "vascular" presentation of a neoplasm. Occasionally the reverse may occur and this is a particular feature of carotid artery occlusion.

CASE REPORT

A 38-year-old female gave a ten-month history of intermittent sensory symptoms affecting the left side, headache, memory impairment, and some personality change. Over a period of five days she developed a moderately severe left hemiparesis. Full investigation showed no sign of cerebral tumour but there was almost complete occlusion of the right carotid artery.

CASE REPORT

A 49-year-old military contracts manager for an aeroplane manufacturer gave a three-week history of episodic tingling and numbness in the left limbs. This had been associated throughout with a dull right frontal headache. Examination revealed a left attention hemianopia, left-sided facial weakness, impairment of sensation over the entire left side but no motor signs in the limbs. A tumour was suspected but a carotid angiogram revealed complete occlusion of the right internal carotid artery.

CASE REPORT

A 58-year-old company director complained of pins and needles in his left hand for two weeks which had been treated by neck traction. This was followed by attacks of clumsiness of the left hand, weakness of the left side of his face and difficulty in articulating, each attack lasting seconds only. Over three weeks things worsened until progressive weakness of the left side was apparent and he became forgetful and drowsy but denied headache. On admission he was extremely drowsy with a left hemiparesis, and a left extensor plantar; sensory testing was impossible. A right carotid angiogram showed complete carotid occlusion. Despite attempts to control cerebral oedema he deteriorated and died several days later.

The similarities in the latter case histories are remarkable and yet when the last patient was seen only six weeks after the second, the diagnosis of carotid artery occlusion did *not* seem likely on the clinical evidence. In the author's view carotid artery occlusion mimics a cerebral tumour so closely that a tumour is almost invariably the suspected diagnosis.

A Steady Improvement of the Neurological Status

Any abrupt neurological event with rapid recovery certainly qualifies for the term "a vascular event" and in the majority of instances it will prove to be due to a vascular accident. Unfortunately, in some instances, as already discussed, recovery is not the rule, and in the case of a middle cerebral artery occlusion the subsequent oedema may lead to deterioration, coma and even death. An intra-cerebral haemorrhage may produce a similar picture. This is discussed later.

Immediate loss of consciousness or an epileptic fit are extremely unusual events in an uncomplicated cerebral vascular accident. A major embolus from a fibrillating heart, an intra-cerebral haemorrhage or a sub-arachnoid haemorrhage should be suspected if either of these events occurs. Loss of consciousness or an epileptic fit should *never* be dismissed as due to a "small stroke". They are so unusual in major strokes that the likelihood of their occurring during an otherwise sub-clinical stroke seems remote.

Headache

Although severe headache of abrupt onset associated with neurological signs is most likely to occur during some form of cerebral haemorrhage, headache of moderate severity is by no means unusual in an uncomplicated occlusive cerebral vascular accident. Occasionally patients with migraine are unfortunate enough to suffer an occlusion during an attack of migraine. This is almost invariably an occlusion of the posterior cerebral artery or its terminal branches.

These problems and illustrative case histories have been included to highlight the fact that however obvious the diagnosis of "stroke" may appear to be, the subsequent physical examination should be performed to answer the question "are these signs compatible with a C.V.A. in a certain vascular territory?" This is essential to avoid compounding an error that may have been due to a misleading history.

Other Types of Cerebral Vascular Accident Thrombotic Lesions

Whenever an occlusive cerebral vascular accident has occurred some basic disease processes that may predispose to intra-vascular thrombosis must be excluded, especially in the young patient. Haematological disorders, including polycythemia rubra vera, thrombotic thrombocytopaenic purpura, disseminated lupus erythromatosus and the heavy protein diseases should be excluded. At any age diabetes mellitus and syphilis should be considered and in the elderly a high sedimentation rate should be regarded as due to temporal arteritis until proved otherwise. All the necessary exclusory tests can be performed quite easily, and should be a routine part of the investigation of any patient with a suspected stroke. Embolisation from auricular fibrillation may be the first evidence of thyrotoxicosis, or indicate a recent myocardial infarction; and sub-acute bacterial endocarditis frequently presents as a C.V.A.

Haemorrhagic Cerebral Vascular Accidents

There are three main types of haemorrhagic cerebral vascular accidents. It is now known that very small vascular lesions previously thought to be thrombotic are small lacunar haemorrhages. Because the blood does not burst into the ventricles or sub-arachnoid space, this type of haemorrhage cannot be distinguished from a small occlusive lesion in the internal capsule or brain stem.

1. Intracerebral haemorrhage

A classical intracerebral haemorrhage usually results from the rupture of one of the more peripheral lenticulo-striate arteries in the region of the external capsule. The haemorrhage rapidly strips the soft tissue under the cortex and may rupture into the sylvian fissure or into the lateral ventricle. In either event the typical clinical picture is of a sudden fulminating headache with rapidly deepening loss of consciousness and tentorial herniation. The ipsilateral pupil and then both pupils dilate and become fixed to light. In a typical case death ensues within fifteen minutes to a few hours of the onset (brain stem haemorrhage is discussed in Chapter 12).

2. Angiomas

A less dramatic form of cerebral haemorrhage is associated with cerebral arterio-venous malformations or angiomas. Many such lesions remain asymptomatic throughout the patient's life. In many cases focal epilepsy is the main problem. In others recurrent subarachnoid haemorrhage occurs and as a rule there is a good recovery between attacks. This is because the haemorrhage is from sinusoidal vessels under low pressure, lacking the destructive power of a jet of arterial blood from a ruptured Berry aneurysm or an artery. Finally an acute intracerebral haemorrhage with the development of signs due to a stable intracerebral haem-

atoma may be the first symptom of an angioma. In the latter case evacuation of the clot is essential but in general the prognosis for cerebral angiomas is extremely good and surgical attack is only indicated for intractable focal epilepsy or intracerebral haematoma. Recurrent subarachnoid haemorrhage may cause dementia due to hydrocephalus. This is thought to occur when the arachnoid villi become blocked by blood products, and C.S.F. resorption is impaired. A shunt procedure will often be of benefit to the patient in these cases.

CASE REPORT

A 52-year-old man had lunch and drinks with friends. A little later while walking his dog he was seen to stumble and fall down a bank. When helped to his feet he was noted to have clumsiness of the right leg. He insisted on going home and for several hours seemed to be well. However the next morning he had a series of Jacksonian fits starting in the right arm and becoming generalised. During one of these he fell and injured the occipital region and remained drowsy. He was admitted to hospital. On examination he was drowsy with a flaccid weakness of the right arm and a spastic weakness of the right leg. He had bilateral extensor plantar responses. The differential diagnostic possibilities were legion but rapid deterioration in his conscious level required urgent surgical help. He was found to have an intracerebral haematoma in the posterior frontal pole associated with two separate arterio-venous malformations. Following evacuation of the haematoma he made a good recovery.

3. Sub-Arachnoid Haemorrhage

Sub-arachnoid haemorrhage due to aneurysms on the vessels traversing the sub-arachnoid space represents a common and frequently lethal cause of intracranial haemorrhage. Although these aneurysms may arise at embryologically weak points on the vessel wall, they are no longer regarded as congenital. Aneurysms are only found in children in association with coarctation of the aorta or hypertension due to renal disease. At all ages the presence of an aneurysm tends to parallel the height of the blood pressure. This is most dramatically demonstrated by the sudden change in sex ratio after the age of 50. Until the age of 50 the ratio of females to males is 3 : 2. Over 50 it rises to 10 : 1. This is thought to be due to the better long-term survival of females with significant hypertension leading to the development of aneurysms in the 50–70 age group.

Less than fifteen per cent of patients have symptoms prior to rupture and these usually consist of premonitory headaches over a few days. Headache, acute nausea and vomiting and neck stiffness are the hallmarks of subarachnoid haemorrhage. Transient cardiac arythmias or glycosuria often occur in a patient who has had a subarachnoid haemorrhage for reasons that are not clear.

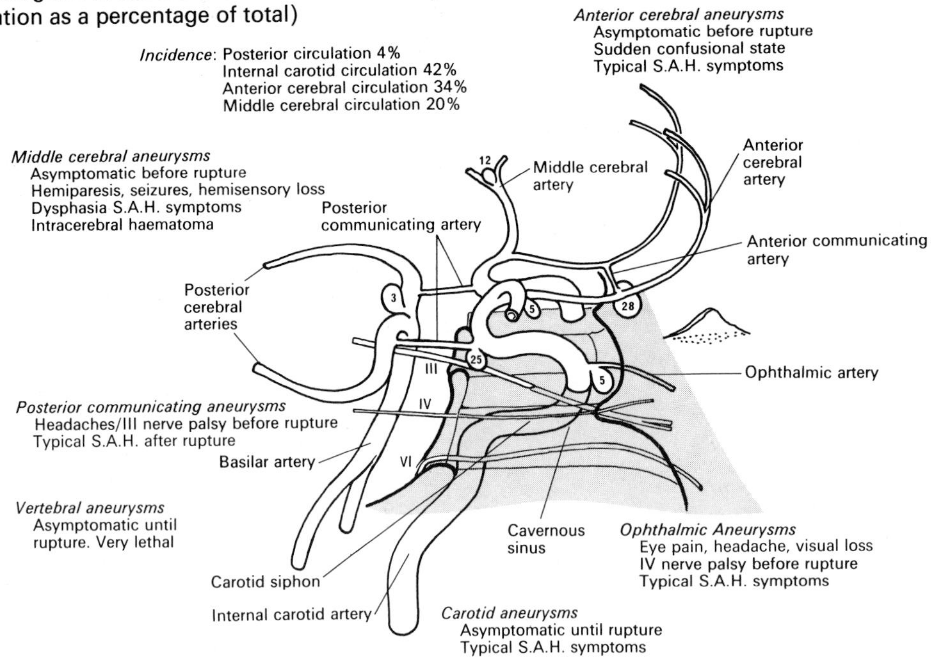

Figure 9.9. Schematic diagram to show the Usual Sites of Aneurysms (Figures on the illustration as a percentage of total)

Incidence: Posterior circulation 4%
Internal carotid circulation 42%
Anterior cerebral circulation 34%
Middle cerebral circulation 20%

Anterior cerebral aneurysms
Asymptomatic before rupture
Sudden confusional state
Typical S.A.H. symptoms

Middle cerebral aneurysms
Asymptomatic before rupture
Hemiparesis, seizures, hemisensory loss
Dysphasia S.A.H. symptoms
Intracerebral haematoma

Posterior communicating aneurysms
Headaches/III nerve palsy before rupture
Typical S.A.H. after rupture

Vertebral aneurysms
Asymptomatic until rupture. Very lethal

Ophthalmic Aneurysms
Eye pain, headache, visual loss
IV nerve palsy before rupture
Typical S.A.H. symptoms

Carotid aneurysms
Asymptomatic until rupture
Typical S.A.H. symptoms

Middle cerebral artery
Anterior cerebral artery
Posterior communicating artery
Anterior communicating artery
Posterior cerebral arteries
Ophthalmic artery
Basilar artery
Cavernous sinus
Carotid siphon
Internal carotid artery

Aneurysm sites and associated symptoms are fully illustrated in Figure 9.9. If there are no signs except those of subarachnoid blood (headache, photophobia, neck stiffness, vomiting, bilateral extensor plantar response) no prediction as to the site of the aneurysm can be made.

The extremely controversial subject of the correct management of subarachnoid haemorrhage is beyond the scope of the present book. Referral to a neurological centre is indicated in all cases and if focal hemisphere signs are present confirmatory lumbar puncture is best deferred. These signs may indicate an intracerebral clot and lumbar puncture may confirm the diagnosis but kill the patient.

4. *Haemorrhage into Tumours*

When a patient with a cerebral tumour develops symptoms very rapidly it is often assumed that there has been a haemorrhage into the tumour. This is a very rare event—the sudden symptoms are usually produced by necrosis and oedema in the tumour as it outgrows its blood supply. The *only* tumour that characteristically bleeds is a metastatic deposit from a malignant melanoma. Many patients with cerebral metastases from malignant melanomas present with what at first sight is a simple sub-arachnoid haemorrhage.

CASE REPORT

A 36-year-old man collapsed while cycling uphill into a head wind. He was found semi-conscious and hemiplegic. On admission he had a stiff neck and a dense left hemiplegia with sensory loss. C.S.F. examination revealed heavily blood stained fluid. Twelve years previously he had had a malignant melanoma resected from his leg. Angiography revealed an avascular mass in the right parietal lobe. Craniotomy revealed a haematoma and the remains of a melanotic deposit into which the haemorrhage had occurred.

THE INVESTIGATION AND MANAGEMENT OF SUSPECTED CEREBRAL VASCULAR DISEASE

The three considerations that should be applied to this clinical situation are:

a. Is the site and extent of the lesion typical of occlusion of an identifiable vessel?

b. Is there any underlying haematological or biochemical disorder that could have predisposed to or mimicked a C.V.A.?

c. Are there any causative factors such as hypertension, auricular fibrillation, vessel stenosis or myocardial infarction that can be identified and treated?

a. This entire chapter has been devoted to the recognition of symptoms and signs that are typical of vascular accident. Anything that casts doubt on this diagnosis should prompt immediate further investigation.

b. Underlying disorders that predispose to cerebral vascular accidents include anaemia, polycythaemia, diabetes mellitus, malignant or severe hypertension, inflammatory vascular disease and in the elderly temporal arteritis. Heavy protein diseases such as myelomatosis should also be excluded.

Careful exclusion of cardiac arrhythmia, cardiac murmurs and subacute bacterial endocarditis by clinical examination, ECG and blood cultures should always be performed. Thyrotoxicosis should be excluded if the patient has auricular fibrillation as in the elderly the clinical evidence of this disorder may be minimal or absent.

Two special conditions related to diabetes mellitus are of great importance. Hypoglycaemia may cause focal signs such as a hemiparesis persisting for twenty-four hours or more with recovery. This possibility should always be considered with an intermittent clinical picture, and it is important to realise that the patient may remain fully conscious throughout the episode. It may occur in patients on oral antidiabetic drugs or insulin and rarely as a presenting symptom of primary hypoglycaemia. The second condition is hyperosmolar non-ketotic coma. The exact relationship of this condition to diabetes is uncertain. The biochemical syndrome consists of marked hyperglycaemia (often a glucose level over 1000 mgms. per cent) with marked dehydration and gross increase in serum osmolarity. Many patients with this condition develop focal neurological signs before becoming comatose. The condition is fatal unless recognised. An important clue is marked dehydration in a patient who has only been ill for a few hours. There is no ketosis which is the main distinguishing feature from diabetic coma.

c. Once it has been established that the patient has had a simple cerebral vascular accident without evidence of underlying disease the difficult problem of further management arises. Management depends on the clinical situation:

1. *The Patient who has a Completed Infarct*

Angiography is unnecessary as the surgical restoration of circulation to the damaged hemisphere usually causes haemorrhage into the infarct. This also may occur if anti-coagulants are used. Investigation is only indicated if other possibilities such as a subdural haematoma or tumour are suspected.

2. *The Patient who has Made a Complete Recovery*

This situation constitutes a "transient ischaemic attack". Definitions of "transient" vary from full recovery in one hour to twenty-four hours, but in general it is accepted that there should be no residual physical signs.

a. Any source of emboli should be excluded as discussed above. It should be remembered that in some series as many as thirty per cent of emboli originated in the heart, often in an area of myocardial infarction. Anti-coagulants are indicated unless there are any specific contra-indications and most physicians are reluctant to anti-coagulate patients over 65 years of age. Within the last two years soluble aspirin 300 mgms. twice daily has been used as an alternative to anti-coagulants. This form of treatment can be safely used in the over 65 age group and is thought to act by reducing platelet stickiness.

b. If the blood pressure is elevated anti-coagulants are contra-indicated and there is evidence that lowering the blood pressure often prevents further attacks. Hypotensive therapy should be pursued aggressively in this situation *whatever* the patient's age. There is no evidence to support a widely held belief that lowering the blood pressure is harmful to these patients. They may well develop symptoms of postural hypotension but this does *not* cause further cerebral vascular accidents.

c. If no source of emboli is found and the patient is normotensive the question of carotid angiography must be considered. Enthusiasm for this procedure is greatly increased if the patient has a bruit over one or other carotid artery. The problem with a bruit is that sometimes it *does* indicate local narrowing of the vessel, sometimes *no* cause is found and sometimes it is due to increased blood flow in the *normal* vessel because the other carotid artery is completely occluded. Angiography therefore carries considerable risks; it may complete a partial occlusion, particularly if the needle is pushed through the narrow area, or cause further cerebral ischaemia if the vessel injected proves to be the *normal* vessel. There are many and varied statistics as to the mortality and morbidity of angiography in this group of patients and even in centres where aggressive angiography is undertaken surprisingly few patients are found who have surgically amenable lesions.

3. *The patient Who is Having a Series of Attacks with Increasing Disability*

This situation is sometimes referred to as a "stuttering hemiparesis" or a "stroke in evolution". In this group of patients a progressive thrombosis of the carotid artery is usually responsible and the risk of *completing* the thrombosis during angiography is high. In the writer's view immediate anti-coagulation by heparinisation is the correct management and even this is often unsuccessful in preventing completion of the stoke.

In the author's view each patient with cerebral vascular disease presents an entirely different set of problems and the statistics of cerebral vascular disease become meaningless when faced with an individual patient. There is no convincing evidence of the advantages of neck vessel surgery and therefore the not inconsiderable risks of angiography in these patients should be seriously questioned. It is small consolation to the patient whose condition deteriorates as a result of investigation to be reassured that no definite abnormality was found. A decade of intensive investigation by retrospective and prospective studies of cerebral vascular disease has done little to advance the actual management of this common and potentially lethal problem. The patient's best chance lies in the discovery of an underlying condition that *is* amenable to specific treatment.

Chapter 10

THE CEREBRAL HEMISPHERES: 3. DISORDERS AFFECTING THE LIMBIC SYSTEM AND HYPOTHALAMUS

There is a borderland area between psychiatry and neurology concerned with acute and chronic disorders of personality and intellect. Patients in these categories present considerable diagnostic problems as in many instances the patient is unable to give a coherent account of his illness. A third party history from friends, relatives and workmates is vital if an accurate account of the course of the illness is to be obtained. It often transpires that an apparently acute illness has been preceded by several weeks' history of altered personality, headaches, speech disorder and loss of motor skills which provide important clues to the presence and site of an underlying lesion. A history of drug or alcohol abuse, previous malignant disease or recent head injury may completely alter the approach to the investigation and management of a patient with altered personality or intellect.

There are four major types of disorder in which particular care must be exercised. In general if the incoherent, confused, aggressive or hallucinating patient is regarded as a diagnostic challenge rather than as a disposal problem errors will be avoided. It is essential that a complete neurological examination and any necessary investigations are performed before the patient is transferred to a mental hospital for custodial care.

1. *Toxic Confusional States*

Toxic confusional states may be due to drug overdose or idiosyncratic reactions to drugs such as anti-parkinsonian agents. Pneumonia may cause a similar picture due to hypoxia, fever or general toxicity. In the elderly an afebrile course is possible and the physical signs of pneumonia are easily missed. Congestive cardiac failure, uraemia, liver failure, meningitis, subarachnoid haemorrhage, or hypoglycaemia may all cause a toxic confusional state. Patients with a history of alcoholism may develop a toxic confusional state with seizures when alcohol is withdrawn, the condition known as delirium tremens. This may happen when the patient is hospitalised for another condition. It is also very important to remember that alcoholics do develop other forms of cerebral pathology and are particularly likely to sustain subdural haematomas from trauma occurring during the drunken state. The author has seen two patients with subdural haematomas and one with a temporal lobe glioma who had been diagnosed as suffering from delirium tremens because of a history of alcoholism. Patients tend to be referred to psychiatrists if hallucinations or paranoid delusions dominate the clinical picture or to a neurologist if the patient becomes stuporose or develops any sort of epileptic disturbance.

2. *Dysphasic Confusion*

Patients who have disease in the dominant parietal lobe present an extremely difficult group of disorders, in which the communication problem is due to receptive or expressive dysphasia or combinations of these problems and where there is a danger that the patient will be classified as "confused" or "demented". A patient recently seen in a mental hospital was unable to carry on a sensible conversation due to the total absence of nouns from her sentences. Formal assessment of speech function revealed a pure and almost complete nominal aphasia.

Tragically, the recognition of dysphasia not only reveals the presence of a focal lesion but often indicates a poor prognosis, as extensive surgical procedures in the dominant parietal lobe are technically impossible. However, this should not preclude full investigation as occasionally a subdural haematoma or a small lesion with massive oedema which maybe amenable to a surgical attack with minimal residual deficit of speech function is found.

3. *Temporal Lobe Automatism*

Prolonged disturbances of temporal lobe function occur in epilepsy (psychomotor attacks) or temporal lobe ischaemia (transient global amnesia, migraine). In both conditions bizarre and totally uncharacteristic behaviour may result; for example patients may undress in public or shout obscenities. The condition known as acute auditory hallucinosis, which complicates alcoholism, is possibly due to a metabolic disturbance in the temporal lobe. In this state non-stop auditory hallucinations are often coupled with paranoid behaviour which may persist for several days in the presence of an otherwise intact sensorium.

Many patients with migraine can recognise an impending attack by a change in behaviour or mood in the hours before the headache develops. This is presumably due to impaired perfusion in the territory of one or both posterior cerebral arteries. An extreme example of this type of transient temporal lobe dysfunction in migraine occurred in a patient recently under the author's care and is worth quoting in detail.

CASE REPORT

A 46-year-old carpenter of previously exemplary character went swimming with his daughter early one Sunday morning. On his return he completed his income tax forms and started to mow his lawn. Shortly afterwards he went indoors and told his wife his vision was "funny" and he thought he was developing a headache. He went to lie down and a few minutes later when his wife took him a cup of tea he complained that he could not see or hear. He then became drowsy and if disturbed became extremely violent. He remained in this state for forty-eight hours. C.S.F. examination to exclude a subarachnoid haemorrhage and blood sugar determination to exclude hypoglycaemia were both normal. At this stage it was discovered that both his father and brother suffered from severe migraine. A tentative diagnosis of a somnolent state with a rage reaction due to medial temporal lobe ischaemia was made. On the third day the patient sat up in bed very bewildered and completely normal mentally. He had no recollection of events after his wife came into the room. He was able to relate that the visual upset was loss of the right visual field and that this had happened on previous occasions and had been followed by a headache. There seems little doubt that these were isolated migraine headaches. Several EEGs taken during the period of confusion were within normal limits.

This case indicates the extremely narrow area between "normal" and abnormal behaviour, not dependent on a gross disturbance of cerebral function but due to quite limited areas of dysfunction, usually in the region known as the limbic system, or its cortical connections.

4. *Dementia*

Dementia is a problem common to neurology and psychiatry and is usually divided into pre-senile dementia (onset before age of 65) and senile dementia. This classification places undue emphasis on the pre-senile group, because at any age dementia is a devastating problem both for the patient and even more so for the distraught relatives. At *any* age *full* investigation to exclude any treatable cause is vital. This is so important that a later section of this chapter is devoted to the causes and investigation of dementia.

The patient is to some extent protected from the full impact of his illness by loss of insight into his condition. There are many diagnostic and management problems in dementia, two of which are worth mentioning at this stage. A previously intelligent patient may react to the onset of dementia by developing obsessional behaviour patterns to avoid embarrassment or by becoming severely depressed. In either case it is easy to overlook the underlying intellectual decline. In the later stages of dementia patients may react with paranoid suspicion, often directed at the closest relatives whose concern is regarded with suspicion by the patient who may alter his will in others' favour. Testamentary capacity in these patients is a difficult medico-legal problem as favoured relatives often become involved in the patient's delusional system.

Although dementia often indicates diffuse loss of cerebral substance occasionally exactly the same situation is produced by quite local lesions particularly in the parasagittal or subfrontal regions. Typical case histories have been quoted in Chapter 8. Symptomatic dementia of this type is often due to interference with the activity of the cingulum or the orbital surface of the frontal lobe, both areas with important connections to the limbic system.

To understand the wide range of clinical features and disturbances of mood and affect that occur in diseases affecting these regions a broad grasp of the anatomy of the interconnections of the cerebral cortex and the limbic system and hypothalamus is necessary.

THE LIMBIC SYSTEM (Figure 10.1)

There are several definitions of the limbic lobe depending on whether anatomical or physiological considerations are paramount. Most current definitions exclude much of the olfactory apparatus and its central connections. The older terms, rhinencephalon, fornicate lobe or "smell" brain are not therefore synonymous with what is known clinically as the "limbic" system.

The limbic system includes the hippocampus and hippocampal gyrus, the uncus, amygdala, cingulate gyrus, part of the insula, the septal area, the isthmus, Broca's olfactory area and the orbital surface of the frontal pole. Embryologically the inner surface of the temporal lobe rolls in on itself, forming the curved groups of cells known as Ammons Horn which lie in the floor of the lateral ventricle as the hippocampus. The hippocampal gyrus is the area overlying the hippocampus which is visible on the surface of the posterior end of the temporal lobe immediately behind the bulge overlying the amygdala. The main fibre tract from the hippocampal area is the fimbria which is joined by other fibres from adjacent areas to form a dense bundle called the fornix which sweeps posteriorly and then up and over anteriorly to distribute to all areas of the hypothalamus but particularly to the mammillary body and parts of the thalamus. Some fibres from the fimbria decussate directly to the

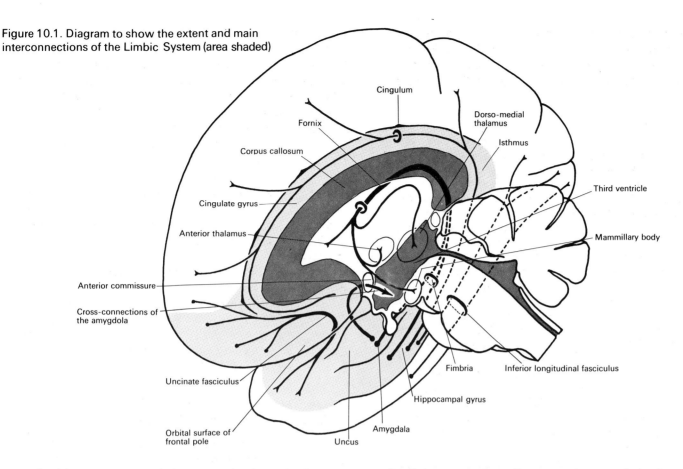

Figure 10.1. Diagram to show the extent and main interconnections of the Limbic System (area shaded)

opposite hippocampus and there are also important cross connections between the amygdala on each side through the anterior commissure.

Damage in the region of the amygdala is associated with rage reactions, hyperphagia (over-eating) and increased sexual activity. Lesions in the region of the uncus are associated with olfactory and gustatory hallucinations sometimes known as "uncinate fits". In fact seizures starting in any part of the temporal lobe have a unique opportunity to spread and involve other areas or both temporal lobes resulting in a wide range of physical and emotional phenomena that may occur during a "psychomotor seizure".

The cingulate gyrus lies above the corpus callosum, its connecting pathways traversing the isthmus posteriorly and extending as far forward as Broca's olfactory area. Operations directed at these pathways and the connections from the cingulate gyrus to the thalamus (see also Figure 10.2) form the basis of psycho-surgical procedures. These include frontal leucotomy and cingulotomy which may be performed in patients with phobic anxiety states and chronic pain syndromes; in the latter case producing blunting of the emotional response to pain although not abolishing the pain

itself. In recent years direct attacks on pain pathways have become more popular than psychosurgical procedures in the treatment of patients with intractable pain.

THE HYPOTHALAMUS (Figure 10.2)

Although the hypothalamus is *not* included in the limbic system from a functional point of view its exclusion is hard to understand as much of the expression of activity in the limbic system occurs via its important connections with the hypothalamus. The main afferent connections of the hypothalamus are derived from the fornix which is distributed to all the hypothalamic nuclei and terminates in the mamillary body. Olfactory information reaches the hypothalamus via the medial forebrain bundle which also receives information from other areas of the limbic system and forms the main longitudinal tract between the various hypothalamic nuclei as it lies along the lateral border of the hypothalamic area. Cortical activity reaches the hypothalamus directly and via the thalamus. From below, the hypothalamus receives visceral and gustatory sensation via both the dorsal longitudinal fasciculus and the reticular formation. Much of this

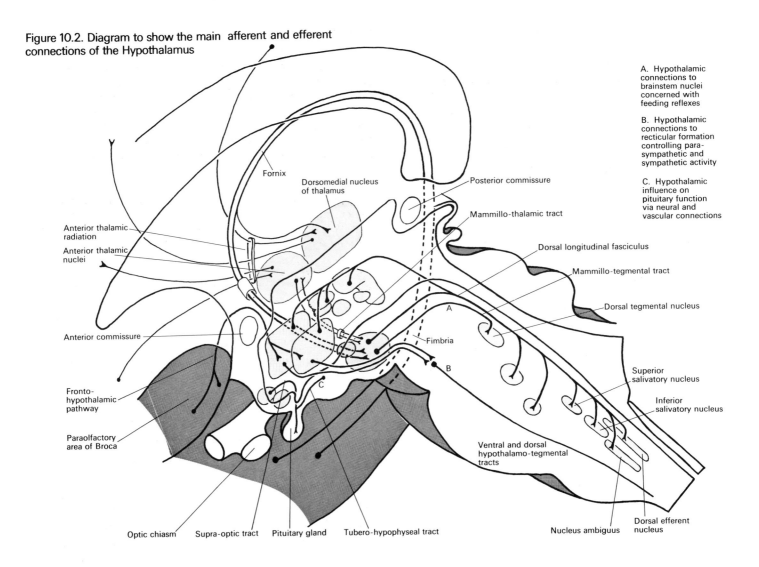

Figure 10.2. Diagram to show the main afferent and efferent connections of the Hypothalamus

A. Hypothalamic connections to brainstem nuclei concerned with feeding reflexes

B. Hypothalamic connections to recticular formation controlling para-sympathetic and sympathetic activity

C. Hypothalamic influence on pituitary function via neural and vascular connections

Fornix

Dorsomedial nucleus of thalamus

Posterior commissure

Mammillo-thalamic tract

Anterior thalamic radiation

Anterior thalamic nuclei

Dorsal longitudinal fasciculus

Mammillo-tegmental tract

Dorsal tegmental nucleus

Anterior commissure

Fimbria

A

B

Superior salivatory nucleus

Inferior salivatory nucleus

Fronto-hypothalamic pathway

C

Paraolfactory area of Broca

Ventral and dorsal hypothalamo-tegmental tracts

Dorsal efferent nucleus

Optic chiasm   Supra-optic tract   Pituitary gland   Tubero-hypophyseal tract

Nucleus ambiguus

visceral sensation is relayed to the cortex via the mammillo-thalamic tract and thalamus.

The efferent connections of the hypothalamus include ascending projections into the limbic system, the cortex, and thalamus and descending projections to the tegmentum, the reticular formation and the cranial nerve nuclei over the pathways already described (note: in the illustration the medial forebrain bundle and both afferent and efferent components of the main tracts are not shown to avoid over complicating the diagram).

Hypothalamic activity is mediated in three ways:

1. by control of the activity of sympathetic and para-sympathetic nervous system including the adrenal medulla.

2. extensive projections into the reticular formation.

3. through control of pituitary function by both direct neural connections (the supra-optico hypophyseal and tubero-hypophyseal tracts) and via the portal vascular system which carries the various releasing factors to the gland which liberate trophic hormones.

Functional Grouping of Hypothalamic Nuclei
(Figure 10.3)

A detailed knowledge of the names and positions of the various hypothalamic nuclei is not essential for clinical purposes, but there are some rough generalisations that can be made as to the functional grouping of the nuclei.

The anterior nuclei including the supraoptic and para-ventricular nuclei are particularly concerned with fluid balance via ADH (anti-diuretic hormone) secretion and control of the thirst mechanism. The central nuclei are concerned with body temperature regulation by control over skin blood vessels and sweating mechanisms. Damage to these areas may cause diabetes insipidus, complete adipsia, hyperpyrexia, pulmonary oedema or acute gastric erosions. This part of the hypothalamus is particularly likely to be damaged by pituitary tumours, craniopharyngiomas, head injuries and intracranial surgery directed at tumours in this region.

Figure 10.3. Clinical Effects of Hypothalamic Lesions

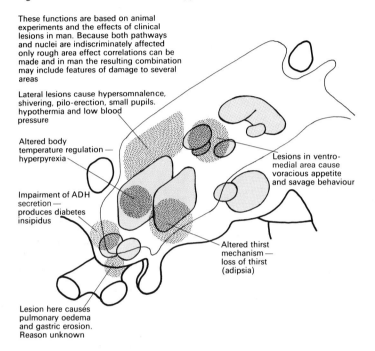

These functions are based on animal experiments and the effects of clinical lesions in man. Because both pathways and nuclei are indiscriminately affected only rough area effect correlations can be made and in man the resulting combination may include features of damage to several areas

Lateral lesions cause hypersomnalence, shivering, pilo-erection, small pupils. hypothermia and low blood pressure

Altered body temperature regulation — hyperpyrexia

Impairment of ADH secretion — produces diabetes insipidus

Lesion here causes pulmonary oedema and gastric erosion. Reason unknown

Lesions in ventro-medial area cause voracious appetite and savage behaviour

Altered thirst mechanism — loss of thirst (adipsia)

The posterior hypothalamus contains the dorsal nuclei, the posterior hypothalamic nucleus, and the supramammillary and mammillary nuclei and is mainly concerned with appetite, satiety, feeding reflexes, peristalsis and the control of the various secretions associated with eating and digestion. Lesions in this region are fortunately unusual and maybe associated with total loss of appetite leading to gross emaciation or gross overeating with obesity and altered personality often characterised by extremely bad temper and aggression.

Study of the lateral hypothalamic area is complicated by the fact that the inter-connecting pathways run through the area so that the clinical signs may indicate damage to either the nuclei or the tracts. Lesions in the lateral area are characterised by somnolence, disturbances of body temperature control and occasionally altered appetite.

The following case histories give some idea of the problems presented by hypothalamic disorders.

CASE REPORT

An 18-year-old boy became obese and somnolent and complained of visual failure. A suprasellar lesion was found which at surgery proved to be an extensive craniopharyngioma. Following surgery he was blind, and developed diabetes insipidus coupled with total loss of the thirst mechanism. Frequent episodes of drowsiness and epileptic seizures paralleled gross changes in hydration which could not be controlled by hormone replacement therapy and careful fluid balance control. He died a few weeks later.

CASE REPORT

A 32-year-old Indian lady flew to England to join her husband who had emigrated two years earlier. The husband had been informed prior to her arrival that she had been unwell with a personality disorder and had needed psychiatric treatment. He did not recognise her at the airport. Her weight had increased by 60 lb. She was apathetic and sleepy and took little interest in her surroundings. It was suspected that she had a visual disturbance of some sort. The optic discs appeared normal but formal field testing was impossible as the patient kept falling asleep. Her body temperature was low at 35°C and she woke up only long enough to eat a meal. Investigation revealed a large suprasellar mass. She died during surgical exploration. Post mortem revealed an extensive craniopharyngioma.

CLINICAL DISORDERS OF THE TEMPORAL LOBE–LIMBIC–HYPOTHALAMIC SYSTEM

Due to the anatomical extent of the limbic system and its widespread cortical connections lesions in many areas can give rise to an unusually complex range of symptoms. Due to the considerable importance of the area in special sense perception and visceral function these symptoms take unusual forms often including hallucinations. The area also has considerable importance in memory function and consciousness and several rare and unusual disorders of memory and sleep may have a basis in disordered limbic function.

1. Temporal Lobe Epilepsy

The most varied range of abnormalities undoubtedly occur in temporal lobe epilepsy and we can now consider some of these in an anatomical setting (see also Chapter 8).

1. Disturbances of hearing and balance. The cortical representation of hearing and balance are found in the upper temporal gyri just below the Sylvian fissure and discharges starting in this area typically produce auditory and vestibular symptoms.

CASE REPORT

For example, a 19-year-old shop assistant complained that for six months he had had brief attacks of a "whirring" noise in the head followed by a sensation as if he were pitching forwards which on several occasions had led to a fall. These attacks had occurred as often as six times a day and had never lasted more than thirty seconds. He had not lost consciousness. An EEG revealed seizure discharges originating in the right temporal lobe.

2. Seizures originating in the visual association areas in the parieto-temporal-occipital region may give rise to complex visual hallucinations. However *déjà-vu* phenomena, in which the patient's surroundings suddenly seem frozen and familiar, may have their origin in memory function abnormalities and are more likely to be due to hippocampal dysfunction.

3. Discharges arising in the region of the amygdala or uncus typically cause olfactory or gustatory hallucinations. These are very brief in duration and usually unpleasant in nature; often likened to "rotting cabbage" or "burning rubber". The brevity of the attack causes difficulty in identifying the odour; patients often complain that before they can take a second sniff the smell has gone. Persistent unpleasant smells are unlikely to indicate temporal lobe dysfunction. Such symptoms are often psychogenically determined or due to chronic suppurative sinus disease (sometimes known as ozena).

4. Altered awareness during the period of an attack or sometimes half-recalled events are characteristic of a temporal lobe attack and are probably related to hippocampal dysfunction, preventing complete sequential memory storage. Often bystanders cannot detect any change in the patient apart from rather deliberate movements frequently described as "zombie-like". Sometimes overtly peculiar behaviour may occur. One of the author's patients came to himself in a bus queue having completely destroyed his umbrella slowly and deliberately in front of bewildered onlookers.

5. The insula cortex deep in the Sylvian fissure is concerned with the involuntary motor activity of visceral function. Common motor accompaniments of a temporal lobe attack are lip smacking or chewing movements, which often provide an important diagnostic clue in episodes that might otherwise be mistaken for petit mal. Occasionally other visceral activity occurs and one of the author's patients frequently terminated her attacks by involuntary defecation which she was quite unable to prevent although fully conscious.

6. Another characteristic feature of temporal lobe attacks are visceral sensations. These commonly include epigastric "rising sensations", nausea, increased peristalsis and colicky pain or peculiar tingling and numbness in the perineum. These are sensations normally relayed through the reticular

formation to the thalamus and hypothalamus and ultimately discharged to the temporal and frontal cortices.

7. A few patients have been reported whose attacks include heightened sexual activity, including masturbation to orgasm. The responsible discharges seem to arise in the medial temporal lobe. A central representation for sexual function in this region may be responsible for impotence in patients with temporal lobe neoplasms.

8. It is important to remember that "temporal lobe" phenomena may occur when cortical areas with close connections to the temporal lobe are damaged. These regions particularly include the orbital surface of the frontal lobe and the parasagittal region. Occasionally tumours quite remote from the temporal lobe may cause "temporal lobe epilepsy".

2. Disorders of Memory

Memory disorders usually follow damage to the medial temporal lobe and its connections to the mammillary body and upper brain stem. It follows that symmetrical lesions are usually responsible and unilateral temporal lobe lesions or surgical extirpation of one temporal lobe should *not* affect memory. Bilateral removal of the anterior temporal lobe produces the Kluver—Bucy syndrome which is characterised by psychic blindness (inability to identify friends and relatives), pathological overeating, heightened sexual activity and altered emotional responses. Some of these features may reflect the memory loss, the continued eating and sexual activity being due to incomplete recollection of previous indulgences.

Because bilateral damage is necessary for disorders of memory metabolic or infective processes are the usual cause, i.e. anoxia, hypoglycaemia and limbic encephalitis (sometimes associated with malignant disease and sometimes due to herpes simplex encephalitis). Bilateral posterior cerebral artery occlusion (due to an embolus lodged at the bifurcation of the basilar artery or sometimes occurring during a migraine attack) may cause transient or permanent memory deficit. Severe head injuries typically cause amnesia for the events of the injury and sometimes for the period immediately preceding the injury. This may be due to acute cell trauma, bilateral temporal lobe bruising, or dysfunction secondary to anoxia due to other injuries or post-traumatic cerebral swelling.

Two particularly interesting causes of amnesia are electroconvulsive therapy and Korsakoff's psychosis. In E.C.T. electric shocks sufficient to provoke an epileptic seizure are applied to one or both frontal lobes. Surprisingly this not only produces amnesia for the E.C.T. but also causes amnesia for events prior to the E.C.T. and following a large series of treatments patients may suffer permanent memory deficits. The explanation of this is unknown. Korsakoff's psychosis occurs in alcoholics usually as a permanent sequel to an attack of Wernicke's encephalopathy. The brain stem symptoms (nystagmus, extraocular nerve palsies and dysarthria) usually respond rapidly to vitamin therapy, but a permanent memory deficit with a particular tendency to upset temporal relationships occurs. This may be the cause of confabulation which is a striking but *not* diagnostic feature of the condition. There is often defective recognition of events and defective sequencing so that the patient often inaccurately relates past events as if they had happened recently. The responsible lesion is thought to be the haemorrhage and atrophy that is found in the mammillary bodies. Significant recovery from this condition is unusual.

Memory deficit is a constant feature of dementia and this problem is discussed in detail later in this chapter.

3. Disorders Affecting Sleep and Eating Habits

There are a few rare and peculiar disorders in which sleep and sometimes appetite are affected. Many have no known pathological basis and yet the association of the clinical features strongly suggests and underlying disorder of hypothalamic/limbic dysfunction.

Various encephalitic disorders cause pathological disorders of sleep including African trypanosomiasis and particularly Von Economo's encephalitis or encephalitis lethargica. In this disorder prolonged sleeping or complete reversal of the diurnal sleep pattern are the dominating features of the acute stage. Survivors later develop parkinsonian syndromes but in acutely fatal cases the bulk of the pathological changes are found in the peri-aqueductal grey matter rather than in the basal ganglia.

A peculiar disorder that usually occurs in young males is the Klein–Levin syndrome. This may follow an infective illness and is characterised by prolonged periods of sleeping coupled with peculiar behaviour and voracious appetite during the periods in which the patient is awake. Attacks lasting days to weeks may occur over several years. At the opposite extreme is the condition known as anorexia nervosa which usually occurs in females, and although a neurotic basis is suspected the combination of altered personality, complete anorexia and amenorrhea strongly suggest a hypothalamic/limbic system disturbance.

The "Pickwickian" syndrome, named after the fat boy in Dickens's novel *The Pickwick Papers* is a combination of extreme obesity, alveolar hypoventilation, carbon dioxide retention and frequent brief attacks of sleep in a setting of continual drowsiness. The sleep component may be a combination of fatigue due to sheer bulk and metabolic factors but the whole syndrome could well start as a hypothalamic disorder. The patient quoted earlier who had a craniopharyngioma represents a minor degree of this syndrome.

Rarely cerebral tumours, particularly pinealomas and midbrain tumours, may produce pathological drowsy states in which the patient may appear to be in a coma but the eyes remain open and the patient may be able to indicate alertness by eye movement. This state is known as "akinetic mutism" and the alert but immobile condition as "coma vigil". The lesions responsible usually damage the midbrain reticular formation and include the tumours mentioned above and vascular lesions, particularly thrombosis of the upper segment of the basilar artery.

Finally we should mention narcolepsy. Although there is no known pathological basis for this disorder the combination of pathological sleepiness, hypnagogic hallucinations, paralysis and sudden collapse of posture all suggest dysfunction in the limbic-basal ganglia region. Narcolepsy should always be carefully distinguished from other causes of pathological drowsiness and full details of the condition are given in Chapter 22.

4. Dementia

In previous chapters we have referred to dementia as a presenting symptom. It is always essential to regard dementia as a symptom and not as a diagnosis. The only exception is in the very elderly in whom dementia is usually due to senile changes in the brain. Dementia should always be regarded as a symptom requiring urgent and complete investigation.

Dementia may be simply defined as failing intellectual function. There are three major components and various admixtures of the three may cause very variable clinical syndromes.

a. *Cognitive Dysfunction*

This includes memory deficit, failing judgement, difficulty in abstract thought and rumination on the past, progressing to total confusion for time and place and failure to identify even close relatives. In the very early stages perseveration of thoughts, losing the thread of conversations and even frank confabulation may occur, the latter not being a specific problem of alcoholism but occurring in any disorder in which memory is impaired.

b. *Disorders of Mood and Affect*

The patients' response to developing dementia varies widely. Some patients become extremely anxious and seek reassurance. Others react in a short-tempered way with relatives who cannot keep up with their disordered thought processes. Patients of an obsessional nature may try to cope by keeping minute-by-minute diaries and check lists and may successfully conceal failing intellect for months or years by this device. Some patients become extremely depressed to the extent that the underlying dementia may be mistaken for gross psychomotor retardation. Visual hallucinations may be a problem particularly when the situation is complicated by the use of drugs such as barbiturates, anti-parkinsonian agents, alcohol or during a fever. One severely demented patient who also took alcohol to excess had frequently attacked his wife during the night while suffering from hallucinations in which he thought he was being attacked by "savage swans".

c. Disorders of Behaviour

Disinhibition is a feature of confusional states due to organic disease, alcohol or drug abuse. Any change in a patient's behaviour such as a previously sober man taking to alcohol or minor criminal acts such as indecent exposure should arouse the suspicion of early dementia. Clergymen may become profane and previously mild-mannered men may become subject to temper outbursts. All these features can occur in psychiatric disease but may also indicate the onset of dementia. Even though the disease is now relatively rare, neuro-syphilis should be excluded in any patient in whom personality change is the main feature. At any age hypoglycaemia should also be considered particularly if the abnormal behaviour occurs in attacks, although an epileptic attack arising in the temporal lobe remains the main diagnostic consideration in this group.

The Investigation of Dementia

The importance of detecting historical and physical evidence of a focal cerebral lesion has been repeatedly stressed. The fact that tumours which typically cause dementia may *not* produce any physical signs should not be forgotten.

In addition to cerebral tumours other causes of dementia include drugs, chemicals (particularly bromides) and alcohol. A complete history of drug use is essential including innocuous "over the counter remedies" that may contain bromides. Remember that alcohol intake may be denied or grossly underestimated by the patient *and* his relatives. Specific infections, diseases such as neuro-syphilis, tuberculous meningitis or fungal meningitis should be considered, particularly in patients with an acute onset. Similarly, metabolic disorders such as renal or hepatic failure, hypercalcaemia, hypoglycaemia and the hyperosmolar non-ketotic coma typically cause confusional states of acute onset in a previously normal patient.

Patients may become demented following head injuries,

repeated subarachnoid haemorrhage, meningitis or recurrent epilepsy. In some cases the dementia may be due to communicating hydrocephalus secondary to the blockage of the subarachnoid C.S.F. pathways and a shunt procedure may be of benefit. Closely related to these disorders is the condition known as normal pressure hydrocephalus; in which the ventricles become enormously enlarged and compress the thinned cortex against the inner table of the skull, so that at pneumoencephalography the air goes into the ventricles and none passes over the surface of the brain. It is very doubtful that this is as specific a pathological entity as was originally suggested.

Specific degenerative diseases which include dementia as part of the syndrome include the following:

a. Huntington's chorea; (dementia coupled with choreiform movement disorders) (see Chapter 12).
b. Jakob–Creutzeld disease; (dementia coupled with parkinsonism and motor neurone disease). This disease has been transmitted to monkeys and is thought to be due to a slow virus infection. The disease is fatal over a period of months to two years.
c. Steele–Richardson–Olzewski syndrome (dementia associated with specific impairment of conjugate eye movements and pseudo-bulbar palsy).

The majority of patients with dementia fall into a non-specific group in which no cause can be established. Post mortem examination may reveal diffuse changes in cerebral neurones and the condition is then called Alzheimer's disease. A more restricted form of degeneration affecting the frontal lobes particularly severely is known as Pick's disease. This is inherited in a dominant way and is the most important of the pre-senile dementias as it may be identifiable by air studies and genetic counselling may be helpful once the diagnosis has been established in a family.

Dementia may occur in the terminal stages of parkinsonism and motor neurone disease. Some patients with extensive multiple sclerosis, particularly those with lesions affecting frontal lobe connections become demented. In fact the majority of patients with multiple sclerosis who are described as "euphoric" are demented and have lost the sense of appreciation of their predicament.

In all demented patients the most important test is formal psychometry to confirm dementia. The typical findings are a fall in the performance I.Q. to 100 or less and a disparity between this and the pre-morbid (verbal I.Q.) which may be 120 or higher. Sometimes in severe dementia the pre-morbid I.Q. can only be judged from the patient's educational, job and social achievements as the patient is too demented for full testing. In some patients the performance I.Q. may be as low as 50. The other importance of psychometry is that it can identify patients who are severely retarded due to depression and the occasional case of "pseudo-dementia" due to a functional nervous disorder.

Physical examination should always include a search for signs of neuro-syphilis, alcoholism, involuntary movement disorders, parkinsonism, motor neurone disease and non-specific signs such as pout reflexes (tap the upper lip and watch the lips pout); the palmar mental reflexes (scratch the palm of the hand and observe wrinkling of the patient's chin on the same side), grasp reflexes and extensor plantar responses. A *unilateral* grasp reflex indicates a lesion affecting the opposite frontal pole.

Arteriosclerosis is often accepted as the basis of dementia and yet this diagnosis should always be subject to very careful review. Many patients with overt cerebral vascular disease do not become demented, making it difficult to accept the suggestion that a normotensive patient with *no* history of cerebral vascular episodes is demented because of arteriosclerosis. However there is one very specific syndrome that is usually acceptable on this basis and is due to small vessel disease. This consists of the combination of dementia, pseudobulbar palsy, emotional lability and the characteristic "marche au petit pas" (short shuffling steps often mistakenly diagnosed as parkinsonism). This may occur as a consequence of several unequivocal cerebral vascular attacks or come on quite acutely.

It is often said that tortuous hardened peripheral arteries or absent pedal pulses indicate cerebral arteriosclerosis but it is obviously unwise to draw any conclusions as to the state of the cerebral circulation from such findings. Many patients diagnosed as "arteriosclerotic dementia" are found to have other disorders when investigations are completed.

Special Investigations

1. Routine haematological and biochemical studies including E.S.R., urea, calcium, fasting sugar, liver function and thyroid tests (to exclude myxoedema in particular).

2. Serological tests for syphilis.

3. Serum B_{12}, folate and drug levels (including bromides and lead if indicated).

4. Routine chest x-rays and skull series (to exclude primary lung neoplasm or obtain evidence of chronically raised intracranial pressure).

5. EEG and gamma scan (to exclude any obvious focal pathology that would preclude pneumo-encephalography and indicate the need for angiographic studies).

6. Pneumo-encephalography including full examination of the CSF taken *before* the procedure (C.S.F. taken *after* the test often shows a mild pleocytosis and raised protein). This should absolutely exclude any local lesion and adequately demonstrate enlargement of the ventricles and or atrophy of the cerebral gyri.

Hopefully within the next few years these neuro-radiological procedures will be superseded by E.M.I. scanning allowing faster and safer investigation of these unfortunate patients. The necessity for careful physical examination and the exclusion of all possible metabolic and toxic causes of dementia will remain the responsibility of the neurologist. The demented patient is demanding of both time and effort but at least fifteen per cent of demented patients are found to have a remediable cause and unless all patients are carefully investigated many will be allowed to deteriorate while under medical care.

Chapter 11

THE BRAIN STEM

The anatomy of the brain stem is very complicated, but the structures that cause most of the complexity, the extrapyraminal, cerebellar and vestibular pathways, produce clinical signs of limited localising value. The functional importance of these pathways cannot be denied and they are briefly detailed in Chapter 12, but for localising brain stem lesions they are of little help.

To localise a brain stem lesion we need to establish the location in the transverse plane using evidence provided by the signs of damage to the long tracts and then determine the level of the lesion in the brain stem by the associated cranial nerve lesions. The findings are then used like a grid reference on a map. To do this effectively one has to be able to visualise the brain stem in three dimensions.

A series of diagrams that can be used to localise a lesion in two planes have been prepared for this chapter. The angle of view of the brain stem is an unusual one which allows the relative positions of all the important structures to be seen in a single view. It is suggested that the reader thoroughly familiarise himself with the basic angle of view in Figure 11.1 before attempting to read further.

THE ANATOMY OF THE BRAIN STEM

The brain stem structures are arranged in layers (Figure 11.2). There is a ventral layer containing motor pathways, an intermediate layer carrying mainly sensory pathways and a dorsal layer containing the nuclei of the cranial nerves. The extrapyramidal, cerebellar and vestibular connections run across all areas and cannot be considered in detail without confusing the basic arrangement, and as noted previously this additional knowledge does not greatly help clinical localisation.

The Motor Pathways

Corticospinal Pathways (Figure 11.4)

As the corticospinal fibres descend into the mid brain they rotate into the medial part of the cerebral peduncle; the fibres carrying information to the leg lying laterally and the fibres to the arm lying medially. At pontine levels the pathways are broken up into a series of bundles by the transverse pontine fibres which cross to the cerebellar hemispheres. In the lower third of the pons the fibres come together again as a preliminary to their decussation in the medullary pyramid.

The anatomy of the decussation is of some importance. The arm fibres lie medially and cross the midline above the leg fibres to assume the medial position in the cortico-spinal tract on the opposite side of the cord. They are then in the ideal position to supply the ventral horn cells which control the muscles of the arm which now lie on the medial aspect of the tract.

As the decussation of the leg fibres is slightly lower than that of the arm fibres it is possible for a discrete lesion to cause weakness of one arm and the *opposite* leg, a clinical condition that might easily be dismissed as hysterical unless this anatomical possibility is realised. Similarly it is possible for weakness of both arms to occur with little or no detectable weakness in the legs with the lesion shown in Figure 11.4.

The majority of the corticospinal fibres cross in the pyramid; those that do not do so decussate in the anterior commisure at cervical level. Ultimately, all pyramidal fibres reach the opposite side of the cord.

Cortico-Bulbar Pathways (Figure 11.5)

These extremely vital pathways are usually given scant attention in anatomical and neurological textbooks. A knowledge of their anatomy and function is essential to an understanding of the physical signs in patients with brain stem lesions.

The cortico-bulbar fibres pass via the genu of the internal capsule to the most medial part of the cerebral peduncle with the rotation of the motor tract. This places them in the ideal position to cross the midline to innervate the cranial nerve nuclei on the opposite side of the brain stem. (The pathways to the nuclei innervating the extra-ocular muscles have already been discussed in Chapter 7, including their important internuclear connections.)

The motor nucleus of the fifth nerve which controls the muscles of mastication derives only half of its innervation from the opposite hemisphere, which means that it is equally innervated from its own hemisphere. This 50:50 innervation ratio means that a unilateral lesion of the supranuclear pathway rarely leads to detectable deficit in these muscles. For example in a C.V.A. affecting the internal capsule, motor power of the jaw is rarely impaired.

The supranuclear innervation of the seventh nerve which

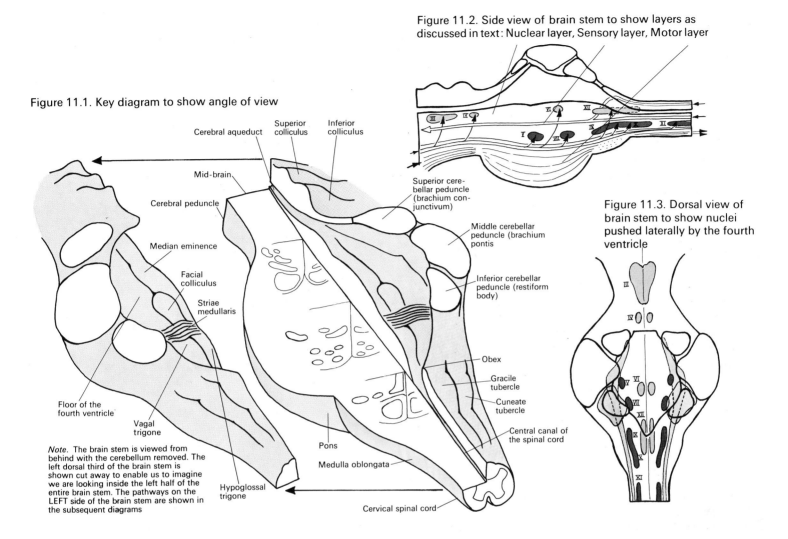

Figure 11.1. Key diagram to show angle of view

Figure 11.2. Side view of brain stem to show layers as discussed in text: Nuclear layer, Sensory layer, Motor layer

Figure 11.3. Dorsal view of brain stem to show nuclei pushed laterally by the fourth ventricle

Cerebral aqueduct
Superior colliculus
Inferior colliculus
Mid-brain
Cerebral peduncle
Median eminence
Facial colliculus
Striae medullaris
Floor of the fourth ventricle
Vagal trigone
Hypoglossal trigone
Pons
Medulla oblongata
Cervical spinal cord

Superior cerebellar peduncle (brachium conjunctivum)
Middle cerebellar peduncle (brachium pontis)
Inferior cerebellar peduncle (restiform body)
Obex
Gracile tubercle
Cuneate tubercle
Central canal of the spinal cord

Note. The brain stem is viewed from behind with the cerebellum removed. The left dorsal third of the brain stem is shown cut away to enable us to imagine we are looking inside the left half of the entire brain stem. The pathways on the LEFT side of the brain stem are shown in the subsequent diagrams

controls the muscles of the facial expression is more complicated. The supply ratio to the forehead muscles is 50:50 so that a unilateral supranuclear lesion will not affect the forehead muscles (U.M.N. lesion, see Chapter 8). The part of the nucleus supplying the lower face is strongly innervated by decussating fibres with little ipsilateral control, similar to the pyramidal fibre distribution to the limbs. Therefore a unilateral supranuclear lesion produces marked weakness of the lower face (see Figure 11.6).

The supranuclear control of the nucleus ambiguus (the motor nucleus of cranial nerves IX, X and XI) is variable. In the majority of patients with a capsular lesion there is no detectable weakness of the palate or vocal cord suggesting that a 50:50 innervation ratio is the rule. In some patients transient weakness is found suggesting that contra-lateral innervation occurs in some people. The same is true of the XII

nucleus (motor to the tongue). Usually there is no weakness of tongue movement in a typical unilateral capsular C.V.A. When there is tongue weakness it is almost invariably combined with weakness of the palate on the same side suggesting that these cranial nerves are usually innervated in a 50:50 ratio but are contralaterally innervated in a few people. This is of clinical importance for two reasons.

a. Tenth and twelfth nerve lesions on the *same* side as a hemiparesis might be thought to indicate *two* brain stem lesions affecting the cranial nerve nuclei on one side and the pyramidal pathway above the pyramidal decussation on the other. An upper motor neurone facial weakness on the *same* side as the hemiparesis should indicate that a single lesion is responsible.

b. The prognosis for the recovery of a L.M.N. cranial nerve lesion due to a brain stem C.V.A. is poor whereas if it is a

Figure 11.4. Corticospinal Pathways

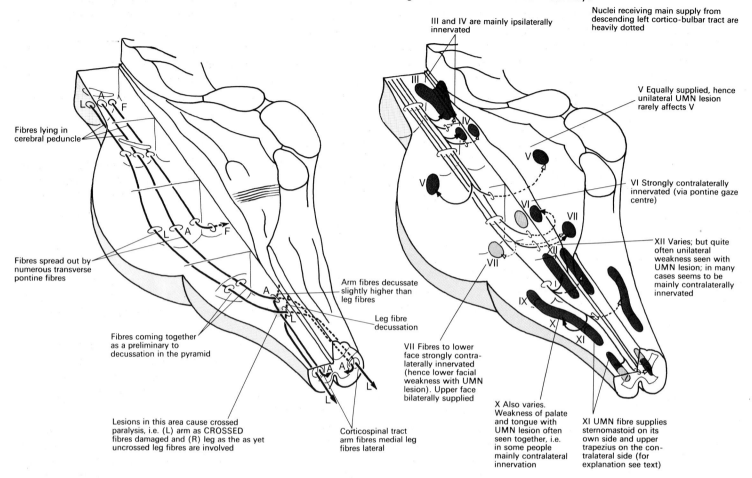

Fibres lying in cerebral peduncle

Fibres spread out by numerous transverse pontine fibres

Fibres coming together as a preliminary to decussation in the pyramid

Arm fibres decussate slightly higher than leg fibres

Leg fibre decussation

Lesions in this area cause crossed paralysis, i.e. (L) arm as CROSSED fibres damaged and (R) leg as the as yet uncrossed leg fibres are involved

Corticospinal tract arm fibres medial leg fibres lateral

Figure 11.5. Cortico-bulbar Pathways

III and IV are mainly ipsilaterally innervated

Nuclei receiving main supply from descending left cortico-bulbar tract are heavily dotted

V Equally supplied, hence unilateral UMN lesion rarely affects V

VI Strongly contralaterally innervated (via pontine gaze centre)

XII Varies; but quite often unilateral weakness seen with UMN lesion; in many cases seems to be mainly contralaterally innervated

VII Fibres to lower face strongly contra-laterally innervated (hence lower facial weakness with UMN lesion). Upper face bilaterally supplied

X Also varies. Weakness of palate and tongue with UMN lesion often seen together, i.e. in some people mainly contralateral innervation

XI UMN fibre supplies sternomastoid on its own side and upper trapezius on the con-tralateral side (for explanation see text)

Figure 11.6. Diagram to show the dual supranuclear innervation of the facial nerve nuclei

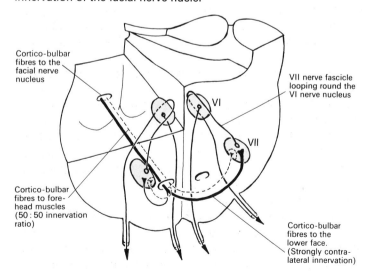

Cortico-bulbar fibres to the facial nerve nucleus

VII nerve fascicle looping round the VI nerve nucleus

Cortico-bulbar fibres to fore-head muscles (50 : 50 innervation ratio)

Cortico-bulbar fibres to the lower face. (Strongly contra-lateral innervation)

"pseudo-bulbar" cranial nerve palsy due to a lesion higher up, the signs usually recede over several days as the hemiparesis improves and as ipsilateral innervation takes over.

Thus diagnostically *and prognostically* the distinction is important.

The supranuclear control of the XI nerve nucleus (spinal part) is also unusual. The hemisphere controls the sternom-astoid muscle on the *same* side and the upper fibres of the trapezius on the *opposite* side. At first sight this might appear to be an unnecessarily complex arrangement, but the func-tional importance is obvious if one realises that the right sternomastoid turns the head to the left side. Were the left sternomastoid active simultaneously with the left limbs, the head would turn in the wrong direction! Thus in a patient with a capsular C.V.A. and a left hemiparesis the right sternomastoid will be weak. This is another finding that may lead an unwary examiner to believe that there are *two* lesions responsible for this combination of signs. Further evidence of this innervation pattern is found in patients during a focal seizure; the head and eyes look *towards* the seizuring limbs, (see also Chapter 7).

The Sensory Pathways (Figure 11.7)

Dorsal Column Sensation (Touch, two point discrimination sense and joint position sense)

Fibres from the dorsal columns of the spinal cord ascend to the gracile (leg) and cuneate (arm) nuclei in the dorsal medulla. The leg fibres lie medially in the dorsal column, but as the fibres decussate in the medulla through the internal arcuate fibres, the leg fibres come to lie laterally, to parallel the motor fibre arrangement. The new tract that is formed by the decussation (the medial lemniscus) is at first vertically disposed and then flattens and spreads laterally merging finally with the spino-thalamic tract in the midbrain, just below the thalamus.

Spino-Thalamic Sensation (Pain and temperature sensation)

Fibres conveying these sensations have already crossed in the spinal cord and ascend into the medulla lying in a lateral position with the leg fibres laterally and the arm fibres medially. The tract maintains its position in the dorsolateral brain stem until the medial meniscus merges with it in the mid-brain. Throughout its course in the brain stem it lies in close association with the descending sympathetic pathways. This leads to the almost invariable association of a Horner's syndrome on one side with pain and temperature loss on the opposite side of the body, whenever the dorsolateral brain stem is damaged.

The Trigeminal Sensory System

The very complex central pathways subserving facial sensation are discussed in detail in Chapter 15 as they are best understood when considering the anatomy of syringomyelia.

Basically, information from the right side of the face (see Figure 11.8) enters the brain stem in the fifth nerve at mid-pontine level. Fibres subserving the corneal reflex and simple tactile sensation enter the nucleus of the fifth nerve in the pons, and decussate at mid-pontine level to the opposite side of the pons. Fibres subserving pain and temperature sensation descend parallel to the descending nucleus of V and enter it to relay to the opposite side in the lower medulla and upper cervical cord. The crossed fibres then become the

secondary ascending tract of V (the quinto-thalamic tract) lying adjacent to the medial lemniscus throughout the brainstem.

A lesion in the dorsolateral medulla on the left will therefore cause numbness of the left side of the face and numbness of the right side of the body. This crossed sensory loss is typical of a dorsolateral brain stem lesion, between midpontine level and C2.

The Cranial Nerve Nuclei (Figure 11.9)

The clinical features of cranial nerve lesions have already been covered in previous chapters. The arrangement of the cranial nerve nuclei is not haphazard and an understanding of their embryological development greatly facilitates learning.

The motor nuclei are derived from two nuclear columns (see Figure 11.3).

1. The nuclei of III, IV, VI and XII are derived from a paramedian nuclear mass. III and IV retain a close relationship in the midbrain but VI is pulled down into the pons when the pontine flexure develops (see Chapter 15). The XII nerve nucleus is a long column of cells lying ventral to the central canal of the cord.
2. The IX, X and XI nerve nuclei arise from a ventro-lateral column, and are splayed laterally by the development of the fourth ventricle.

The positions of the nuclei greatly influence the course of the cranial nerves in the brain stem. The fascicles of the III, VI, and XII nerves must traverse the entire depth of the brain stem (fascicles are those parts of the nerve that course through the substance of the brain stem) to exit just lateral to the midline on the ventral surface. The IV nerve solves the problem in a unique way by escaping from the dorsal aspect of the brain stem after decussating in the superior medullary velum and then passing forwards around the cerebral peduncles.

The V nerve passes laterally to exit from the lateral surface of the pons.

The VII nerve fasciculus follows a peculiar course at first heading towards the floor of the fourth ventricle, passing round the VI nerve nucleus and then turning back on itself to cross the entire depth of the brain stem in the opposite direction to exit from the ventral surface. This peculiar arrangement means that a brain stem lesion in this area almost invariably damages both the VIth and VIIth nerves.

Cranial nerves IX, X and XI have complicated nuclei. The main motor nucleus of all three is the nucleus ambiguus. The main parasympathetic motor nuclei (to the lacrimal and salivary glands) are the inferior salivatory nucleus to the IXth

Figure 11.7. Sensory Pathways

Fibres all come together in upper outer quadrant in mid-brain

Fibres from (R) V nerve distribution entering brain stem then descend as shown to as low as C3

Spinothalamic tract

Medial lemniscus flattens and moves laterally

2° ascending tract of V (trigeminal sensation from the opposite side)

Internal arcuate fibres —dorsal columns decussating to opposite medial lemniscus

Decussation of dorsal column pathways in gracile and cuneate nuclei

Decussation of trigeminal fibres to form 2° ascending tract of V

Spinothalamic tract (pain and temperature sensation) decussate IN the cord (leg lateral, arm medial)

Dorsal columns (joint position sense, accurate light touch) (leg —medial, arm —lateral)

Figure 11.9. Cranial Nerve Nuclei

Note. The different tones on the nuclei are the same for nuclei derived from the same embryological nuclear columns i.e. (a) III IV VI & XII
(b) V VII & nucleus ambiguus
(c) Sup. Inf. salivary nuclei and dorsal efferent nucleus

Motor nucleus of V

Main sensory nucleus of V

Vestibular nucleus

Cochlear nucleus

Nucleus of the descending tract of V

Dorsal efferent nucleus (autonomic motor to viscera)

Superior and inferior salivary nuclei (to salivary glands via VII and IX)

Nucleus of tractus solitarius (taste sensation and efferent reflexes)

Nucleus ambiguus (motor to phyarnx larynx etc.)

Spinal nucleus IX continuous with nucleus ambiguus

XI (cranial)

(spinal accessory)

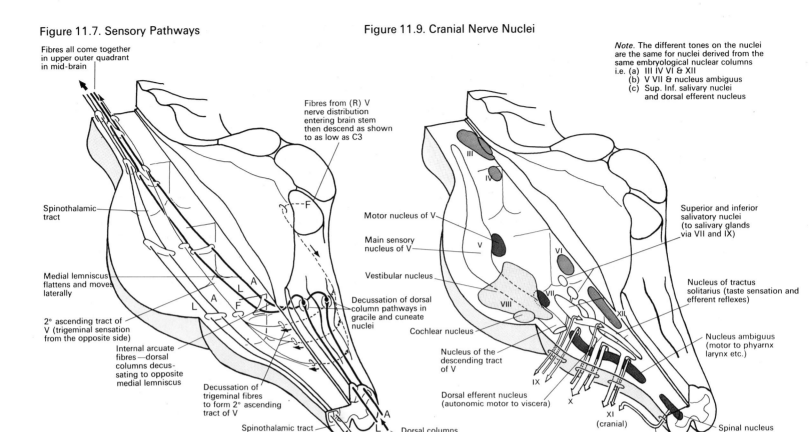

Figure 11.8. To show the Trigeminal Sensory Nucleus and the Sensory Supply of the Face

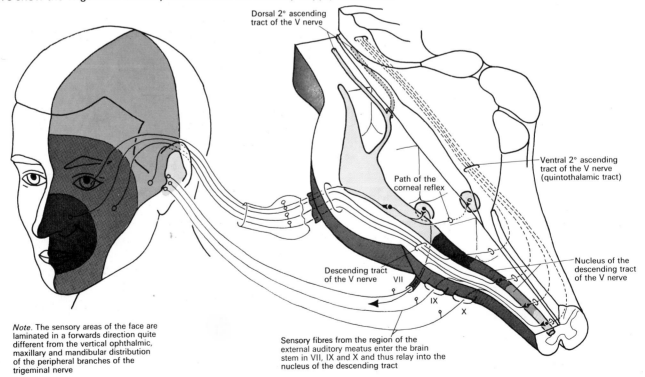

Dorsal 2° ascending tract of the V nerve

Ventral 2° ascending tract of the V nerve (quintothalamic tract)

Path of the corneal reflex

Nucleus of the descending tract of the V nerve

Descending tract of the V nerve

Note. The sensory areas of the face are laminated in a forwards direction quite different from the vertical ophthalmic, maxillary and mandibular distribution of the peripheral branches of the trigeminal nerve

Sensory fibres from the region of the external auditory meatus enter the brain stem in VII, IX and X and thus relay into the nucleus of the descending tract

nerve and its anatomical continuation, the dorsal efferent nucleus to the Xth nerve.

Gustatory reflex activity and taste sensation are relayed through the long spoon-shaped nucleus of the tractus solitarious.

The vestibular nuclei occupy almost the entire lower lateral pons with ramifications over the entire brain stem from the midbrain down to the cervical spinal cord. For this reason vestibular symptoms and signs are almost always present in brain stem disease but are of limited localising value.

The Blood Supply of the Brain Stem (Figure 11.10)

Vascular lesions have always been important causes of brain stem disease. Forty years ago syphilitic vascular disease was extremely common and numerous eponymous brain stem syndromes were described. Syphilis is now a rare cause but degenerative arterial disease has assumed increasing significance and produced a relatively new syndrome, known as "vertebral-basilar ischaemia". Therefore there is a continuing need to have a basic idea of the blood supply of the brain stem in order to understand the constellations of symptoms and signs that may result from a brain stem vascular accident.

The main blood supply is derived from the paired vertebral arteries which join at the pontomedullary junction to form the basilar artery. The blood supply of the medulla is mainly derived from the vertebral arteries. From its medial side each vertebral artery gives rise to a branch that joins with its fellow to form the anterior spinal artery. This vessel supplies part of the central medulla, and the bulk of the spinal cord down to D1. Laterally each vertebral artery gives off a variable branch, the posterior inferior cerebellar artery. This vessel is absent in twenty-five per cent of people. When the vessel is present it runs a tortuous course along the side of the medulla, which it supplies.

The other brain stem vessels follow the same pattern of distribution; these are, from below upwards, the anterior inferior cerebellar artery, the transverse pontine arteries, the

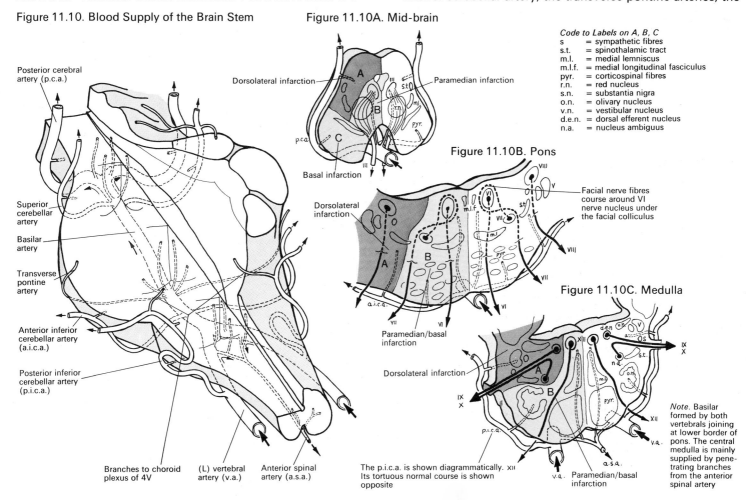

Figure 11.10. Blood Supply of the Brain Stem

Figure 11.10A. Mid-brain

Code to Labels on A, B, C
s   = sympathetic fibres
s.t. = spinothalamic tract
m.l. = medial lemniscus
m.l.f. = medial longitudinal fasciculus
pyr. = corticospinal fibres
r.n. = red nucleus
s.n. = substantia nigra
o.n. = olivary nucleus
v.n. = vestibular nucleus
d.e.n. = dorsal efferent nucleus
n.a. = nucleus ambiguus

Posterior cerebral artery (p.c.a.)

Dorsolateral infarction

Paramedian infarction

Basal infarction

Figure 11.10B. Pons

Facial nerve fibres course around VI nerve nucleus under the facial colliculus

Dorsolateral infarction

Superior cerebellar artery

Basilar artery

Transverse pontine artery

Anterior inferior cerebellar artery (a.i.c.a.)

Posterior inferior cerebellar artery (p.i.c.a.)

Paramedian/basal infarction

Figure 11.10C. Medulla

Dorsolateral infarction

Note. Basilar formed by both vertebrals joining at lower border of pons. The central medulla is mainly supplied by penetrating branches from the anterior spinal artery

Branches to choroid plexus of 4V

(L) vertebral artery (v.a.)

Anterior spinal artery (a.s.a.)

The p.i.c.a. is shown diagrammatically. Its tortuous normal course is shown opposite

Paramedian/basal infarction

superior cerebellar arteries and the posterior cerebral arteries. Each gives off a long penetrating paramedian branch that supplies the central area of the brain stem to the floor of the ventricle, and a series of short branches that supply the basal area of the brain stem, while the main trunk of the vessel passes round the brain stem to supply the dorsolateral quadrant of the brain stem and part of the cerebellum. The superior cerebellar artery supplies all the deep structures of the cerebellum including the nuclei. The anterior inferior cerebellar artery usually gives off a named branch called the internal auditory artery that supplies the inner ear and the vestibular apparatus.

Clinical Aspects of Brain Stem Disorders

Brain stem disorders unfortunately represent one aspect of neurology in which an often voiced criticism, that neurologists make the diagnosis but have no treatment to offer, has some substance. There are some relatively rare but treatable conditions. As is often the case in neurology, it is the ability to recognise unusual features or signs that do not make anatomical sense that enables such cases to be diagnosed correctly.

The differential diagnosis of brain stem disease is complicated by an unusual feature of the symptomatology. The most frequent symptoms such as diplopia, dysarthria, vertigo, nausea and vomiting are by their very nature acute symptoms. For example, a patient either has double vision or he does not; although it may vary in degree the onset must be abrupt. Unless this is recognised all lesions will appear to be due to vascular disease because of the abrupt onset of symptoms. Progression of a brain stem lesion can be established only if new acute symptoms appear or if clinical evidence of damage to previously unaffected structures is found. Occasionally, the situation is so critical that the necessary period of observation, which so often indicates the nature of the neurological disorder, may prove a harmful or even fatal course of action.

In general a vascular lesion produces a defined area of damage in an identifiable vascular territory. If the lesion appears to be patchy or to involve both sides of the brain stem a vascular lesion becomes less likely. We shall start by considering the vascular syndromes and we can then compare the clinical pictures produced by multiple sclerosis, pontine gliomas and other brain stem disorders in further discussion.

Brain Stem Vascular Syndromes

In the diagrams of the midbrain and pons three vascular territories are indicated and in the medulla only two. This is because the central area of the medulla is supplied by penetrating branches from the vertebral, basilar and anterior spinal arteries. Occlusion of any of these main vessels, with consequent occlusion of their penetrating branches may lead to extensive unilateral or even bilateral infarction of the central medulla.

Mid-Brain Vascular Lesions (Figure 11.10A)

Dorsolateral Infarction

Infarction of the dorsolateral area will cause a Horner's syndrome on the same side and *total* loss of sensation on the opposite side of the body as all the sensory pathways have come together at this level. There will also be a severe cerebellar deficit on the *same* side if the superior cerebellar peduncle is damaged.

Paramedian Infarction

A third nerve palsy will be produced by damage to the nucleus itself or the nerve fascicle. Because of the long vertical extent of the occulomotor nucleus incomplete IIIrd nerve lesions may occur. Damage to the red nucleus interrupts the dentato-rubro-thalamic tract from the opposite cerebellar hemisphere and this will cause severe cerebellar signs in the limbs *opposite* the IIIrd nerve palsy. This is referred to as Benedikt's syndrome.

Basal Infarction

The IIIrd nerve fascicle will be destroyed causing a complete IIIrd nerve palsy. The damage to the cerebral peduncle will result in hemiplegia of the opposite limbs including the face. This is called Weber's syndrome. Combinations of paramedian and basal infarctions may occur but in these cases the hemiplegia will usually mask the cerebellar signs.

Pontine Vascular Lesions (Figure 11.10B)

Dorsolateral Infarction

A Horner's syndrome on the side of the lesion will be found. This will be coupled with loss of pain and temperature sensation in the limbs on the opposite side of the body. The face will be spared and touch and proprioception will be intact as the medial leminiscus is too deeply placed at this level to be damaged. Below mid-pontine levels there is an increasing likelihood of finding loss of sensation over the face on the same side because the lesion damages the entering and descending fibres of the Vth nerve. At all levels some degree of cerebellar involvement on the same side will be found. At mid-pontine level the lateral gaze centre may be affected with loss of conjugate lateral gaze towards the side of the lesion. The VIth nerve itself will be spared. In the lower pons the vestibular and cochlear nuclei are likely to be damaged causing severe vestibular symptoms, nystagmus and deafness. This will almost invariably be combined with loss of pain and temperature sensation over the face on the side of the lesion and loss of the same modalities on the opposite side of the body.

Paramedian Infarction

Identifiable lesions occur at the level of the VIth nerve nucleus. There will be a VIth nerve palsy often combined with a conjugate gaze palsy to the same side as the connections to the opposite IIIrd nerve are also damaged. The VIIth nerve fibres will be interrupted as they sweep round the VIth nerve nucleus. If the medial lemniscus is affected there will be loss of touch and proprioception on the opposite side of the body.

Basal Infarction

The fascicles of the VIth and the VIIth nerve are likely to be damaged together with the pyramidal pathways. In an extensive lesion a full hemiplegia will result and this coupled with the VIth and VIIth nerve lesions is known as the Millard–Gubler syndrome. As the pyramidal pathways are spread out at this level an incomplete hemiplegia may occur and a VIth nerve palsy coupled with weakness of the opposite arm may be found. In most cases conjugate gaze will be intact. Therefore although the eye on the side of the lesion will be unable to abduct because of the VIth nerve palsy, the opposite eye will move normally on attempted lateral gaze towards the side of the lesion. There may be a complicated combination of facial weakness in some cases. The facial nerve on the side of the lesion may be damaged at fascicular level causing a lower motor neurone lesion on that side. In addition the upper motor neurone fibres to the opposite VIIth nerve may be affected leading to an upper motor neurone VIIth nerve lesion on the opposite side. Bilateral facial weakness of this sort can be very hard to detect and may easily be overlooked! Combinations of infarction in areas B and C may be seen. These are sometimes referred to as Raymond's syndrome and Foville's syndrome.

Medullary Vascular Lesions (Figure 11.10C)

Dorsolateral Infarction

The clinical picture resulting from damage in this area is known as Wallenberg's syndrome. Because of the variability of the blood supply it is incorrect to regard this as necessarily synonymous with posterior inferior cerebellar artery occlusion. In many cases it is an occlusion of the parent vertebral artery that is responsible. A Horner's syndrome and loss of pain and temperature sensation on the opposite side of the body will be found. The descending tract and nucleus of the Vth nerve are invariably affected with loss of pain and temperature sensation over the face on the side of the lesion. The lower vestibular nuclei are involved with severe vertigo, nausea, vomiting and nystagmus. Damage to the inferior cerebellar peduncle causes ataxia of the limbs on the side of the lesion. The IXth and Xth cranial nerves are affected and this often causes intractable hiccups and serious difficulty in swallowing. Some authorities state that VIth, VIIth and XIIth nerve lesions and hemiplegia can occur as part of the syndrome. Clearly, such a combination of signs indicates infarction of the entire half of the medulla and is inconsistent with a pure dorsolateral lesion. To use the term Wallenberg's syndrome for such a combination of signs renders the eponymous syndrome invalid as a synonym for dorsolateral medullary infarction.

Paramedial/Basal Infarction

As noted earlier, extensive unilateral or bilateral infarction of the central medullary area may occur on a vascular basis. In the upper brain stem vascular lesions tend to produce strictly unilateral lesions that do not transgress the midline; an important diagnostic point. Central lesions in the medullary area cause combinations of a XIIth nerve palsy on one side with hemiplegia and sensory loss to touch and joint position sense on the other side. A bilateral lesion renders the patient mute and quadriplegic with impaired sensation over the entire body. This has been called the "locked-in" syndrome, as the patient is quite unable to communicate although fully conscious. In addition there may be bilateral loss of sensation over the face as the decussating fibres of the trigeminal system may be damaged as they cross to their respective quintothalamic tracts.

Transient Brain Stem Ischaemic Attacks

Transient brain stem ischaemic attacks are particularly likely to affect the medulla. Vertigo, dysarthria and tingling around the mouth suggest central medullary dysfunction. At pontine levels vertigo, hearing abnormalities, tingling, numbness or weakness of the limbs and diplopia are frequent symptoms. Mesencephalic ischaemia may cause diplopia, sudden loss of consciousness, weakness of limbs and subsequently transient hemianopia if the calcarine cortex becomes ischaemic from impaired flow in either posterior cerebral artery.

CASE REPORT

A 63-year-old man visited his son in Cyprus. During a meal in a mountain-top restaurant at 6,000 feet he suddenly felt very dizzy and his speech became slurred. He thought it was the altitude and staggered outside for fresh air but found he could barely walk and his right leg was weak. He was driven down the winding mountain road with steadily increasing vertigo, slurred speech and vomiting. He made a steady recovery over the next two days and when he became mobile he noticed that he was bumping into things on his right side. When examined a week later the only residual physical sign was a right macular sparing hemianopia typical of a posterior cerebral artery occlusion.

It seems likely that this is an example of a large embolus or shower of emboli producing an on-going brain stem ischaemic episode with the final lodgement of the clot in the terminal reaches of the territory as discussed above.

Brain Stem Dysfunction Caused by Intracranial Haemorrhage

There are several ways in which intracranial haemorrhage can affect the brain stem.

An acute haemorrhage into the pons itself causes a very characteristic clinical picture. The patient becomes unconscious, and develops periodic respiration, pin-point pupils, loss of reflex eye movements and a spastic tetraplegia. Death may occur within hours, but should the patient survive for several days the body temperature steadily rises to about 106°F (42°C) before death. Haemorrhage into the cerebral hemisphere may track down the cerebral peduncle and produce a midbrain lesion. If the haematoma ruptures into the ventricular system the rapid rush of blood into the fourth ventricle may produce acute brain stem dysfunction with cardiac and respiratory arrest.

A primary haemorrhage into the cerebellum produces its lethal effect by brain stem distortion. Surgical evacuation offers a significant chance of recovery and it is vital to recognise this condition immediately. The onset is acute with occipital headache, vomiting and ataxia. Within a variable period consciousness becomes impaired with the onset of gaze palsies, bilateral pyramidal signs and periodic respiration. Death follows rapidly unless surgical evacuation of the clot is attempted.

Subarachnoid haemorrhage may produce a very similar picture. The onset is heralded by sudden headache often associated with nausea, vomiting and vertigo. These features occur so frequently that the bleeding is often mistakenly thought to come from an aneurysm in the posterior fossa. The similarity between this and the previously discussed condition should indicate that it is unwise to rush into performing a lumbar puncture in a case of suspected subarachnoid haemorrhage. An intracerebral haematoma is "space occupying" in the same way as a tumour. The risks of lumbar puncture are the same, and in the case of a cerebellar haematoma the risk is considerable. Lumbar puncture is *never* a life-saving procedure in subarachnoid haemorrhage and should not be allowed to become a life-threatening investigation. Expert neurological advice should be obtained before performing a lumbar puncture when the patient is rapidly deteriorating.

Multiple Sclerosis and the Brain Stem

Multiple sclerosis often affects the brain stem. In an established case of multiple sclerosis the diagnosis is easy. If it is the first event the diagnosis can be very difficult. Fortunately there are certain features that strongly suggest that the cause of a brain stem lesion is multiple sclerosis. The medial longitudinal bundle is extremely vulnerable and any form of internuclear ophthalmoplegia is very likely to be caused by demyelination in the brain stem. Isolated VIth nerve palsies are another common manifestation. Bilateral vestibular pathway damage with rotatory nystagmus on lateral gaze and vertical nystagmus on upward gaze is unlikely to be cause by any other disorder. The subsequent spontaneous recovery of any of these findings makes the diagnosis almost certain. The hallmark of brain stem multiple sclerosis is probably the combination of bilateral cerebellar and pyramidal signs. The patient may only complain of ataxia and slurring of speech, but examination often reveals that in addition to the anticipated cerebellar signs there are bilateral pyramidal signs. These include a brisk jaw jerk, pathologically brisk reflexes and bilateral extensor plantar responses. Although these signs strongly suggest the diagnosis of multiple sclerosis, it is always worth remembering that nothing can be regarded as absolutely pathognomonic of this condition.

Pontine Glioma

If a young child or a patient with neurofibromatosis develops brain stem signs the possibility of a brain stem glioma should be considered. In other situations or age groups this diagnosis is extremely difficult to make and multiple sclerosis is usually suspected. Any delay in diagnosis is potentially serious as many pontine gliomas are radiosensitive and early diagnosis and treatment may offer some hope of a prolonged remission. Many of these tumours start in the region of the VIth nerve nucleus and any combination of a VIth and VIIth nerve palsy should be regarded with suspicion. Minimal motor signs, brisk reflexes and extensor plantar responses are often present but hemiplegia is not an early symptom. The sensory pathways seem to be extremely resistant to infiltration by these tumours and patients often die of the disease without detectable sensory loss. Careful documentation of the signs and the recognition of new lesions in the brainstem should indicate the correct diagnosis if there is initial uncertainty. In spite of gross enlargement of the pons, blockage of the aqueduct is unusual and therefore headache is not a constant feature of the clinical picture.

Other Posterior Fossa Tumours

Cerebellar tumours in childhood produce rapidly progressive cerebellar signs and raised intracranial pressure. Medulloblastomas may infiltrate the brain stem via the cerebellar peduncles. Ependymomas arising in the floor of the fourth ventricle produce unheralded vomiting and the presence of papilloedema usually excludes the diagnosis of a primary pontine tumour. Cystic astrocytomas do not invade the brain stem but may threaten the viability of the brain stem by mechanical distortion if the diagnosis is long delayed. Posterior fossa tumours other than metastases are relatively rare in adulthood. They also tend to be slow-growing producing a much less florid clinical picture than in childhood and differential diagnosis may be extremely difficult. Pineal tumours produce raised intracranial pressure and evidence of upper midbrain compression such as Parinaud's syndrome. Acoustic nerve tumours usually produce signs of a cerebellopontine angle lesion. Rarely the signs of brain stem distortion dominate the clinical picture (see Chapter 6) Chordomas, cholesteatomas and meningiomas may arise in front of the brainstem. All may produce intermittent brainstem symptoms mimicking multiple sclerosis or transient ischaemic attacks. Transient VIth nerve palsies, ataxia and pyramidal signs may be found. Even vertical nystagmus, often held to be diagnostic of an intrinsic brain stem lesion, can occur with extrinsic compression of the brain stem. Tumours in the region of the foramen magnum, usually meningiomas or neurofibromas, are notorious for producing recurrent episodes of tetraparesis and ultimately tetraplegia. A careful myelographic search in the region of the foramen magnum should always be made before ascribing such symptoms to multiple sclerosis.

Metabolic Brain Stem Dysfunction

The toxic effects of alcohol and many drugs are caused by reversible metabolic effects on the brain stem. Severe vertigo ataxia, dysarthria, and nystagmus are common side-effects of anticonvulsant drugs. Diphenylhydantoin (Epanutin) (Dilantin U.S.P.) may even cause a reversible internuclear ophthalmoplegia. The diagnosis of deliberate or accidental overdose of Epanutin should be suspected in any patient having repeated attacks of drowsiness, ataxia, dysarthria and nystagmus. An overdose of glutethimide causes drowsiness, widely dilated pupils and brisk reflexes stimulating a brain stem lesion. Extensor plantars may occur transiently during

drug overdosage and deflect attention from the desirability of obtaining blood samples for drug levels in *any* drowsy or unconscious patient.

Wernicke's encephalopathy is a serious complication of alcoholism. In addition to the characteristic mental change of gross confusion with memory loss there is a potentially fatal disturbance of brain stem function. Extra-ocular nerve palsies, usually VIth nerve palsies, conjugate gaze palsies, nystagmus and ataxia are the main features. These signs are readily reversible following parenteral therapy with Vitamin B_1. It should be remembered that this condition can also occur in patients who are malnourished for medical reasons such as malabsorption or following postoperative vomiting.

Central pontine myelinolysis is a rare lethal condition closely related to Wernicke's encephalopathy, occurring in the same clinical setting and with the same signs. The diagnosis is usually made at post mortem when the patient has failed to respond to Vitamin B_1 therapy.

Brain stem angiomas and brain stem encephalitis are exceptionally rare and usually gain more prominence in differential diagnostic discussions than they deserve. In the majority of cases where either diagnosis is entertained the patient is eventually found to have another condition. Encephalitis of the brain stem caused by herpes simplex virus has recently been reported and a rhomboencephalitis associated with Listeria monocytogenes meningitis also occurs.

Congenital anomalies of the foramen magnum may lead to the development of brain stem problems in later life. The syndrome of vertebrobasilar ischaemia may be caused by an anomalous odontoid peg or basilar invagination and syringomyelia and syringobulbia are probably related to congenital abnormalities of the foramen magnum. These conditions are fully discussed in Chapter 15.

Brain stem lesions occur quite frequently and may represent an immediate threat to the patient's life or a delayed threat from complications such as aspiration pneumonia. Prompt accurate diagnosis is essential and this can best be achieved with a sound anatomical knowledge and an idea of the common causes of brain stem disease and their clinical behaviour.

The investigation of a lesion distorting the brain stem is difficult. Vertebral angiography is assuming increasing importance both in diagnosis and pre-operative assessment of the vascular supply of extrinsic tumours such as acoustic neuromas. Pneumo-encephalography causes little risk if the lesion *is* in the brain stem itself and often reveals characteristic displacement of the aqueduct and fourth ventricle. If it transpires that the lesion is in the cerebellum the risk of this procedure is so great that it is absolutely contra-indicated. In such cases ventriculography, in which the air or contrast medium is introduced through a burr hole into one or other lateral ventricle, is used. The risks of this procedure and potential complications are only acceptable when a lesion is known to be present; it cannot be regarded as a routine screening test. In most instances it is performed in theatre as a prelude to surgery. Simple isotope scanning is not very useful; if a lesion is seen it helps, but small lesions can easily escape detection. Computerised axial tomography (E.M.I. scanning) can detect lesions as small as 1 cm. in diameter and holds promise for the future for investigation of the posterior fossa but facilities are so limited at present that availability is the determining factor for performing the test. Myeloencephalography, in which myodil, introduced through the lumbar route, is allowed to run into the head, has some use particularly in extrinsic lesions such as neurofibromas, meningiomas and acoustic nerve tumours but unfortunately only indicates the site and extent of the lesion. It cannot indicate the possible pathology and carries all the risks of lumbar puncture *if* intracranial pressure is raised (Investigation techniques are discussed in greater detail in Chapter 25.)

Chapter 12

THE EXTRAPYRAMIDAL SYSTEM AND THE CEREBELLUM

There are anatomical, pathological and clinical reasons for considering disorders of the extrapyramidal system and cerebellum together.

Anatomical knowledge of the architecturally homogenous cerebellum has always been in advance of clinical knowledge. There are few physical signs of cerebellar disease and direct clinico-anatomical correlation is rarely possible. Often the resulting physical signs and symptoms are due to distortion of the brain stem and interference with the circulation of the C.S.F.

In contrast many disorders were long thought to be due to lesions in the extrapyramidal system and yet pathological findings were minimal or absent. Even now the anatomical extent of the extrapyramidal system is disputed, hence the expression "extrapyramidal system" rather than the more restrictive title "basal ganglia disease".

Since the relatively recent demonstration that many of these disorders have a neurochemical basis an entirely different concept of the functioning of the system has emerged. It is now apparent that far from the cerebellum being the "head ganglion of the proprioceptive system" with direct control over movement it merely serves as an integrating centre for postural information which it relays to the cerebral cortex and the basal ganglia. This explains the similarities of the symptoms and signs of extrapyramidal and cerebellar disease which may cause diagnostic confusion. Disease in both areas causes abnormalities of gait and unwanted additional movements either at rest or on attempted movement.

Unfortunately, such dynamic clinical disorders do not readily lend themselves to an illustrative approach. Instead an attempt has been made to provide a clear description of the various clinical signs and a disease classification based on clinical similarities and the age of the patient. The latter is particularly important in cerebellar disease in which the diagnostic possibilities are quite different in the child and adult.

ANATOMICAL CONSIDERATIONS (Figure 12.1)

Movement is initiated through the direct cortico-spinal or pyramidal system which is very highly developed in man. At the same time the continual postural adjustments that under-

lie smooth and co-ordinated movement are initiated by the cortico-pallidal system which projects mainly into the putamen. To complete the volitional side of activity there are the important cortico-ponto-cerebellar projections, which enter the cerebellum through the very large brachium pontis (middle cerebellar peduncle). Therefore all three parts of the C.N.S. concerned in movement are simultaneously alerted to the onset, intended direction and aim of a movement.

It is only in disease states that the extent and importance of the non-pyramidal mechanisms become apparent.

The main sensory input to the system comes from the muscle, tendon and joint position sense nerve endings, mainly via the spino-cerebellar tracts, and from the vestibular apparatus via the vestibular nuclei. Information from both sources enters the cerebellum through the inferior cerebellar peduncle (the restiform body).

The cyto-architecture of the cerebellar cortex is uniquely arranged to allow the projection of a vast amount of information on to the extensive dendritic net of each purkinje cell and models explaining this in computer and mathematical terms have been made. The large axon from each purkinje cell projects to the central cerebellar nuclei; mainly to the dentate nucleus on the same side. This nucleus relays the information to the opposite ventral-lateral thalamus and cortex via the dentato-rubral, rubro-thalamic, dentato-thalamic and thalamo-cortical projections. These pathways leave the cerebellum in the brachium conjunctivum (superior cerebellar peduncle) and decussate through the region of, or relay in, the red nucleus. The information reaching the thalamus is then projected to the extrapyramidal cortical areas and direct to the basal ganglia particularly to the putamen, caudate and external globus pallidus. This completes a group of circuits involving cortical, basal ganglia and cerebellar components; the cortex initiating the activity and the cerebellar input providing the necessary feed-back information.

In addition to these outer circuits there is a very important inner loop which appears to have an inhibitory feed-back effect on the globus pallidus. This is a relay through the subthalamic nucleus (of Luys). Damage to this circuit literally unleashes one of the most dramatic conditions in neurology, the syndrome known as hemi-ballismus.

The other efferent pathways from the basal ganglia

Figure 12.1. Scheme of Extrapyramidal/Cerebellar System

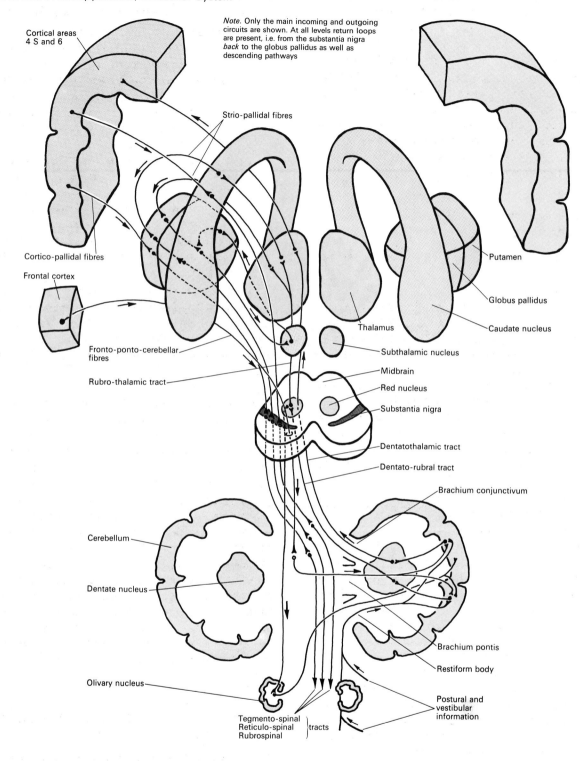

Cortical areas
4 S and 6

Note. Only the main incoming and outgoing
circuits are shown. At all levels return loops
are present, i.e. from the substantia nigra
back to the globus pallidus as well as
descending pathways

Strio-pallidal fibres

Cortico-pallidal fibres

Frontal cortex

Putamen

Globus pallidus

Caudate nucleus

Thalamus

Fronto-ponto-cerebellar
fibres

Rubro-thalamic tract

Subthalamic nucleus

Midbrain

Red nucleus

Substantia nigra

Dentatothalamic tract

Dentato-rubral tract

Brachium conjunctivum

Cerebellum

Dentate nucleus

Brachium pontis

Restiform body

Olivary nucleus

Postural and
vestibular
information

Tegmento-spinal
Reticulo-spinal   tracts
Rubrospinal

remain uncertain. Certainly an important pathway to the substantia nigra is known to exist but the exact routes of extrapyramidal activity below this level are unknown. The projections probably include tegmento-spinal, rubro-spinal, reticulo-spinal and olivo-spinal tracts. The relay through the olivary nucleus includes a circuit back into the cerebellum. Damage in this pathway has been implicated in disorders characterised by myoclonic phenomena.

The pathways described and illustrated represent only a fraction of the total neuronal circuitry involved in normal extrapyramidal function. Those included provide the best framework for clinical discussion.

PATHOLOGICAL AND BIOCHEMICAL CONSIDERATIONS

Parkinsonism was the first recognised and certainly the most studied disease of the extrapyramidal system. In spite of intensive pathological study the only constant finding was depigmentation and loss of neurones in the substantia nigra. In the period 1918–1927 a pandemic of a viral disorder known as encephalitis lethargica (Von Economo's encephalitis) occurred. This was associated with very gross disturbances of sleep, behaviour and every possible combination of abnormal movement. In patients dying of the disorder no constant pathological findings that could account for the physical signs were obtained. In recent years the severe and occasionally irreversible facial dyskinesias and dystonias caused by phenothiazine tranquillisers provided further evidence of obvious clinical disease in the absence of pathological abnormalities.

It is only in the last twenty years that histochemical studies of the brain have produced the dramatic breakthrough that indicated that these conditions are due to neurochemical disorders in the absence of neuronal damage. The normality of the underlying neural pathways has been adequately confirmed clinically by the dramatic restoration of near normal function to patients immobilised by parkinsonism for decades, by the oral administration of transmitter precursors such as L-Dopa. Acetylcholine, nor-adrenaline, dopamine and serotinin are the known transmitters but only the acetylcholine/dopamine system is understood. It would appear that it is not a simple matter of stimulatory and inhibitory transmitters in balance. There is evidence that both acetylcholine and dopamine have stimulant effects in some areas and inhibitory effects in others. However, some rough generalisations in the present state of knowledge indicate the possible relationship of the two systems:

In normal extrapyramidal function it would seem that a balance between cholinergic and dopaminergic pathways exists, whether these be inhibitory or stimulatory.

1. A decrease in activity in the cholinergic pathways *or* an increase in dopaminergic pathway activity causes choreiform movements. For example in Huntington's chorea severe degeneration of the caudate nucleus, in which most cholinergic neurones are concentrated, is a prominent feature. Conversely, if an excessive dose of L-Dopa is given to parkinsonian patients they develop choreiform movements.

2. An increase in cholinergic activity *or* a decrease in dopaminergic activity causes parkinsonism, a combination of tremor, rigidity and slowness of movement. Hence atropine-like drugs which block cholinergic neurones are of benefit in parkinsonism, and drugs that deplete or block dopaminergic neurones will worsen or cause parkinsonism. Such drugs include reserpine and the phenothiazines.

It follows from these therapeutic and biochemical considerations and the fact that depression often complicates parkinsonism and that antipsychotic drugs produce parkinsonism that there is a possibility that mental disorders are related to similar but as yet unidentified alterations in the neurotransmitters.

The complexity of these pathways which are actually closed loops with different transmitters at different synapses certainly explains the peculiarities and paucity of pathological findings. For example, histochemically and clinically it is clear that in parkinsonism the main problem lies in the dopaminergic synapses in the pallidum and yet the main pathological change is found in the synaptic area of the substantia nigra. It also explains why a lesion in one site does not necessarily indicate a specific function for that area. For example it would be incorrect to assume that because chorea occurs if the caudate is damaged that the normal function of the caudate is to prevent chorea. However, the assumption that damage to one circuit leads to an inbalance that could be corrected by deliberately destroying another circuit formed the theoretical basis for the moderately successful stereotactic operations for parkinsonism which enjoyed a vogue before the introduction of L-Dopa. There is still a place for such surgery in some conditions and this will be indicated in a later discussion.

CLINICAL FEATURES OF EXTRAPYRAMIDAL DISEASE

There are a wide range of movement disorders and physical signs associated with disease in the extrapyramidal system.

To avoid lengthy descriptions a terminology for these signs has been developed which ought to have simplified their documentation. However, because of varying use of these terms the situation has become even more confused and attempts are now being made to combine certain signs into fewer major groups. It is probably best to define carefully all terms in current use to enable the beginner to find his way through this particularly difficult neurological "jargon". A table is provided which indicates the major clinical causes of the various movement disorders which will be amplified in later discussion (Table 4). Many of these are extremely rare diseases. From the neurological novice's point of view the main problem is recognising that a movement disorder is organic.

Tremor

The most important feature is that the rhythm is constant, producing a steady oscillation, although the amplitude of the movement may vary. From the outset it is important to stress that tremor is *not* always due to parkinsonism. Although parkinsonism often starts as a tremor there are numerous other diagnostic possibilities. There are three clinically distinct forms of tremor:

1. *Rest Tremor*

Tremor due to any of the causes shown in the table may be present at rest and is invariably accentuated when the hands are held outstretched.

2. *Action tremor (or Intention tremor)*

It is so often stressed that action tremor is typical of cerebellar disease that the fact that nearly all sorts of tremor including parkinsonian tremor tends to be worse on action is frequently overlooked. The feature that distinguishes cerebellar action tremor on finger/nose testing is the inaccuracy of the movement and the tendency for the tremor to be accentuated just before the finger touches the nose (terminal intention tremor) unlike a parkinsonian tremor where the movement is accurate and the tremor constant. The most extreme degree of terminal intention tremor is sometimes seen in Wilson's Disease and is called a "Batswing tremor" because the oscillations are so violent and over such a wide range that there is a real risk that the patient will injure his face or eye.

3. *Peduncular or Red Nuclear Tremor*

This is the most violent form of tremor and almost invariably occurs in patients who have multiple sclerosis. The tremor is often present at rest causing jerking extension movements of the head and inarticulate speech. The slight-

est attempt to move the arm is followed by severe wide amplitude tremor. For example the patient may take several minutes to release the hand brake of his wheel chair, often bruising his arm in the process. He is quite unable to feed himself and attempts to open his mouth are often accompanied by such violent head jerking that the food or drink is spilled. This type of tremor may respond to stereotactic surgery.

Hemiballismus

This rare condition is considered at this point because it is so similar clinically to peduncular tremor and also responds to stereotactic surgery. It is very rare and is usually of abrupt onset following haemorrhage, infarction or damage to the subthalamic nucleus. It is invariably unilateral. If the patient lies at complete rest the movements may be minimal but any attempt to move is followed by wild flinging movements, particularly of the upper limb. One of the writer's patients broke her arm against a cot side at the onset; a measure of the violence of the disorder. Untreated the patient may die of exhaustion. In the author's limited experience of this condition chlorpromazine 25 mgm. I.V.I. has given almost immediate relief and controls the condition thereafter with a tendency for the movements to subside over a few weeks. If it fails to subside stereotactic surgery may be successful. Some classify this disorder as severe hemichorea but in the writer's opinion the clinical features and the discrete pathological lesion responsible warrants its classification as a separate entity.

Chorea

Choreiform movements are sudden rapid involuntary and purposeless jerks or fragments of movements that continually intrude into the patient's normal activity. They are particularly prominent in the face and distal muscles and the over-all impression obtained of a patient with mild chorea is that the patient is "fidgety". The eyebrows may raise and lower, the mouth distort to produce half smiles and half grimaces. The patient repeatedly crosses and uncrosses his legs and may sit with his arms tightly folded. Occasionally an arm may jerk out of place, the patient often attempting to disguise the movement by stroking his chin or smoothing his hair. When fully developed the gait may be altered by abrupt sudden jerks of the trunk and flinging movements of the arms and legs. The movements are exhausting and are at a minimum while the patient is lying quietly. Any active movement will provoke further jerking. In an extremely mild case the movements are best seen in the outstretched hands or in the feet as sudden flexion or extension movements of

Table 4

MOVEMENT DISORDERS

Movement disorder	Diseases responsible	Pathology
TREMOR		
(a) At Rest	Parkinsonism	Dopamine synthesis failure
	Anxiety	
	Alcohol and drugs	Increased physiological tremor
	Thyrotoxicosis	
	Benign essential tremor	Unknown often familial
	Wilson's disease	Abnormal copper metabolism
	Mercury poisoning (Hatter's shakes)	Basal ganglia damage
	Neurosyphilis	Infective, ? lesion responsible
(b) Action Tremor	Severe parkinsonism	
	Severe essential tremor	
	Cerebellar disease	
	Cerebellar connections	Lesion in red nucleus
CHOREA		
(a) Localised	Sydenhams Chorea	Rheumatic fever
	Posterior capsular C.V.A. (rare)	Lesion in posterior thalamic region
	Tumour in basal ganglia	
	Post-thalamotomy	
(b) Generalised	Sydenhams Chorea	Rheumatic fever
	Birth control pill chorea	? related to previous rheumatic fever
	Chorea gravidarum	
	Thyrotoxicosis	
	Disseminated lupus erythematosus	Unknown
	Polycythaemia rubra vera	
	Huntington's Chorea	Heredo familial degeneration
	Senile chorea	Associated with dementia

Movement disorder	Diseases responsible	Pathology
HEMIBALLISMUS		
	Haemorrhagic damage	Lesion in the subthalamic nucleus
	Embolic infarction	
	Post-traumatic	
ATHETOSIS		
	Cerebral palsy	Very common. Birth trauma
	Wilson's Disease	Abnormal copper metabolism
	Juvenile Huntington's Chorea (Rigid form)	Heredo-familial disease (very rare type)
	Hallevorden–Spatz disease	Demyelinating condition, (cause unknown)
	Following cerebral anoxia	Anaesthetic accident Drowning, etc.
	Alpers disease	Demyelinating condition
	Ataxia telangiectasia	Degenerative disease
DYSTONIAS		
(a) Generalised	Encephalitis lethargica	Viral infection
	Lesch–Nyhan syndrome	Abnormal urate metabolism
	Phenothiazines	Idiosyncratic drug reaction
	Butyrophenones	
	Dystonia musculorum deformans	Inherited metabolic disorder
	Paroxysmal choreo-athetosis (reflex epilepsy)	Inherited disease
(b) Localised	Post-hemiplegia	Basal ganglia damage, but quite rare complication
	Post-thalamotomy	
	Post-traumatic	
	Spasmodic torticollis	probably metabolic disorders
	Writers cramp	
	Blepharospasm/ blepharoclonus	
	Oral facial dyskinesias	Phenothiazines Senility Mental subnormality

CAUSES OF MYOCLONUS AND MYOCLONIC EPILEPSY

(a) *Generalised:* Idiopathic epilepsy
Familial essential myoclonus
Progressive myoclonic epilepsy: Familial type
Lafora body type
Lipoidosis
System degenerations
Spinocerebellar degeneration
Ramsay Hunt syndrome
Myoclonic encephalopathy of infancy
Infantile spasms (hypsarrythmia)

Epilepsia partialis continua
Jones–Nevin Syndrome
Post-cerebral anoxia
Subacute sclerosing panencephalitis
(b) *localised:* Subacute spinal neuronitis
Spinal cord tumours
Palatal myoclonus
Hemifacial spasm
Facial myokymia

Note: Many of these disorders are extremely rare. This list has been prepared to show the wide range of underlying disorders and to emphasise the need for skilled evaluation of all patients with myoclonus.

the fingers or side-to-side movements of individual fingers or toes which are virtually impossible to imitate.

Athetosis

Athetoid movements are slow, writhing sinuous movements of the arms and legs. There is an increasing tendency to include athetosis with dystonia but from a descriptive point of view there is some advantage in describing what is still referred to in the majority of texts as athetosis. In common with many of the movement disorders the condition occurs on attempted movement. Typically the arm becomes extended and externally rotated, the wrist hyperextended or fully flexed with the fingers extended. The foot is inverted and plantar-flexed and the leg extended. These peripheral movements are often associated with dystonic movements of the trunk. It occurs most often in children with an infantile hemiplegia following cerebral palsy and typically develops between five and ten years of age.

Dystonia

Dystonic movements are due to slow prolonged contractions of the trunk muscles which may be regarded as proximal athetosis. They may cause retraction of the head and hyperextension, twisting or lateral flexion of the spine eventually pulling the patient into an extremely uncomfortable, unnatural and maintained posture.

Included in the dystonic group of disorders are localised slow contractions of different muscle groups. These include the conditions known as spasmodic torticollis in which the head is pulled to one side, writer's cramp in which the shoulder muscles go into spasm as the patient attempts to write, blepharospasm in which the eyes shut tightly and remain closed for minutes at a time and various facial distortions including forced tongue protrusion with contraction of the facial muscles and platysma. The latter variety is easily mistaken for tetanus.

Myoclonus

Myoclonus consists of sudden brief shock-like jerks of a group of muscles, a single muscle or part of a muscle. In its most severe form the violence of the movement may throw the patient to the ground, especially as the jerk is often followed by an equally brief inhibition of muscle contraction. If continual, such myoclonus may simulate cerebellar ataxia. At the opposite extreme minute myoclonic twitches in relaxed muscles may be mistaken for fasciculation. Myoclonus may occur physiologically as "sleep starts" or indicate the onset of severe progressive brain disease. The causative conditions are fully discussed in a later section.

Tics

Tics are defined as brief contractions of a muscle or group of muscles, repetitive in the same place. The patient is usually able to mimic the movement and suppress it by intense concentration. They usually occur in children and may take the form of sniffing, grunting, snorting, pouting, clearing the throat, shoulder shrugging, winking, grimacing or appearing to try and bite one or other shoulder and may become so frequent that medical advice is sought. A typical feature is that from time to time the movement alters and for a few months persists in another form. Eventually recovery occurs and no consistent psychopathology is responsible. The most dramatic tic is known as the syndrome of Gilles de la Tourette. In these patients the tic movements are accompanied by the utterance of a four-letter word. This particular variant may respond to phenothiazines, suggesting an organic basis for the disorder.

Other physical signs of extrapyramidal disease including rigidity, reflex changes and associated specific signs of certain disorders will be discussed in the appropriate clinical section.

EXTRAPYRAMIDAL DISEASES
1. Benign Essential Tremor

This condition occurs sporadically or is inherited as an autosomal dominant. It may start at any age but in the inherited varieties the onset is typically in the teens in some families and in senility in others.

The upper limbs are most severely affected by a fine tremor which is present at rest but dramatically increased by stress or embarrassment. One of the most striking and even diagnostic features of the disorder is a dramatic response to alcohol. This may be so effective at controlling the symptoms that some sufferers have become alcoholics. Half the patients also suffer from titubation (a fine nodding movement of the head) and a third have some movement of the trunk and legs.

In most cases the disability is a purely social one and many patients deliberately avoid social functions and may become very depressed. The main importance of the condition lies in the frequency with which it is mistaken for parkinsonism. In the elderly the use of anti-parkinsonian drugs for senile familial tremor may cause gross confusion and compound the error. Diazepam, chlordiazepoxide and propranalol are helpful in severe cases but in mild cases the social use of alcohol will often control the symptoms adequately.

The differential diagnosis includes simple anxiety states, thyrotoxicosis and alcohol induced tremor. Parkinsonism is excluded by the absence of *any* other signs of the disorder (see below).

2. Parkinsonism

There are three features common to idiopathic, post-encephalitic and drug induced parkinsonism. So-called arteriosclerotic parkinsonism is discussed separately.

Tremor

Tremor has already been described. In parkinsonism it may also involve the facial, jaw and tongue muscles, but primarily affects the hands producing the very characteristic "pill-rolling" tremor. This results from the posture of the hand—it is flexed at the wrist with the fingers extended and the thumb abducted. The oscillations of the fingers and thumb in two planes produces the "pill-rolling" effect. The tremor is worse during anxiety and is supposed to decrease on activity, but in many patients with well-developed tremor it persists, producing an intention tremor easily mistaken for cerebellar disease.

Rigidity

All muscle groups are rigid in parkinsonism producing stiffness of movement throughout the entire range. This has been likened to the sensation experienced when bending a lead pipe. In some patients phasic decreases in tone produce "cog-wheel" rigidity, a sensation as if turning a sticking cog wheel. This is best felt while passively flexing and extending, or supinating and pronating the patient's wrist. It is markedly increased if the patient clenches the opposite fist while the test is performed. It is difficult to detect rigidity in the legs in a mild case, but it is sometimes first detectable at the hip by gently rolling the leg from side to side.

Bradykinesia

Bradykinesia is the most disabling component of the disease, affecting mainly the face and axial muscles which when combined with rigidity and tremor makes simple tasks such as writing, dressing or doing up buttons almost impossible. The slowness of postural adjustments coupled with the forward flexed posture and shuffling of the feet greatly increases the risk of the patient tripping and falling. This is known as a "festinant" gait. Patients often find they can run more easily than they can walk.

Presenting symptoms are varied and frequently dismissed as due to "old age", "arthritis", "rheumatism", "depression" or "one of those things". Occasionally, if one side is predominantly affected, particularly by bradykinesia, the patient may be suspected of having suffered a stroke or of developing a cerebral tumour. Occasionally the presenting symptom is a head injury or a fractured hip resulting from one of the many falls. In some patients slurring or hesitation of speech are prominent features. Excessive salivation and dribbling may be prominent in such patients and may suggest the diagnosis of dementia. In fact the production of saliva is no greater than in a normal patient, it is the infrequency of swallowing that allows it to accumulate and dribble from the mouth. Infrequent blinking also occurs and is one of the useful confirmatory diagnostic clues. It gives the patient rather an intense staring look. The loss of facial expression and infrequent smiling—the "mask facies" is indistinguishable from the uncompromising miserable face of a patient with severe retarded depression and this is another frequent diagnostic trap, compounded by the fact that many patients with parkinsonism *are* severely depressed.

A series of very useful questions will often confirm the diagnosis:

1. What has happened to the patient's writing? Invariably it has become so difficult that they have stopped writing altogether, but they always mention that their writing became very small before they did so.
2. Can they manage to get in and out of the bath? This is usually a serious problem and many patients relate being stuck in the bath for hours while waiting for help.
3. Can they turn over in bed? This apparently simple but technically very difficult manœuvre, is an early problem and the spouse will usually recall being woken up to assist the patient.
4. Can the patient, depending on sex, do ironing, peel potatoes, wring out washing, use a screwdriver etc?
5. If gait difficulties are a problem, does the patient ever find himself "stuck to the floor"? This is the situation in which the patient just cannot move, and for some reason often happens when going through a doorway or a gate. A useful tip is to advise the patient to imagine they have to step over a brick or log rather than move forward; this often enables them to get moving again. Perhaps for the same reason some patients notice they can walk better on uneven ground, where walking is a deliberate "pyramidal" function, than on the flat where walking is a purely automatic "extrapyramidal" function. One patient likened this difficulty to his "automatic pilot being switched off"!

Specific Types of Parkinsonism

The features discussed above are applicable to parkinsonism in general and especially the idiopathic variety which is now known to be due to an abnormality of dopamine synthesis or release in the globus pallidus.

Parkinsonism also occurs in patients exposed to manganese (a major industrial problem in manganese miners) and following carbon monoxide poisoning (leaking car exhaust, unsuccessful suicide bid).

Drug-induced parkinsonism causes little tremor but considerable cogwheel rigidity and bradykinesia. A full list of drugs that may cause parkinsonism is included in Chapter 24. Oculogyric crises are the only additional feature in drug-induced disease. Very rarely parkinsonism follows a head injury. The rarity probably reflects the fact that a head injury of sufficient severity to damage the basal ganglia is likely to prove fatal.

Postencephalitic Parkinsonism

This condition occurs as an immediate and delayed complication of Von Economo's encephalitis. The peak incidence of this condition has now passed but isolated patients manifesting some of the features very typical of the post-encephalitic variety are still seen. Historically, there have been several pandemics of this disorder over several hundred years and it may well appear again.

These features are:

1. Reversed-Argyll–Robertson pupils (see Chapter 2)
2. Oculo-gyric crises (see Chapter 8).
3. Seborrhoeic dermatitis of the forehead and face.
4. Severe sialorrhoea (drooling of saliva).
5. Respiratory tics, intractable hiccoughs.
6. Behavioural disturbances.

Arteriosclerotic Parkinsonism

In the writer's opinion this is *not* parkinsonism; arteriosclerotic rigidity is a better term. The patient or relative usually gives a history of the abrupt onset of mental and physical slowing coupled with slurred speech, drooling of saliva, difficulty chewing and swallowing and immobility.

There is no tremor, the main physical findings are very marked rigidity and slowness of movement without features typical of parkinsonian bradykinesia such as the feet getting stuck. In fact the gait consists of quick short, shuffling steps known as "Marche au petits pas".

On physical examination pseudo-bulbar dysarthria, a brisk jaw jerk, brisk reflexes and bilateral extensor plantars provide evidence of diffuse cerebral damage. In idiopathic parkinsonism the reflexes are unaffected and the plantar responses are usually flexor.

This diagnosis has great practical significance. The use of anti-parkinsonian drugs in these patients almost invariably provokes severe confusion and visual hallucinations without any beneficial effect on their physical disabilities. Only diazepam seems to be of some help to these patients.

Intellectual Function and Depression in Parkinsonism

It was previously held that parkinsonism was not associated with intellectual deterioration. Since the advent of the marked physical improvement produced by L-Dopa it has become apparent that at least half the patients with parkinsonism have a moderate to severe degree of intellectual impairment. Although at first it was thought that this had been unmasked by L-Dopa there is growing concern that in some cases the therapy is in some way responsible for the sometimes abrupt dementia that may occur in patients on L-Dopa.

Depression has always been recognised as a part of the parkinsonism syndrome and lately the suspicion that it is an integral part of the disease rather than a reaction to the disease has been raised. This is discussed further in Chapter 24.

Varying degrees of parkinsonism complicate several rare disorders including Shy–Drager syndrome. In this disease a combination of parkinsonism, autonomic neuropathy and motor neurone disease occurs more or less simultaneously. It is a very rare but an exceedingly unpleasant and lethal disease. Nearly all reported patients have presented with micturition disturbances, either retention or incontinence of urine and severe constipation. Postural hypotension causes frequent syncopal attacks and careful physical examination will usually detect evidence of both parkinsonism and motor neurone disease. The normal course of the disease is death within two to four years of the onset.

CASE REPORT

A 48-year-old female was admitted to hospital with a history of unsteadiness of gait, severe constipation, urinary retention and syncopal attacks. She was discharged with the diagnosis of hysteria. When reviewed in the clinic only six months later she had obvious parkinsonism with gross bradykinesia, a postural hypotensive drop from 120/80 to 60/0 and severe sphincter disturbance. She steadily deteriorated over the next few months developing widespread muscle wasting and fasciculation. This is a classical example of the Shy–Drager syndrome.

Parkinsonism associated with dementia and motor neurone disease constitutes the syndrome known as Jakob–Creutzfeld Disease (see Chapter 10).

The treatment of parkinsonism is detailed in Chapter 24.

Sydenham's Chorea

This condition has become a rare disease with the decreased incidence of rheumatic fever. It typically occurs within three months of an attack of rheumatic fever in patients between 5 and 20 years of age. It has an insidious onset and in half the patients is unilateral. It is frequently dominated by an emotional upset that very easily leads to a mistaken diagnosis of hysteria. The typical choreiform movements subside in three to six months. Occasionally an unusual variant of this condition in younger children produces a flaccid hemiparesis.

Chorea gravidarum probably represents a recurrence of Sydenham's chorea during a subsequent pregnancy, and has also declined in frequency. Some doubt has been thrown on this explanation by the recent recognition of typical chorea syndromes produced by the birth control pill. Furthermore one of the author's patients with chorea due to the pill developed the condition three months after the completion of a chorea-free pregnancy, making an underlying neural deficit unlikely.

Other Rare Causes of Chorea

Chorea has been reported in association with systemic lupus erythematosus, polycythaemia rubra vera, thyrotoxicosis, diphenylhydantoin (epanutin) intoxication, phenothiazine hypersensitivity and as a complication of excessive doses of L-Dopa. Some elderly patients develop choreiform movements spontaneously which may raise the possibility of Huntington's Chorea. This is usually senile chorea without genetic significance.

Huntington's Chorea

Huntington's chorea is certainly one of the most unpleasant diseases known. This is not only because it is inherited as an autosomal dominant with complete penetrance but because of the nature of the disease itself.

Rarely the disorder may manifest itself in childhood and is then somewhat atypical with considerable rigidity and even parkinsonian features rather than chorea; even epilepsy may occasionally be the first symptom. Family studies have suggested a high incidence of anti-social, alcoholic or psychopathic behaviour as a premorbid personality change in patients with this disease, but it has been argued that these phenomena merely reflect the young person's knowledge of the possibility that he will get the disease that has killed so many of his family. When one realises that the death often involves ten years of relentless generalised choreiform movements with progressive dementia this alternative explanation seems reasonable. Apart from the movement disorder and dementia which usually begins in the third decade there are no physical signs. Reflexes are usually normal, plantar responses are flexor and continence is only impaired with the onset of severe dementia. In some cases dementia may precede the movement disorder by several years or vice versa.

Perhaps the greatest hope lies in the recently devised test which may enable future sufferers to be detected before they can have children. This is based on the demonstration that low doses of L-Dopa induce choreiform movements in a certain percentage of relatives of patients with Huntington's chorea and does not do so in control patients. The predictive value of the test will have to await proof that these L-Dopa sensitive patients go on to develop the disease. Although genetically this will be a valuable advance the ethical dilemma that will result when discussing the test results with the patient is obvious.

Some symptomatic relief from the movements may be achieved with haloperidol or thiopropazate but relentless progression is the rule.

Athetoid and Dystonic Diseases

Dystonia is a feature of many rare diseases and their rarity justifies only a brief description of some of the clinical and biochemical features.

1. *Kernicterus*

Children who have had kernicterus (neonatal jaundice) may develop athetoid posturing of the limbs later, between the ages of 5 and 15. This problem has been greatly reduced by the treatment of Rhesus negative babies by exchange transfusion and latterly prevention in utero by immunisation procedures.

2. *Wilson's Disease*

This is a rare inborn error of copper metabolism in which copper is deposited in the basal ganglia and liver. A wide range of tremors, athetoid and dystonic movements develop but cirrhosis of the liver is the most serious feature. One of the diagnostic clinical features is a fine brown dust-like ring around the edge of the limbus of the cornea called a Kayser—Fleischer ring. The serum copper and caeruloplasmin levels (the copper transport protein) are greatly decreased. The disorder is now treatable with penicillamine but early recognition of the disorder is essential for complete control.

3. *Hallevorden-Spatz Disease*

This is a rare degenerative disease of children that causes progressive dystonia, hyperkinetic movements and retinitis pigmentosa. The aetiology is unknown; the course is one of progressive physical and mental deterioration.

4. *Lesch—Nyhan Disease*

Lesch—Nyhan Disease is the most recently recognised of these disorders. It is associated with severe athetoid/dystonic movements and self-mutilation. The latter is not uncommon in mentally defective children but is particularly severe in this disorder in which the children will eat their lips, tongue and fingers unless all the teeth are removed. It is associated with very high serum uric acid levels but the relationship of this finding to the movement disorder is unknown.

5. Dystonia Musculorum Deformans

This condition is inherited either as an autosomal recessive or dominant gene. The recessive variety is particularly common in Jewish families and usually produces severe disability. The dominant variety demonstrates variable penetrance with very mild disability in some affected members of the family. In the fully developed form the patient's body is pulled into grossly abnormal dystonic postures and jerked by frequent choreiform movements.

6. Paroxysmal Choreoathetosis (Reflex Epilepsy)

This is also often inherited as an autosomal dominant. In typical form sudden brief choreoathetoid postures or movements follow a sudden movement. One young male patient of the author's dreaded fielding in cricket. If he had to run for the ball his first few strides were dominated by bizarre writhing movements of his right limbs. His brother and mother had the same problems although his mother had outgrown the problem and was a first class pianist.

The commonest types of dystonia are known as the segmental torsion dystonias as opposed to the disorders discussed above which involve all or most of the body.

7. Spasmodic Torticollis

This extremely unpleasant and disabling condition affects the middle aged of either sex. The head is turned to one or other side and typically the shoulder on the same side is slightly hunched up as if to meet the chin. Initially the movement is spasmodic often occurring when the patient reaches out for something but later the spasm is continual with severe cramp-like pain in the contracting muscles and aching in the neck. In some cases the patient or preferably *someone else* can easily get the head back to the normal position by gentle pressure applied to the side of the chin. For years this was regarded as a psychological disorder but the overwhelming opinion amongst neurologists is that this is an organic syndrome related to the torsion dystonias.

8. Writer's Cramp

Writer's cramp was previously regarded as a neurotic syndrome in pre-retirement clerical workers. Current opinion now recognises that this occurs in many patients as an organic extrapyramidal syndrome and in fact many patients go on to develop parkinsonism or other dystonic syndromes.

9. Blepharoclonus and Blepharospasm

This condition occurs in an older age group and consists of frequent and prolonged episodes of forced eye closure. As in the case of writer's cramp it may be an early feature of parkinsonism.

10. Facial Dyskinesias

This group of disorders have been increasingly recognised as a complication of phenothiazine therapy but in fact these chewing, chomping movements of the face, lips and tongue often occur in elderly demented patients and in patients with mental subnormality. It is possible that the self-mutilation of the lips in the latter group and in the Lesch—Nyhan syndrome is merely a gross aberration of these movements. In addition to the facial movements repeated swallowing or tongue protrusion may occur.

11. Drug Induced Dystonias

The commonest cause of dystonic syndromes at the present time is drug hypersensitivity. The drugs responsible include all the phenothiazines, tricyclic antidepressants, benzo-diazepines and L-Dopa. In fact it is the recognition that all the syndromes described above and formerly thought to be due to neurosis, occur during drug reactions that has completely altered medical opinion to the general acceptance that these are organic disorders.

Drug-induced disorders include blepharospasm, oculogyric crisis, facial spasms, tongue protrusion, webbing of the neck due to muscle contraction, torticollis, antecollis, retrocollis, hyperextension of the back, lateral flexion of the spine, dystonic postures of the limbs and fine jerking restless movements of the limbs (sometimes called peripheral akathisia).

Although drug therapy is generally ineffective in the organic disorders, in drug-induced cases, increasing the dose of the offending drug or treatment with an alternative phenothiazine may prove as effective as withdrawing the drug. In fact on occasions the movement disorder may develop *after* the offending drug is withdrawn (tardive dyskinesia). This is particularly true of the facial movement group.

There are important differences between the different types of phenothiazine and extrapyramidal syndromes.

Piperazine side chain drugs: tri-fluo-perazine (Stelazine), fluphenazine (Modecate), perphenazine (Fentazine), prochlorperazine (Stemetil), are particularly likely to produce *acute* onset dystonia—often after a single dose in young females. It is interesting that it is the anti-emetic effect that is often the indication for the use of the drug, and that metoclopramide (Maxalon) an anti-emetic drug unrelated to the phenothiazines, may also produce acute dystonic syndromes. These are hypersensitivity reactions.

The chloro-substituted agents such as chlorpromazine are more likely to produce parkinsonian syndromes after many years of use, and are usually responsible for the tardive dyskinesias. Clearly these drugs are not producing hypersensitivity reactions but chronic alterations in transmitter substances.

Myoclonic Disorders

In Infancy and Childhood

Myoclonic jerking and myoclonic epilepsy are features of several conditions in infancy. These range from the progressive lipoidosis of Krabbe causing dementia and ultimately death to non-progressive and remitting conditions such as the myoclonic encephalopathy of infancy. In this condition brief shock-like muscle contractions follow startle or attempted movement. This condition may respond to ACTH and remit without sequelae. Infantile myoclonic spasms or "salaam" attacks are more serious and associated with a classical EEG appearance known as hypsarrythmia. The attacks start in the first year of life and consist of a cry followed by trunk flexion or a brief "lightning jerk" of the entire body with extension of the legs and upturned eyes. Eventually, after two to three years, the attacks cease but are usually superseded by other forms of epilepsy and almost invariably the child is found to have suffered considerable cerebral damage.

In the second decade another group of disorders occur. These include simple myoclonic epilepsy with occasional grand mal attacks and myoclonic jerks complicating petit mal or idiopathic grand mal. A highly lethal variant is known as Lafora-Body disease. In this condition what starts as myoclonic epilepsy is rapidly followed by cortical blindness and increasing dementia. Lafora bodies are mucopolysaccharide cellular inclusions found in nerve cells, and in the supra-renal glands and kidneys. All patients die within six years of the onset. Another important disorder, which is usually fatal, has been recently recognised as due to an abnormal immune response to the measles virus. This is the condition known as subacute sclerosing leucoencephalopathy and occurs in the age range 5–20 years. The affected patient has usually had measles very early in life (before 2 years of age). The onset includes intellectual or behavioural problems, myoclonic jerking, spasticity, rigidity and increasing dementia leading to death over a period of one to two

years. The C.S.F. globulins are markedly elevated and immunological evidence suggests that an abnormal immune response to intra-neuronal measles virus is responsible. The EEG is characterised by an extremely flat tracing with occasional bursts of high voltage spikes associated with visible myoclonic jerks. In recent years a few patients who have apparently recovered from this condition have been reported.

In the Adult

Myoclonic jerking preceding an epileptic fit occurs in some 10 per cent of epileptic patients. It is particularly likely to occur in the first hour or two after waking and often warns the patient that an attack is pending.

Myoclonic jerking occurs in some families with Friedreich's ataxia and as a specific component of Ramsay—Hunt cerebellar degeneration (dyssynergia cerebellaris myoclonica), which is discussed in detail in the next section. Some families have been reported in which parkinsonism and myoclonus appear in different members and some patients with myoclonic epilepsy may develop a parkinsonian state in later life.

A rare disorder known as Jones—Nevin syndrome (subacute spongiform encephalopathy) is also associated with myoclonus. Patients with this condition develop rapidly progressive dementia and myoclonic jerking, usually between the ages of 50 and 70. The aetiology is unknown but there is considerable overlap with Jakob—Creutzfeld syndrome and it is thought that the two disorders may be variants of the same condition. Jakob—Creutzfeld disease has been shown to be due to a virus infection.

There are many other disorders in which myoclonic jerking may occur of even greater rarity than those already mentioned. As a general rule in view of the possible serious implications any patient with myoclonic jerking should be referred for an expert opinion.

THE CEREBELLUM

For clinical purposes there is little to be gained by attempting to learn the complicated anatomy of the cerebellum with its confusing double nomenclature.

Basic Anatomy

The anatomy of the cerebellum and its connections is shown in Figures 12.2, 12.3 and 12.4.

There are two basic regions, the midline structures and the cerebellar hemispheres. The midline groups include the lingula anteriorly, the vermis in the middle and the flocculonodular lobe posteriorly. The lobes are divided into a small

Figure 12.2. Schematic diagram of the Cerebellum in relation to the Brain Stem

This is the same angle of view as
in the brain stem illustrations in
chapter 11

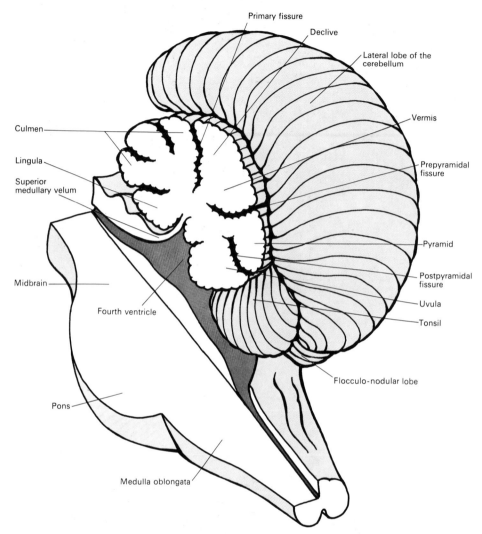

anterior lobe and a large posterior lobe. Each hemisphere contains a large main nucleus, the dentate, through which the bulk of efferent cerebellar information is discharged. There are smaller roof nuclei which are mainly concerned with vestibular reflexes and occular movements.

Clinically lesions affecting the midline group produce severe ataxia. Lesions in the lingula extend into the superior medullary velum producing fourth nerve palsies or into the superior cerebellar peduncle producing severe tremor of the arm on the same side. Lesions in the vermis cause severe ataxia; often making it impossible for the patient to sit or stand unsupported. Lesions in the flocculo-nodular region

cause ataxia, vertigo (due to damage to vestibular reflex pathways) and vomiting if they extend into the floor of the fourth ventricle. Tumours at all midline sites tend to cause early obstruction of the aqueduct or fourth ventricle resulting in headache and papilloedema.

The signs of a lesion in the lobes depend on the symmetry. A unilateral lesion produces classical cerebellar signs in the limbs on the same side (see later). Symmetrical involvement of both hemispheres, as happens in some of the cerebellar degenerations may produce quite mild symmetrical signs with moderate gait ataxia.

The most dramatic "cerebellar" signs are found in diseases

Figure 12.3. The Cerebellum—Main Afferent Connections

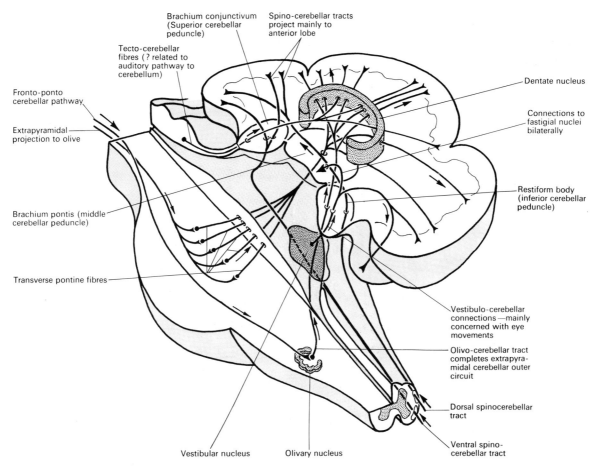

Brachium conjunctivum (Superior cerebellar peduncle)

Spino-cerebellar tracts project mainly to anterior lobe

Tecto-cerebellar fibres (? related to auditory pathway to cerebellum)

Fronto-ponto cerebellar pathway

Extrapyramidal projection to olive

Brachium pontis (middle cerebellar peduncle)

Transverse pontine fibres

Dentate nucleus

Connections to fastigial nuclei bilaterally

Restiform body (inferior cerebellar peduncle)

Vestibulo-cerebellar connections—mainly concerned with eye movements

Olivo-cerebellar tract completes extrapyramidal cerebellar outer circuit

Dorsal spinocerebellar tract

Ventral spino-cerebellar tract

Vestibular nucleus

Olivary nucleus

Figure 12.4. The Cerebellum—Main Efferent Connections

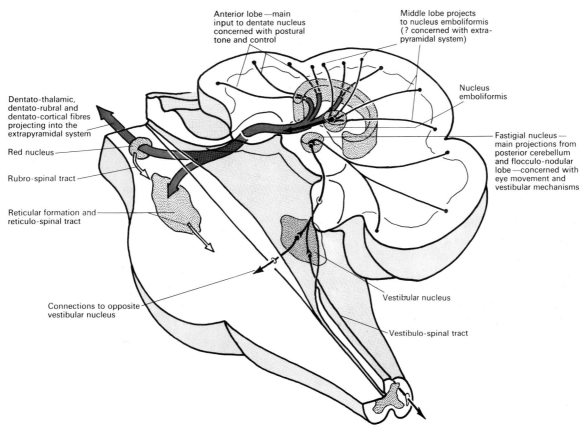

Anterior lobe—main input to dentate nucleus concerned with postural tone and control

Middle lobe projects to nucleus emboliformis (? concerned with extra-pyramidal system)

Dentato-thalamic, dentato-rubral and dentato-cortical fibres projecting into the extrapyramidal system

Red nucleus

Rubro-spinal tract

Reticular formation and reticulo-spinal tract

Connections to opposite vestibular nucleus

Nucleus emboliformis

Fastigial nucleus—main projections from posterior cerebellum and flocculo-nodular lobe—concerned with eye movement and vestibular mechanisms

Vestibular nucleus

Vestibulo-spinal tract

which damage cerebellar connections in the brain stem, either the main efferent pathways in the superior cerebellar peduncle or the inflow pathways in the inferior and middle cerebellar peduncles. One of the most difficult false-localising signs in neurology may result from a lesion affecting the fronto-ponto-cerebellar pathway.

CASE REPORT

A patient seen recently by the writer, a 50-year-old female had a known history of carcinoma of the breast. She presented with a short history of headache, vomiting and drowsiness. On examination she had marked papilloedema, left-sided cerebellar signs and bilateral extensor plantar responses. A confident clinical diagnosis of a left-sided cerebellar metastasis was made but on further investigation a right frontal metastasis was found!

CLINICAL SIGNS OF CEREBELLAR DISEASE

The most important physical sign of cerebellar disease is ataxia. This is best defined as inco-ordinated or inaccurate movement *which is not* due to paresis, alteration in tone, loss of postural sense or the intrusion of involuntary movements. For this reason the majority of neurologists do *not* test cerebellar function until they are certain that the patient has normal power, tone and sensation.

In children there are three common findings that may easily be mistaken for ataxia. These are the intrusion of choreiform movements, myoclonic jerks or minor status epilepticus (status petit mal). In the latter variety the child will sit drooling, with a blank expression on its face and all voluntary movements are performed with little pauses and sudden jolts. The EEG is diagnostic.

In the adult there are also three common clinical errors. Mild pyramidal weakness may easily produce "ataxia" on cerebellar testing unless allowances are made for the weakness. Many extrapyramidal disorders in their early stages produce "pseudo-paresis" or "pseudo-ataxia" unless the rigidity and involuntary movements are identified. Extremely anxious patients frequently perform very badly on formal cerebellar function tests due to tremulousness.

1. Gait Ataxia

A patient who has gait difficulty due to a cerebellar disorder is frightened to stand. He spreads his feet apart and will hold on to any support that is available. He will not fall but may reel from side to side even when supported and consistently to the same side if a unilateral lesion is present. Minimal degrees of gait ataxia are best detected by asking the patient to walk on a line. After one or two inaccurate steps the patient refuses to go further and reverts to a wide based stance. Although patients in this position tend to

wobble even more when they close their eyes they do not fall. This is often referred to as a positive Romberg Test, but as discussed in Chapter 6 this is not strictly accurate.

An important gait abnormality also often misdiagnosed as ataxia occurs in elderly females. It has been called the 3F syndrome (Fear of Further Falling). It typically occurs after an elderly female has had an attack of vertigo, syncope or a drop attack. They will only walk in a bizarre posture, pushing one foot forward tentatively while leaning right back on the other. The arms are held at 90° to the body, slightly forward with the hands facing downward. They insist on a relative walking behind them, and insist on reaching forward to sit on a chair long before they reach it. They do *not* fall. This seems to be an entirely functional disorder that is extremely difficult to cure. Even prolonged physiotherapy seems to provide little reassurance and as soon as they attempt to walk alone they revert to the classical and ridiculous posture.

2. Truncal Ataxia

Truncal ataxia is a particular feature of midline cerebellar lesions. The patient may be unable to sit or stand without support with a tendency to fall backwards. Unless the flocculo-nodular lobe is involved there may be no other definite symptoms or signs. Limb ataxia is minimal or absent.

3. Limb Ataxia

Cerebellar function in the limbs is tested in several ways. In Chapter 9 we have discussed the value of observing the patient's outstretched hands as a screening test for disorders of pyramidal and proprioceptive function. In pure cerebellar disease the outstretched hand on the affected side tends to hyperpronate so that the palm faces outwards, and rises, often to 12" above the level of the other hand. In severe cerebellar disease some tremulous movements appear. If the examiner presses down gently on the patient's outstretched hands and suddenly releases the pressure the affected hand flies up completely out of control.

When these tests have been performed the patient's ability to touch the tip of his nose and then the examiner's index finger is tested. This is known as the finger/nose test. if postural sense has already been tested there is *no need* for the patient to attempt the test with his eyes closed. In fact, the value of the test is greatly enhanced if the examiner moves the target finger, varying both the direction *and* distance from the patient's nose. In this way quite mild inco-ordination, terminal intention tremor and dysmetria (over-shooting) can be detected.

The equivalent test in the legs is the heel/knee/shin test. The patient is asked to place the tip of the heel (not the sole of the foot) on the tibial tubercle of the other leg and run the heel down the shin. The heel is then *lifted* off and replaced on the tibial tubercle. The foot is *not* rubbed up and down the shin. If the sole of the foot is allowed to sit astride the shin the foot slides up and down with the tibia acting as a guide! Some mild inco-ordination is within normal limits for this test, particularly in the elderly with painful hips or knee joints. The test must be performed properly and over-interpretation of minor abnormalities should be avoided.

Unilateral ataxia is a reliable indication of disease affecting the cerebellar hemisphere on the same side. If severe, it could indicate disease affecting cerebellar input on the same side, the decussated dentato-rubro-thalamic pathway damage or even a lesion in the opposite frontal pole. When one adds the possibility of subtle ataxia produced by pyramidal lesions and posture sense loss the clinical difficulty occasionally experienced in diagnosing a cerebellar lesion with confidence is understandable.

4. Rapid Alternating Movements

On completion of the ataxia tests a variety of simple rapid movement tests are performed. These detect fragmentation of movement or inaccuracy of movement which is accentuated by the speed at which the movement is attempted. This is known as dysdiadochokinesia. The most useful tests are those in which the patient taps himself on the back of one hand as fast as he can or taps his foot on the floor or against the examiner's hand. This test is also subject to the proviso that there should be no pyramidal deficit. Finally, the patient is asked to make a fist and with his elbow half flexed tries to pronate and supinate the fore-arm as fast as possible. In an abnormal situation the movement is slow and irregular and the shoulder joint will start to abduct and adduct wildly as the whole arm becomes involved in the effort.

5. Other Signs

The signs already discussed, difficult as they are to elicit, are definite evidence of cerebellar dysfunction. There are a variety of other signs that are occasionally even more difficult to elicit and less certain in their interpretation.

Tone: In cerebellar disease the tone of the muscles is reduced on the side of the lesion. Reduced tone is a highly subjective phenomena and although occasionally it is unequivocally reduced this is by no means invariably true.

Reflexes: In parallel with the decrease in tone the reflexes tend to be less brisk and rather slower in rise and fall producing what is known as a pendular jerk. Again, this is highly subjective and in the majority of patients no definite abnormality of the reflexes is found.

Nystagmus: As discussed in Chapter 8, nystagmus is not

an essential feature of cerebellar disease, and if found usually reflects involvement of the flocculo-nodular lobe. If present the nystagmus is maximal towards the side of the lesion.

Dysarthria: Cerebellar disease affects the auto-regulation of breathing and particularly its integration with speech. This tends to produce spluttering staccato speech. So-called scanning dysarthria is more typical of combined pyramidal-cerebellar lesions and usually occurs in multiple sclerosis.

Writing: Writing is often affected and typically the patient enlarges his writing to make it more legible—quite the reverse of parkinsonism in which the writing becomes smaller.

Head Posture: there are three ways in which head posture may be altered by cerebellar disease. All produce a head tilt to one side. Lesions in the superior medullary velum may cause a fourth nerve palsy and lead to head tilt to compensate for diplopia. A cerebellar hemisphere lesion may unbalance postural tone, leading to a head tilt towards the side of the lesion. Lesions in the flocculo-nodular lobe causing raised intracranial pressure may directly irritate the dura in the posterior fossa, causing neck stiffness and tilting and retraction of the head to one side.

Vomiting: In view of the difficulties encountered in making a definite diagnosis of cerebellar disease on clinical evidence the considerable significance of vomiting in patients with cerebellar tumours deserves special mention. The characteristic features may be remembered as the 3 P's; postural, positional and projectile vomiting. The vomiting is typically very sudden without nausea and hence tends to be projectile. It typically occurs if the patient is in a certain position and very commonly if the patient attempts to sit up suddenly. The writer would regard the latter feature as diagnostic of a cerebellar tumour *even* in the absence of other physical signs.

CASE REPORT

A 36-year-old self-employed builder had been under a great deal of pressure and developed mild headaches and attacks of sudden vomiting. There were absolutely no physical signs but if he suddenly sat up from lying he almost invariably vomited. An E.M.I. scan revealed a cystic midline tumour, confirmed by operation. The patient and his medical advisers thought his symptoms were due to anxiety.

In summary pure cerebellar disease may produce very definite symptoms, particularly unsteadiness of gait, but remarkably subtle physical signs often dominated by a single feature, such as truncal ataxia. Patients with very florid physical signs usually have involvement of cerebellar connections in the brainstem. For the same reason extensive surgical resection of part of the cerebellum may produce remarkably little residual deficit, and even metastatic lesions may be treated surgically in anticipation of an acceptable end result.

CEREBELLAR DISEASE IN CHILDHOOD

In childhood there are five main categories of disease that may affect the cerebellum. Some of these are detailed elsewhere and will not be discussed in detail here.

Congenital Lesions

These conditions include various maldevelopments of the cerebellum, often associated with Arnold–Chiari malformation or the Dandy–Walker syndrome (see Chapter 15). Often the associated meningocoele or raised intracranial pressure are the presenting symptoms, but mild cases of Arnold–Chiari syndrome may not produce symptoms until two years of age. As in the case of extrapyramidal disorders it is worth remembering that ataxia cannot become fully manifest until the pyramidal system becomes functional. Apparently "acute" movement or gait disorders starting in the second year of life are frequently found to be due to congenital abnormalities or neonatal brain damage. One condition that genuinely causes a delayed presentation dominated by ataxia is congenital aqueduct stenosis. Some patients with this condition may present in their teens, with symptoms which include ataxia, VI nerve palsies, enlargement of the head, papilloedema with visual failure and declining intellectual function. The onset may be very insidious and the condition is easily misdiagnosed as a cerebellar tumour.

Metabolic Disorders

There are several metabolic disorders which may cause cerebellar dysfunction and ataxia. These include metachromatic leucodystrophy, Bassen–Kornzweig disease and Refsum's syndrome, which are discussed in Chapter 16. There are five additional disorders.

1. Ataxia in children may be due to drugs, especially anticonvulsants and in particular diphenylhydantoin and primidone. Occasionally acute ataxia and drowsiness may be found to be due to alcohol if the child has had access to spirits.

2. Ataxia, papilloedema and drowsiness may be due to lead poisoning and consequent cerebral swelling. This is easily misdiagnosed as a cerebellar tumour.

3. Maple Syrup urine disease. This is one of the rare disorders of amino-acid metabolism in which episodic ataxia occurs, often precipitated by infection. During attacks increased amounts of valine, leucine and isoleucine are excreted in the urine. Between attacks there is no abnormality.

4. Hartnup disease. This disease is due to impaired absorption of Tryptophan. Episodic ataxia precipitated by infection and usually associated with a dry, scaly red pellagra-like skin rash occurs. Variable amino-aciduria is found even between attacks.

5. Ataxia—Telangiectasia (Louis–Bar syndrome). The main features of this progressive disorder are telangiectasia of the conjunctivae (usually misdiagnosed as chronic conjunctivitis), progressive cerebellar degeneration and a tendency to infection in those patients who have agammaglobulinaemia which is occasionally associated with this disorder. Progressive ataxia and mental impairment, and early death from infection is the usual course of the disease.

Infectious Disorders

Acute viral infection of the cerebellum has been reported, or at least patients in whom the signs of viral encephalitis have been dominated by ataxia.

An acute ataxic syndrome may occur after *any* of the exanthemata of childhood and infectious mononucleosis. There is a specific association with chicken pox; in which severe ataxia may start within three weeks of the initial infection and almost always subsides over several months. Chicken pox "cerebellitis" usually occurs in children under two years of age and is rare in older children. In all cases of "post-infectious" ataxia in childhood it is important to exclude the metabolic disorders that can be triggered by infection (see above).

Children with Guillain–Barré syndrome may appear to be ataxic on initial examination. This is due to proximal motor weakness or sensory deficit and re-emphasises the importance of being certain that ataxia is not "pseudo-ataxia".

Degenerative Disorders

The commonest inherited form of spino-cerebellar degeneration is Friedreich's ataxia which usually causes symptoms between the ages of 5 and 10. It is fully discussed in Chapter 14. The majority of inherited cerebellar degenerations present in adulthood and are certainly the longest delayed in onset of all "inherited" disorders. Two varieties may cause symptoms in childhood. Olivo-ponto-cerebellar atrophy which causes dysarthria and ataxia in the adult may cause progressive spastic paralysis and death in the child. Ramsay–Hunt syndrome (dyssynergia cerebellaris myoclonica), in childhood causes a mild progressive ataxia complicated by sudden myoclonic jerking which may be sufficiently severe to throw the child to the ground in addition to falls directly due to the ataxia.

Tumours

Tumours have been considered in Chapter 8. It is pertinent to recall that the majority of cerebral tumours in childhood occur in the cerebellum and that there are two types; the highly malignant medulloblastoma which produces a "midline" picture with gross truncal ataxia and the benign cystic astrocytoma which may start in the midline but later spreads laterally as a large cystic extension into one or other hemisphere and produces a typical unilateral cerebellar syndrome.

The presenting symptom of cerebellar tumours in the child is usually ataxia, closely followed by headache, vomiting and papilloedema. The main differential diagnoses are lead poisoning and aqueductal stenosis. Pontine gliomas do *not* cause C.S.F. obstruction and are more likely to produce cranial nerve palsies (see Chapter 11).

CEREBELLAR DISEASE IN THE ADULT

In the adult the causes of cerebellar disease are quite different. Vascular disease is a rare cause of cerebellar dysfunction except that due to involvement of cerebellar pathways in a brainstem lesion. Acute intracerebellar haemorrhage has been described in Chapter 11. Several hereditary disorders typically cause their first symptoms in late adulthood. Tumours are rare if one excludes acoustic nerve tumours, and are usually metastatic, the one exception being the cerebellar haemangioblastoma. Finally, there are several "toxic" causes of cerebellar disease, alcohol being the main offender.

Inherited Cerebellar Disease

Friedreich's ataxia has already been discussed and usually causes symptoms in childhood. There are three major inherited cerebellar degenerations.

1. *Ramsay–Hunt syndrome* (dyssynergia cerebellaris progressiva or myoclonica). This consists of the insidious development of cerebellar ataxia often associated with myoclonus. It usually begins in the third decade of life and upper limb ataxia of severe degree rather than gait ataxia is the rule. This is consistent with the main pathological lesion which is in the dentate nucleus and its pathway to the thalamus.

2. *Olivo-Ponto-Cerebellar Atrophy* (of Dejerine–Thomas). This disorder is dominated by dysarthria, and for reasons that are not clear sphincter dysfunction occurs with incontinence of urine and impotence. Generalised jerking at rest rather than a pure ataxia occurs with rigidity rather than hypotonia. The pathology varies but degeneration of the olivary and pontine nuclei and loss of cerebellar Purkinje cells are the usual histological findings.

3. *Cerebellar Ataxia with Spasticity* (Marie and Sanger-Brown). This is a late onset disorder which is strongly hereditary and is dominated by ataxia. Unlike other heredofamilial degenerations, the reflexes are brisk and there is severe spasticity of the lower limbs. Optic atrophy is a frequent finding and the disorder is easily misdiagnosed as multiple sclerosis unless the progressive nature is recognised or a positive family history is obtained.

In all these disorders some decline in intellectual function is common even though the brunt of the damage falls on the cerebellum. The familial nature may be obscured by the early death of parents (before they could develop the disease) or separation from siblings by the time the disease occurs. Careful family tracing may reveal several siblings in different parts of the country with the same disease masquerading under different diagnostic labels.

"Toxic" Cerebellar Degeneration

There are a variety of possible causes of "toxic" cerebellar degeneration, characterised by loss of Purkinje cells and in some cases confined to fairly discrete areas of the cerebellum. Alcohol is the commonest cause and may produce very severe but reversible acute ataxia during intoxication, slowly worsening ataxia or severe acute irreversible ataxia during an attack of Wernicke's encephalopathy. The brunt of the damage falls on the anterior lobe and severe gait ataxia is the result.

Anticonvulsant drugs cause reversible ataxia in acute overdosage but there is no doubt that chronic and occasionally acute overdoses of diphenylhydantoin can produce irreversible cerebellar damage.

Carbon monoxide poisoning may produce acute destruction of the cerebellar cortex.

CASE REPORT

An elderly man attempted suicide in a gas oven. He was found and taken to hospital semiconscious. He was given oxygen and within twenty-four hours appeared normal. Ten days later he became acutely ataxic, dysarthric and dysphagic. He was tube fed but his condition deteriorated and he died a few days later. At post mortem the cerebellum had a jelly-like consistency and was completely destroyed.

Malignant disease usually causes metastatic cerebellar disease but cerebellar degeneration complicating carcinomas, and malignant lymphomas *without* direct metastasis does occur—but rather less often than the impression that is sometimes given in discussion. In general a patient with malignant disease who develops cerebellar signs is much more likely to have a metastasis in the cerebellum than a degenerative disorder.

Neoplastic Involvement

Metastatic malignant disease accounts for the majority of cerebellar tumours in the adult. Carcinoma of the lung and breast are usually responsible but a surprisingly high proportion are metastatic from large bowel tumours, particularly those in the descending and recto-sigmoid colon.

Primary tumours are rare although occasionally medulloblastomas may occur in the adult. Primary gliomas are also rare. The most frequent tumour is the benign haemangioblastoma—often a very small vascular nodule associated with a large cyst. The prognosis is excellent although recurrences are quite frequent. Occasionally these tumours produce erythropoietin and are associated with polycythaemia. Extrinsic compression of the cerebellum by acoustic neuromas has been considered in Chapter 6.

Multiple Sclerosis

"Cerebellar" signs in multiple sclerosis are common but in the majority of cases the lesions are in the brain stem cerebellar pathways and the cerebellar signs are almost invariably associated with internuclear ophthalmoplegia, long tract signs and evidence of bilateral pyramidal lesions.

Cerebellar disease can be difficult to diagnose, but having made the diagnosis there are a wide range of diagnostic possibilities. In the adult a very detailed family history and enquiry into drug and alcohol intake is essential. In the child urgent investigation to exclude a tumour should take priority.

DISEASES AFFECTING THE SPINAL CORD

The next three chapters cover diseases affecting the spinal cord. We will consider not only intrinsic disease of the cord, but also damage due to lesions of the spinal cord coverings, the vertebral canal and the spinal cord blood supply.

The subject is dealt with in three main sections and these should ideally be read in sequence for full understanding, as the clinical features are fully described in the first chapter and referred to in subsequent chapters to avoid repetition.

The most important anatomical feature of the spinal cord is rarely appreciated and that is the relationship of the cord to the vertebral column. The cord extends from the foramen magnum to the first lumbar vertebra. Too often, a lesion causing very high cord compression may be missed at myelography if the contrast medium is not followed up to the foramen magnum. At the opposite extreme a lesion below L1 vertebral level *cannot* compress the spinal cord and can only damage the cauda equina. Yet frequently the first investigation performed in a patient with a spastic paraparesis is an X-ray of the lumbar-sacral spine! This also explains why there is no risk of impaling the spinal cord during a lumbar puncture, provided that an interspace below L1/2 level is used. (See also Chapter 25.) These extremely important practical points will all be amplified in later sections.

Chapter 13

THE ANATOMY, PHYSIOLOGY AND CLINICAL FEATURES OF SPINAL CORD DISEASE

PRACTICAL ANATOMY OF THE SPINAL CORD PATHWAYS

1. Motor Pathways (Figure 13.1)

Damage to the motor pathways is the most frequent and easily recognised part of the clinical picture produced by conditions affecting the spinal cord. Clinically, the constellation of findings are known as "pyramidal signs", although it is likely that many of the typical features are produced by damage to non-pyramidal pathways. The main

problem is that with the exception of the vestibulo-spinal tract the exact anatomy of these pathways below cervical level is uncertain. The pyramidal pathway (the cortico-spinal tract) is easily identified in the cord at all levels including the conus.

2. Sensory Pathways (Figures 13.1, 13.2)

The sensory pathways are more complicated than is generally appreciated but for clinical purposes the traditional descriptions still form a useful frame-work for discussion.

Figure 13.1. Touch, Joint Position Sense and Pyramidal Pathways

Figure 13.2. Pain Pathways

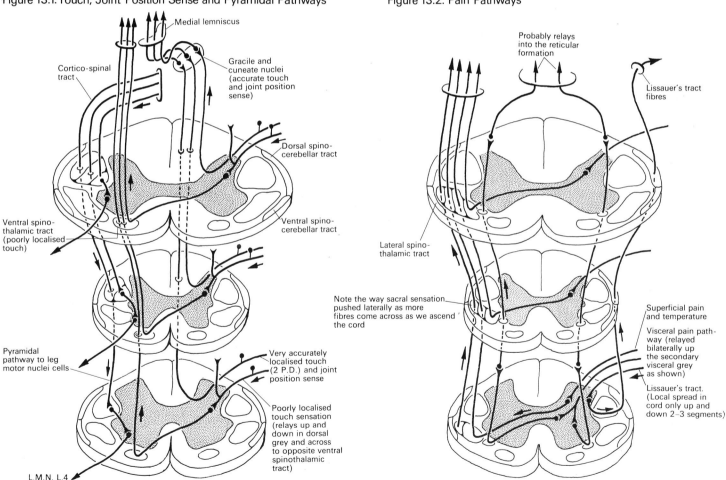

139

a. *Tactile Sensation*. Tactile sense includes accurate localisation of a light touch, two-point discrimination and poorly localised touch sensation. Accurate touch and two-point discrimination (referred to as 2 P.D. in discussion) are relayed to the brain in the gracile (leg) and cuneate (arm) fasciculi on the *same* side of the spinal cord. As the leg fibres enter the cord lower down they are pushed medially as incoming fibres join the cord at higher levels. Clinically the gracile and cuneate fasciculi are referred to as "the dorsal columns", and the sensations conveyed in them as "dorsal column sensation". Poorly localised sense of touch is relayed across the spinal cord to the opposite *ventral* spinothalamic tract and joins the accurate touch pathway, the medial lemniscus, in the brain stem. Because there are two pathways for touch, unless the cord is *totally* transected it is unusual for gross touch sensation to be completely abolished in any form of cord disease.

b. *Joint Position Sense*. Joint position sense (clinically referred to as J.P.S.) is also conveyed in the dorsal columns and is often impaired in cord disease. This only applies to that part of joint position sense that reaches consciousness. Most joint position sense is utilised in the reflex control of posture and is conveyed to the cerebellum via the dorsal and ventral spino-cerebellar pathways. The considerable importance of this insensible joint position information is seen in Friedreich's ataxia, a disease in which the spino-cerebellar pathways degenerate and gross ataxia results.

c. *Vibration Sense*. This is an artificial sensory modality that for many years was thought to be conveyed by the dorsal columns. In recent years considerable doubt has developed and there is much evidence that it is conveyed in several pathways. For this reason impaired vibration sense should not be regarded as specific evidence of a dorsal column lesion.

d. *Pain and Temperature Sensation*. Pain and temperature sensation are traditionally considered together although only one of the several pain pathways also conveys temperature sensation. Pain is conveyed in both fast pathways, allowing immediate and accurate appreciation of a painful stimulus and in slow multi-synaptic pathways which ascend in the central grey matter of the spinal cord. These latter pathways are of great, and yet incompletely understood, importance in several serious and painful clinical disorders including causalgia, the pain that may follow a peripheral nerve lesion.

The classical pain pathway is the lateral spino-thalamic tract and this pathway also carries temperature sensation. Pain afferents enter the spinal cord and ascend two to three segments before they cross the cord anterior to the central canal. This may cause misleading clinical signs. For example,

a lesion at D3 level may damage fibres only from as low as D6, three segments lower down causing false localisation of the level of the lesion. As the fibres cross the cord the lowest entering fibres are progressively pushed laterally as more and more fibres come across the cord at higher levels. Fibres from the lateral spino-thalamic tract may then project back into the central grey matter after crossing the cord. This accounts for the failure of surgical transection of the spino-thalamic tract to completely block pain sensation from the opposite side of the body, especially pain of the deep visceral type. Such pain could only be blocked by complete transection of the cord, clearly not a practical form of treatment! Temperature sensation is also conveyed in this pathway although there is some doubt as to whether the topographical anatomy of the temperature fibres is identical to that of the pain fibres. Hence different sensory levels to pain and temperature sensation may be found when the tract is damaged.

THE SYMPTOMS OF SPINAL CORD DISEASE

Motor Pathway Damage

Lower motor neurone lesions cause wasting and weakness in the appropriate muscle groups. When the spinal cord is damaged the local motor units, arranged as pools of ventral horn cells, are affected. Whether this is clinically detectable depends on the location of the damage. If the damage is at D1 cord level the weakness and wasting of the small hand muscles is readily appreciated by the patient and at L5 level a foot drop can scarcely escape notice. Yet at almost all other levels the damage may pass unrecognised by the patient and only detected by the most diligent examiner. Wasting or fasciculation of the abdominal or intercostal muscles may be difficult or impossible to detect. As a rough generalisation, evidence of a lower motor lesion may be found by the examiner when unnoticed by the patient and this is quite the reverse of an upper motor neurone lesion, in which the patient notices symptoms long before any clinical abnormality can be found.

Damage to the upper motor neurone is usually responsible for the first symptoms of a cord lesion, especially spinal cord compression. The earliest symptom is a subtle stiffening of the legs, often noticed by the patient as a tendency to trip over minor undulations and an inability to walk on rough ground. If the patient attempts to walk quickly or to run the disability is even more pronounced. Patients in England often use the expression "tripping over matchsticks" to describe this symptom. Increasing difficulty in managing stairs, due to weakness of hip flexion and dorsiflexion of the foot, is then noticed. While stepping down a step or kerb spontaneous ankle clonus may occur due to the spasticity of the plantar flexors of the foot. The patient may describe his foot as "vibrating". Finally, it becomes apparent to everyone that the patient's feet are dragging, that he has a peculiar stiff-legged gait, keeps tripping over and is wearing out the toes of his shoes. The whole symptom complex may develop to its full extent over a matter of days in cord compression due to a neoplasm or be prolonged over one or two years in the case of cervical spondylosis or the degenerative condition known as progressive cervical myelopathy. Too often the early symptoms of cord compression or degenerative cord disease are dismissed as normal "ageing" or "arthritis".

It must be stressed that the symptoms of an upper motor neurone lesion may occur long before definite clinical evidence is detectable. It is extremely dangerous to attach facile explanations to such symptoms and the patient should be kept under close observation until the situation is resolved by recovery or the development of physical signs.

The Physical Signs of Motor Pathway Damage

Lower motor neurone lesions are extensively covered in Chapters 16, 18 and 19, and will not be considered further other than to point out that a lower motor neurone lesion causes wasting and weakness of muscles and loss of the local reflex. Therefore if a patient with cord compression presents with bilateral weakness of the legs due to an upper motor neurone lesion, and on examination the triceps muscle on one side is found to be wasted and weak and the triceps jerk absent, there is a strong probability that the compressive lesion is at C7 level.

Upper motor neurone lesions produce the signs of a "pyramidal lesion". The doubtful accuracy of this term has already been mentioned but for clinical purposes it is a useful abbreviation indicating as it does a constellation of symptoms and signs. These signs usually occur in combination and in a sequence which consists of reflex changes, tone changes and weakness developing in specific muscle groups.

In the early stages the reflexes below the level of the lesion are enhanced. This finding is always difficult to evaluate as reflexes are so often enhanced by anxiety. In an extremely anxious patient a few beats of clonus may also occur, further compounding the difficulty. For more certain evidence of a pyramidal lesion one must look to the abdominal reflexes and plantar responses. In the writer's opinion these are two of the most difficult signs in neurology to elicit and interpret. The abdominal reflexes are cutaneous reflexes, elicited by gently stroking the skin over the abdominal wall and observing the contraction of the underlying muscles. In simple terms these reflexes are abolished by an upper motor neu-

rone lesion above D9 level. In practice they are often difficult or impossible to detect in obese, multiparous or multi-scarred abdomens. Only in the young, slim unscathed abdomen can absent abdominal reflexes can be regarded as pathological. The abdominal reflexes are best used as a cross check on a possible extensor plantar response. For example, if the right plantar response appears to be extensor and the right abdominal reflexes are absent and those on the left can be easily elicited this is certain evidence of a pyramidal lesion affecting the cortico-spinal pathway on the right side.

Figure 13.3. Diagram to illustrate the "Babinski" Response

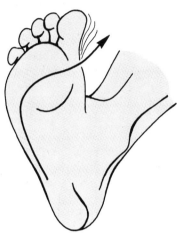

Stimulus must come up the lateral border of the foot and
not touch flexor crease of toes.
not touch big toe at all.
In a classical response the big toe
extends as the stimulus leaves the foot

The plantar responses are often referred to incorrectly as "Babinski's". The Babinski response is the pathological extension of the big toe produced by stroking the sole of the foot. There is no such thing as a "negative" Babinski response. In neurological discussion a Babinski response is frequently referred to as an "up-going toe". The reflex is very difficult to elicit correctly. It is said that a skilled neurologist can make the big toe extend or flex as he wishes and this is certainly true if the examiner wishes to be dishonest! If the very tender palm of the foot is stimulated the big toe will always flex and the whole leg will withdraw. If the stimulus is applied to the lateral side of the foot and then allowed to touch the flexor aspect of any of the toes, especially the big toe, extension of the big toe will be produced, mimicking a Babinski response (see Figure 13.3). The correct way to elicit the reflex is to scrape gently along the lateral border of the sole and then across to the ball of the foot and off *without* touching the toes. The normal response is flexion of the big toe and an abnormal response (a Babinski reflex) is extension of the big toe. What the other toes do is not important, it is usually difficult enough to see which way the big toe is moving without worrying about the movements of the other toes. It is also the *first* movement of the big toe that matters. In patients with extremely sensitive feet the initial normal flexion response is quickly followed by a mass extension of the toes and withdrawal of the entire leg.

These problems have been dealt with at length as many think that an extensor plantar is a very ominous sign in neurological disease and that a flexor plantar virtually excludes neurological disease. Neither view is correct and when one considers the difficulty in performing the test reliably, the potential danger of misdiagnosis is obvious.

As the signs discussed above become established the tone in the affected limbs increases—in clinical parlance, "the limbs become spastic". This term means there is an increased resistance to passive movement of the limbs. Again evaluation may be difficult in a very tense or elderly patient. The elderly, in particular, have great difficulty in relaxing and often try to move the leg to help the examiner. This can make the evaluation of the tone extremely hard work and often quite impossible. The more the patient is asked to relax the more he fights the examiner! A useful trick is to talk to the patient and very gently roll the leg from side to side with a hand placed under the knee and when the leg is rolling freely quickly flick the knee up in the air. The normal leg will passively flex at the knee; a mildly spastic leg will remain stiff and jerk up into the air. Tone in the arm can be tested by holding the patient's hand as if shaking hands and by gently flexing and extending the elbow and wrist joints. It is often easier to detect increased tone in the arm than in the leg.

Tone is increased in those muscles that remain strong; in the arm these are the shoulder adductors, elbow flexors, wrist flexors and finger flexors. The ultimate expression of this tone increase is a stiff flexed arm with flexion contractures of the wrist and hand as seen in patients with chronic spasticity. In the leg the hip extensors, knee extensors and plantar flexors of the foot are affected producing a stiff extended leg with forced plantar flexion of the foot.

At some stage in the development of a pyramidal lesion weakness will appear. The secret of neurological examination in the early stages is knowing where to look for the weakness. Non-neurologists are usually content to test the hand grips and quadriceps muscles and if no weakness is detectable, assume that power is normal. In almost all neurological disorders these two functions are those *least* likely to be affected in the early stages. In a pyramidal lesion the weakness is to be found in the extensor groups in the arm and flexor groups in the leg. This can easily be remembered if

one visualises a patient with a spastic hemiparesis; with a flexed arm and an extended leg, this posture being maintained by the *strong* groups of muscles. A useful screening test for assessing pyramidal function is the ability of the patient to hold his arms extended and to play a piano in mid-air, and then wiggle the toes. Very early pyramidal motor deficit may show as slowing of these movements. The strength in the arms should be tested and it is important to think in terms of movements and not individual muscles. The correct method of testing each group is shown in Chapters 16 and 17. On testing the arm, shoulder abduction, elbow extension, wrist extension and finger abduction (fanning of the fingers) will be weak. In the leg, weakness of the hip flexors, hamstrings and dorsiflexors of the foot will be found.

The patient's gait becomes progressively abnormal. At first there may be a tendency for one or other foot to scrape the ground, later the leg will drag and feel stiff until finally the patient can barely drag one leg past the other.

Sensory Pathway Damage

Radicular or root symptoms occur at the level of a spinal cord lesion especially in the diseases that affect the dorsal roots. These are very important symptoms as they often indicate the level of the disease process extremely accurately. Radicular or root symptoms are readily recognised when they occur in the arm or the leg but when they occur in the thoracic dermatomes this possibility is often completely forgotten. Cardiac, respiratory or intra-abdominal disease may be suspected and serious diagnostic errors may be made. The sensations produced may vary widely from a dull ache in the affected dermatome to a severe knife-like pain; from a warm glow to a sensation like an icy cold bandage around the area. Sometimes soreness or hypersensitivity of the affected area may be described, likened by the patient to "the skin feels as if sandpapered". The important clue is that the pain extends round from the back and along an identifiable dermatome. The description and the localisation of the pain should make recognition possible.

Damage to the central pathways also results in typical, but variable symptoms. Dorsal column damage causes fine tingling paraesthesiae in the extremities below the level of the lesion. At times these assume a vibrating quality that may be likened to touching an electric typewriter or the vibration felt when standing on the deck of a ship. Dorsal column damage also seems to be responsible for the well-known "band sensations". These are feelings described by the patient as if a cold bandage were being pulled tight around the thorax or abdomen, or at the knee and ankle joints. Related disorders of touch and joint position sense produce feelings as if the skin were too tight or as if the skin were covered with a thick layer of cotton wool or encased in plaster.

Spino-thalamic pathway damage causes altogether different and extremely unpleasant symptoms. The earliest symptom of damage consists of very deep, poorly localised aching pain with a nagging quality. The description may be likened to "being kicked in the shin", "as if the flesh were being torn from the bones", "as if my bones were on fire" or "icicles being stuck in my leg". These are entirely typical descriptions and yet because they are somewhat bizarre, the patient is often suspected of malingering. These are often the earliest symptoms of an intrinsic spinal cord tumour and the average delay between first symptoms and diagnosis of an intrinsic cord tumour is over four years, much of this delay being due to the failure to recognise the organicity of such symptoms.

Superficial spino-thalamic abnormalities may also occur. The patient may describe a feeling as if warm or icy water were trickling over the surface of the limb or as if the whole limb had turned into a block of ice. Patients rarely complain that an area has gone "numb". When patients use this expression they nearly always mean the heavy sensation that occurs when a limb is *weak*. This is a descriptive term that should never be accepted as indicating sensory loss until the meaning has been carefully discussed with the patient and if necessary after careful examination to exclude sensory loss

has been performed. Perhaps the most frequently encountered example of this is in the case of Bell's Palsy. This is a purely motor disturbance of movement of one side of the face and yet repeatedly patients will say that the side of the face feels "numb", when they really mean the stiff sensation on the weak side of the face.

Signs of Sensory Pathway Damage

Some of the finer points of sensory examination are best discussed in the next chapter on clinical disorders of the cord. We will confine ourselves at this stage to a few general points.

Because there are dual sensory pathways a casual examination of the "can you feel me touching your leg" type rarely has any value. In fact, one might as well dispense with sensory testing altogether! It is worth remembering that as a general rule patients often have sensory symptoms in the absence of detectable sensory signs whereas motor signs are often found in the absence of motor symptoms. Therefore if there are no sensory symptoms it is unlikely that any sensory signs will be detectable. There are important exceptions to this.

When testing pain sensation it is important to test *pain*. This is *not* a printing error! In conditions specifically affecting pain sensation, touch sensation is preserved. Unless such patients happen to cut or burn themselves by accident they may be quite unaware of extensive areas of loss of pain sensation. During testing the patient must be aware of *both* the touch of the pin *and* the pain produced by it.

Accurate temperature sense testing is virtually impossible on a routine basis and is rarely necessary as temperature loss will not be found if pain appreciation is normal.

Vibration sense has limited clinical value, not only because of the anatomical uncertainty of the pathways involved but also because most patients over 60 have impaired vibration sense to the knees. Vibration sense testing is really only of value in young persons suspected of having multiple sclerosis who often lose vibration sense and in any patient suspected of suffering from a peripheral neuropathy. In peripheral neuropathy vibration sense may be one of the earliest modalities to be impaired (see Chapter 16).

Joint position sense testing is a quick and useful test of dorsal column function. Technique is very important. The terminal inter-phalangeal joint of either the finger or toe being tested should be held at the sides and the tip of the digit in the same way. It is wrong to hold the tip of the digit by the nail and pulp. This provides a push/pull stimulus and will give a clue as to the direction of movement. If the finger or toe is held at the sides, *only* the joint movement can be

Figure 13.4. Diagram to show normal dermatomes
(For comparison with Figure 13.5)

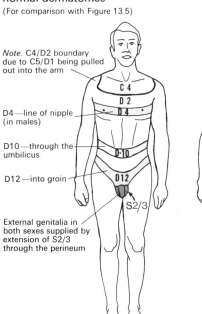

Note. C4/D2 boundary due to C5/D1 being pulled out into the arm

D4 —line of nipple (in males)

D10 —through the umbilicus

D12 —into groin

External genitalia in both sexes supplied by extension of S2/3 through the perineum

Figure 13.5. Diagram to show "physiological" sensory levels

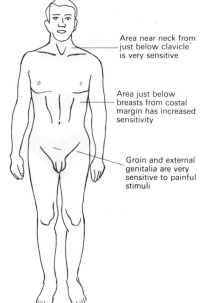

Area near neck from just below clavicle is very sensitive

Area just below breasts from costal margin has increased sensitivity

Groin and external genitalia are very sensitive to painful stimuli

detected. It is usually worth showing the patient what is required with his eyes open and then going on to do the formal test with the eyes closed or averted. Very small movements over a range of 1 mm. should be detectable at the fingers and larger movements of 3–4 mm. at the toes. With severe impairment even movements of the wrist and ankle joints may not be detected by the patient.

Finally, a note on sensory levels. As will be seen in later sections, it is important to search for a level below which cutaneous sensation is impaired. One can only do this with a good appreciation of the various physiological sensory levels that exist. These are indicated in Figure 13.5. It will be seen that these occur at the groin, the costal margin and just below the clavicle. It is very easy to mistake these physiological transitions to more sensitive areas of the body as sensory levels if one is not aware of their existence.

Chapter 14

METABOLIC, INFECTIVE AND VASCULAR DISORDERS

In many textbooks the discussion of spinal cord disease centres around conditions such as tabes dorsalis and sub-acute combined degeneration of the cord. These conditions are now so rare that to base a whole chapter on them would not be representative of either their frequency or the author's familiarity with these conditions. In this chapter we will consider cord disorders in order of clinical importance. Certainly the most frequently encountered spinal cord disease at this time is the rather poorly understood condition known as progressive cervical myelopathy, which in some instances may be associated with cervical spondylosis. Cord lesions related to fracture dislocations of the spine are covered in Chapter 23.

Progressive Cervical Myelopathy

This condition may be encountered in either sex, usually between the ages of 30 and 70. In fact, it is a negative diagnosis; it is the label attached to those patients who have a clinical picture suggestive of compression of the cervical spinal cord with negative myelographic studies and nothing in the history or cerebro-spinal fluid to enable a diagnosis of multiple sclerosis to be made. The condition may be an abortive or localised form of spinal cord demyelination occurring in an older age group and occasional patients may go on to develop other manifestations to suggest that this is a mild form of multiple sclerosis.

Typically the patient attends hospital with the symptoms of a mild to moderately severe paraparesis. In most instances there are no sensory symptoms and bladder function is unimpaired. The signs are often confined to the motor system and in general all reflexes are brisk and both plantar responses are extensor, but the weakness is confined to the legs. Weakness of the arms is a late and minor problem if the arms become involved at all. In the older patients in this group physiological loss of vibration sense to the knees may be an additional feature and the only sensory finding.

One of the main diagnostic problems is the role of cervical spondylosis. In this older age group about half the patients would be expected to have a moderate degree of cervical spondylosis and whether this is playing a role in patho-genesis is a debatable point. There is little doubt that cervical spondylosis may cause cervical cord compression and in any patient with a complete block on myelography decom-

pressive surgery is indicated, and occasionally beneficial. With lesser degrees of spondylosis operation is usually unhelpful. In these instances, rather than regarding surgery as a failure, it is probably more accurate to accept that the diagnosis was incorrect in the first instance. For the same reason there is no convincing evidence that the use of a cervical collar has any beneficial effect in these patients and in many instances the added discomfort seems to make them less able to cope with the problems presented by the paraparesis. In the author's opinion myelography should always be performed for reasons exemplified by the following two case reports.

CASE REPORT

A 53-year-old man developed a slowly progressive paraparesis over two years. There were no signs to indicate damage to the nervous system outside the spinal cord. His plain cervical spine x-rays were normal and myelography was performed with consider-able reluctance. Complete spinal block at C7 was demonstrated and was due to a neuro-fibroma. Surgery cured all his symptoms.

CASE REPORT

A 58-year-old woman had been observed in the neurology clinic for nearly three years as a case of cervical spondylosis with myelopathy. On routine review it was felt that the spondylosis was relatively mild as judged from the plain x-rays and that the signs were those of a spastic tetraparesis with fine lateral nystagmus and a very brisk jaw jerk, suggestive of a very high cord compression. Myelography was therefore performed and a meningioma in the foramen magnum was demonstrated.

However skilled the clinician there are *no* clinical features that allow confident exclusion of spinal cord compression to be made on clinical grounds alone. Myelography is man-datory even if one is then left with the rather unsatisfactory diagnostic label of progressive cervical myelopathy. (Myelopathy due to cervical spondylosis is discussed in greater detail in the next chapter.)

Multiple Sclerosis (Figure 14.1)

In Europe and North America multiple sclerosis is another frequent cause of spinal cord disease. As in the case of progressive cervical myelopathy the clinical picture may be indistinguishable from spinal cord compression and often

PATHOLOGICAL ANATOMY OF CORD LESIONS

Figure 14.4. Sub-acute Combined Degeneration of the Cord

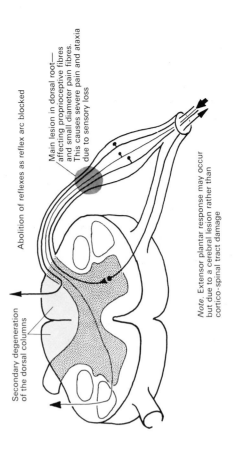

Peripheral nerve symptoms dominate the early picture with ataxia later due to sensory loss. Extensor plantar response but absent reflexes due to peripheral nerve damage

Cortico-spinal tract lesion

Dorsal column degeneration

Peripheral nerve damage

Figure 14.5. Tabes Dorsalis

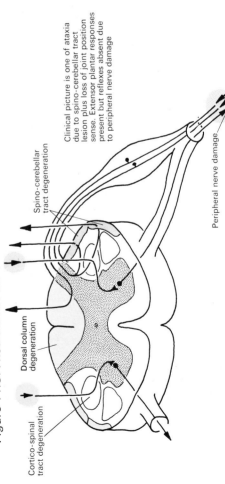

Main lesion in dorsal root—affecting proprioceptive fibres and small diameter pain fibres. This causes severe pain and ataxia due to sensory loss

Abolition of reflexes as reflex arc blocked

Secondary degeneration of the dorsal columns

Note. Extensor plantar response may occur but due to a cerebral lesion rather than cortico-spinal tract damage

Figure 14.1. Multiple Sclerosis

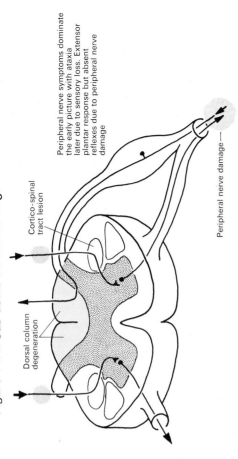

Dorsal column lesion causes tingling paraesthesiae in all limbs—to loss of J.P.S. causing ataxia

Cortico-spinal tract lesion

Mixed lesion causes weak spastic legs and deep unpleasant spino-thalamic sensations or sensory loss

Spinothalamic tract lesion

These are the tracts usually affected

Dorsal column lesion

Figure 14.2. Motor Neurone Disease

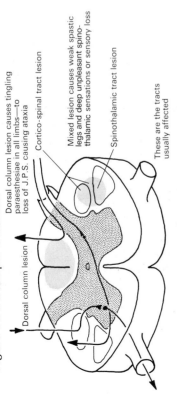

Cortico-spinal tract degeneration

Whether U.M.N. or L.M.N. dominates depends on type (see text). A useful guide to this diagnosis is the preservation of reflexes in the presence of wasting and weakness

Loss of ventral horn cells

Figure 14.3. Friedreich's Ataxia

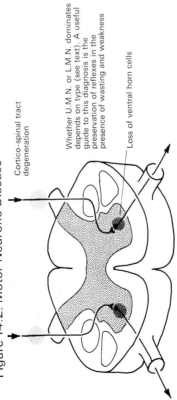

Spino-cerebellar tract degeneration

Clinical picture is one of ataxia due to spino-cerebellar tract lesion plus loss of joint position sense. Extensor plantar responses present but reflexes absent due to peripheral nerve damage

Cortico-spinal tract degeneration

Dorsal column degeneration

Peripheral nerve damage

myelographic exclusion of this possibility is necessary. This is always a difficult decision to take because there is little doubt that occasionally myelography may lead to a rapid and disastrous deterioration in patients with multiple sclerosis. Yet the reverse situation is equally tragic. On one occasion in one ward of a neurological hospital there were three patients with paraplegias and severe bed sores. None had had myelography because a confident clinical diagnosis of multiple sclerosis had been made. All three had subsequently been shown to have operable compressive spinal cord lesions, unfortunately inoperable by the time the lesion was demonstrated. Some neurologists would argue that examination of the C.S.F. alone is adequate; however, not only is the C.S.F. diagnostic only in some twenty per cent of patients with multiple sclerosis, but in many patients with cord compression the C.S.F. and manometric studies are normal so that compressive lesions cannot be excluded. It is probably best to run the risks of myelography if cord compression seems a possible diagnosis. There are three types of clinical presentation of cord lesions in multiple sclerosis. In order of severity these are (a) the "neuropathic" type, (b) sub-acute cord compression type and (c) acute transverse myelitis.

a. "Neuropathic" Type

In this type sensory symptoms predominate and consist of fine, tingling peripheral parasthesia. These may be spontaneous or provoked by touch. They are identical to the symptoms occurring at the onset of peripheral neuropathy. Numbness is minimal and the patients complain that there is no actual numbness, but that the tingle seems to blot out normal sensation. When touched by the examiner the patients often have difficulty in describing exactly what is abnormal about the sensation. They may say that they can feel, but it feels as if there is a layer of cotton wool between the touch and the skin. These feelings will usually be confined to the distal arms and legs and do not involve the area around the mouth. This is an important differential diagnostic point when the differential diagnosis between multiple sclerosis of this type and the symptoms of hyperventilation are being considered (see Chapter 22). Occasionally these symptoms are associated with other evidences of minimal cord damage, such as micturition disturbance or stiffness of the legs. Very often the picture is exclusively sensory. The clue to the diagnosis often lies in the reflexes. Patients who have peripheral sensations of this type due to peripheral neuropathy will have decreased or absent reflexes and usually well-marked peripheral sensory loss. In multiple sclerosis the reflexes are not only preserved but are almost invariably extremely brisk, often the abdominal reflexes are absent and the plantar responses are extensor,

even in those patients without definite motor symptoms. If there is any sensory deficit it is often loss of vibration sense to the level of the costal margins, even though the symptoms are confined to the periphery. The patients' own comments on how they feel are also very instructive and important in this disorder. In the author's opinion hyperventilation syndrome is the most important differential diagnosis. This occurs in anxious patients and produces tingling parasthesia in all four limbs and the reflexes are usually brisk because of the anxiety. Pathological reflexes are not present and the patients often complain of tingling and numbness around the mouth. Patients who read about multiple sclerosis in the press often get anxious and promptly produce these symptoms, reinforcing their own view that they have this disorder! The prognosis for multiple sclerosis of this type is really very good and although these symptoms may continue for months the symptoms usually remit without sequelae although motor signs, if present, tend to persist. The picture is very much a feature of young patients with multiple sclerosis in the 18 to 30 age group and often marks the onset of the disease.

b. Sub-acute Cord Compression Type

This picture is very similar to progressive cervical myelopathy and there is reason to suspect that in some cases the latter condition is actually a variant of multiple sclerosis, occurring in an older age group. In some patients, often with evidence of multiple sclerosis in other areas of the central nervous system and with a history of previous attacks of the disease, a slow decline in walking occurs, often affecting one leg and later both legs over a period of months to years. There are few sensory symptoms and the picture is essentially an asymmetrical progressive spastic paraparesis. In the absence of previous attacks of multiple sclerosis myelography is indicated. If the diagnosis of multiple sclerosis is to be made on clinical grounds alone the history and evidence of previous attacks of multiple sclerosis *should be conclusive*. It is not sufficient to query a little nystagmus or question pallor of an optic disc. In this group myelography does not seem to carry as much risk and it is in this slightly older age group (30–50) that other lesions are most likely to occur. The possibility of making a serious error is at its greatest in this type. It is often the relentless progression of this particular clinical picture that leads to significant disability and eventually a wheelchair existence for patients with multiple sclerosis, although a period of four to five years may elapse before the disability is fully developed.

c. Acute Transverse Myelitis

This type is in every way the most difficult and the most

serious presentation of spinal cord demyelination. The clinical picture is identical to acute cord transection. The onset is abrupt and causes a stage of spinal shock. There is an acute flaccid paralysis of the lower limbs with retention of urine. A sensory level can usually be demonstrated and the onset is often marked by quite severe pain, in and around the chest or abdomen at the level of the lesion. This pain may be so severe as to mimic a myocardial infarction or an intra-abdominal catastrophe and it is only a few hours later that the paraplegia occurs. If the condition occurs in a setting of known multiple sclerosis, if, for example, a past history of retro-bulbar neuritis can be obtained, myelography is unnecessary. If it is the first episode of multiple sclerosis myelography *must* be performed *immediately*, as if this picture *is* due to a compressive lesion, immediate surgery is indicated, and even then the prognosis is poor. However, it is in this group that the myelography carries the greatest risk. There may be a dramatic worsening of the clinical picture with involvement of other areas of the nervous system in the hours following negative myelography if acute transverse myelitis due to multiple sclerosis proves to be the diagnosis.

In some patients, especially children, an attack of acute transverse myelitis may be associated with simultaneous or delayed bilateral retro-bulbar neuritis. This combination is known as Devic's disease and appears to be a sub-variant of multiple sclerosis, in which further attacks are extremely unusual and remarkably complete recovery is the rule.

Motor Neurone Disease (Figure 14.2)

Motor neurone disease can produce a variety of clinical pictures as it is a process which affects both the ventral horn cells and the upper motor neurone. Hence some patients may have overwhelming evidence of a lower motor neurone lesion while others develop a purely upper motor neurone picture with a spastic paraparesis simulating cord compression. In the classical variety a mixture of both upper and lower motor neurone lesions produces the picture known as amyotrophic lateral sclerosis. Typically, in this condition the hands are affected first by progressive wasting and weakness with evidence of a mild spastic paraparesis in the legs. This picture may closely simulate the findings in cervical spondylosis and as this is a disease of the older age group the co-existence of cervical spondylosis often presents diagnostic problems. In some cases the co-existence of lumbar and cervical spondylosis may further confuse the picture by producing root symptoms and areas of sensory loss in the leg or hands. As the disease has a fatal prognosis it is always vital to absolutely exclude other diagnostic possibilities and if possible confirm the diagnosis with electromyographic studies.

Familial Spastic Paraplegia

This is a relatively rare condition causing spastic paraplegia. It is inherited either as a dominant or recessive gene. The recessive variety tends to have an earlier onset (7–10 years of age) and runs a more severe course, whereas the dominant type often starts after the age of 20 and has a benign course. Even those cases that start in childhood tend to have a slower course if they are inherited in a dominant way. The disease is progressive and starts in the legs; arm involvement is late and relatively minor. Significant bladder involvement is very unusual and would be strong evidence against this diagnosis. Furthermore, although called a "paraplegia" in fact, "spastic" is the dominant feature. The patient's power is often near normal but it is the gross spasticity of the extensor groups that is so disabling. Not only are the legs rigid, adducted and plantar flexed, but the active muscles have to overcome the spasticity in order to move the limbs, hence the very peculiar dragging type of gait, the patient often appearing to be about to topple forwards as he drags one leg past the other. The reflexes are very brisk but in some patients the spasticity is so great that the reflexes cannot be elicited at all and are incorrectly documented as being absent. The plantar responses are strongly extensor and often the big toe wears a hole in the top of the patient's shoes, due to its permanently extended position, even at rest. The abdominal reflexes are very often preserved and this coupled with normal bladder function is an almost certain indication that a spastic paraplegia is of the familial type. Sensory loss does occur, but is usually a late feature and invariably takes the form of joint position sense loss. Relatively few patients become confined to a wheel chair and most are able to cope with surprisingly severe disabilities and hold down a job or run normal households, for the bulk of their lives.

Friedreich's Ataxia (Figure 14.3)

For completeness it is worth including Friedreich's ataxia in this section although extensive damage to peripheral nerves and brainstem pathways also occurs. The disease is familial and usually inherited as a recessive. In a given family the age of onset is usually constant and ranges from 8 to 16 years of age. Similarly the clinical picture may be extremely variable but usually constant for that family. At birth a high arched foot with hammer toes may be present; this is known as "Friedreich's foot" and may also be found in family members who do *not* develop a full-blown picture and is then regarded as "forme fruste" of the disease. The pathological lesions are widespread and include the spino-cerebellar pathways, depriving the cerebellum of joint position sense information and causing the ataxia which is a constant feature of the illness. The other lesion that dominates the physical signs is the damage to the peripheral nerves and total absence of reflexes (areflexia) is a constant finding. The plantar responses are usually extensor, presumably due to damage to the cortico-spinal pathways, but the reflexes are unable to become brisk as they are abolished by the peripheral nerve damage. This is one of several conditions that can cause this combination of absent reflexes and extensor plantar responses.

Sub-Acute Combined Degeneration of the Spinal Cord (Figure 14.4)

This is a metabolic disease due to vitamin B_{12} deficiency and/or folate intoxication. It was a frequent complication of pernicious anaemia before liver or B_{12} treatment were available, but in recent years has become a rare condition, with the early recognition and treatment of pernicious anaemia. Nevertheless, patients may present in the neurological clinic with this condition and it is always worth considering this possibility in the differential diagnosis of patients with cord lesions. However, the symptoms that dominate the early picture are almost certainly related to damage to the peripheral nerves rather than the spinal cord. Symptomatically fine tingling peripheral parasthesiae are the first manifestation and are the symptoms most likely to respond to Vitamin B_{12} therapy. Loss of reflexes is the main motor feature and could not be caused by the lesion in the dorsal columns. The areflexia is thought to be due to the coexistent peripheral nerve damage. The first evidence of the cord lesion is the appearance of extensor plantar responses. As in the case of Friedreich's ataxia, the development of the upper motor neurone lesion cannot cause brisk reflexes as they are already abolished by the peripheral nerve damage. In a full-blown case subsequent degeneration of the corticospinal tract and dorsal columns leads to paraplegia in addition to the peripheral weakness and very severe ataxia due to loss of joint position sense. There is also considerable difficulty with bladder function due to loss of bladder reflexes and the patient's sense of bladder fullness. The bladder problems are discussed in Chapter 15. The cord damage is not significantly benefited by Vitamin B_{12} therapy and may be made dramatically worse if folic acid is given instead of B_{12}. It is therefore essential to diagnose the condition before significant cord damage has occurred and Vitamin B_{12} studies should be performed routinely in any patient with peripheral parasthesiae or absent reflexes. Note that this is another condition in which absent reflexes are coupled with extensor plantar responses. Paradoxically there is increasing evidence that an identical clinical picture can be caused by folate deficiency.

Tabes Dorsalis (Figure 14.5)

This classical neurological disorder has become an exceedingly rare disease. This is undoubtedly due to better epidemiological control and effective treatment of syphilis. The exact relationship of the disease to the syphilitic process has never been established although the relationship is an undoubted one. Spirochaetes have not been demonstrated in the dorsal roots or dorsal columns and typically the disorder occurs some ten or twenty years after the primary infection, often at a time when other evidence suggests that the disease is "burnt out". Negative serological tests in the blood were often found in the days before more specific testing for treponemal anti-bodies. The lesion initially affects the dorsal roots and damages the dorsal columns as a secondary phenomena. The pain fibres seem to be particularly vulnerable and the classical "lightning" pains of this disorder, which are described as "electric-shock" like sensations, usually in the distribution of the sciatic nerve, are probably due to damage to these pathways. Later loss of deep pain sensation occurs and the patient's Achilles tendon or testis can be squeezed without producing any discomfort. As the root damage continues the reflex arc is blocked and loss of reflexes occurs. This also leads to considerable hypotonicity of the muscles. This combination of extreme hypotonicity, allowing an excess range of joint movement, coupled with loss of deep pain sensation, is thought to be responsible for the progressive joint destruction known as "Charcot's joints". Completely painless destruction and dislocation of both the knee and ankle joints, can occur. In the later stages of the disease severe secondary degeneration of the dorsal columns leads to virtual abolition of joint position sense. The patient then complains that he cannot feel his feet hitting the ground and feels as if he is walking on cotton wool. He develops a high stepping gait to avoid tripping over, and has no awareness of the position of his legs. This problem is greatly accentuated in the dark or with the eyes closed and is the basis of one of the classical tests in neurology:

Romberg's Test

When anyone stands with their eyes shut, they sway slightly—this has the effect of increasing the sensory input to the cerebellum. In cerebellar disease this swaying is greatly accentuated and the patient may swing wildly from side to side, but will not fall. In the presence of gross posture sense loss, while standing with the eyes open, the patient is perfectly stable, but the moment the patient shuts his eyes he will fall as he is suddenly deprived of all sensory input. Romberg's test is therefore more a test of dorsal column disease rather than cerebellar disease.

In the majority of patients with tabes dorsalis there are also evidences of disease elsewhere. Nearly all patients have Argyll–Robertson pupils and many have optic atrophy with peripheral visual field loss. Damage to the upper motor neurone is revealed by extensor plantar responses (again the reflexes cannot become brisk because they are already abolished by the root damage). If extensor plantar responses are present it is presumed that long tract damage has occurred and the condition is then known as taboparesis. This is the third condition that may cause this combination of absent reflexes and extensor plantar responses.

Radiation Myelopathy

This is a subject of considerable and increasing importance. It is almost exclusively a complication of radiation to the thorax, particularly that directed at the bronchi or oesophagus, rather than the smaller doses used in treatment of the mediastinal lymph nodes, in Hodgkins' disease. Better techniques with rotating portals can do little to limit the dose received by the cord when the oesophagus is irradiated as it lies in the centre of the field. The critical dose may be as low as 1,800 rads. Characteristically, there is a nine- to eighteen-month delay before the onset of the cord damage. Sensory symptoms are prominent with spino-thalamic sensory loss coupled with a mild spastic paraparesis. It is difficult to distinguish from rapidly developing cord compression due to metastatic disease unless sensory symptoms dominate the early picture which is very unusual in cord compression as discussed later. This provides an important clue to the diagnosis of radiation myelopathy. The distinction is extremely important as further radiation directed at a presumed metastasis carries the serious risk of worsening the situation if radiation myelopathy is the actual diagnosis.

Finally, we must consider the important differences between the diseases listed above with intrinsic tumours of the spinal cord and spinal cord compression.

1. SPINAL CORD COMPRESSION

Spinal cord compression may be caused by lesions arising on the nerve roots, the coverings of the spinal cord, in the extra-dural fat or from lesions of the vertebral column itself. At this stage we will consider only the features of the history and the clinical signs that suggest that the patient is suffering from spinal cord compression.

The clinical feature of cord compression that must be emphasised is that the symptoms and signs are dominated by motor pathway damage. The reasons for this are not entirely clear, but may be related to the blood supply of the spinal cord and in particular to the venous drainage. This is discussed in more detail later in this chapter, but basically any impairment of venous drainage will tend to lead to oedema and poor capillary circulation in the watershed zone of the spinal cord, which includes the cortico-spinal pathways. The earliest symptoms are those of a mild spastic paraparesis. The patient may complain of slight dragging of the feet and heaviness of the legs as described in the previous chapter. These symptoms may develop over a period of months in some instances or in a matter of hours in the case of acute lesions and occasionally instantaneously. Impending irreversible cord damage is indicated by either the onset of micturition disturbance or sensory symptoms. Difficulty in initiating micturition or urinary retention may occur quite suddenly, and usually indicates that rapidly progressive deterioration is about to occur. Sensory symptoms have a similar significance and may start as a tingling sensation in the soles of the feet which then ascends. This may reach a fixed level in a matter of hours or advance slowly over several days. In either event it is unwise to delay action until the level becomes fixed.

In summary therefore, spinal cord compression is dominated in the early stages by motor symptoms and signs and the onset of sensory features heralds a phase of rapid deterioration leading to irreversible cord damage. The clinical sequence and signs at the various stages are summarised in Figure 14.6.

2. INTRINSIC TUMOURS OF THE SPINAL CORD

The clinical history and signs of an intrinsic lesion in the spinal cord are quite the reverse of cord compression. The anatomical feature that determines the sequence of events is the course of the pain and temperature pathways in the central spinal cord. These are the fibres most likely to be damaged in the early stages. Initially, a lesion in the central spinal cord (ependymoma, glioma or syringomyelic cavity) will irritate and destroy pain and temperature fibres as they cross the cord, but *only* at the level of the lesion.

No long tract damage can occur at this stage so that a narrow segment of pain and temperature loss is produced. The pain is of deep spino-thalamic type, but the sensory loss may not be detected unless pain sensation is carefully tested. Occasionally, a patient accidentally discovers the sensory loss when he drops a lighted cigarette on the skin or notices an area of impaired sensation while bathing in warm water.

Later as the lesion extends laterally the reflex arc is blocked and the reflexes disappear. This rarely produces any symptoms as far as the patient is concerned, but any patient with

Figure 14.6. Cord Compression (A lesion at D9 on left side is shown)

Note. Although sensory loss is shown developing in sequence, it must be stressed that in most cases the motor signs dominate the clinical picture

A
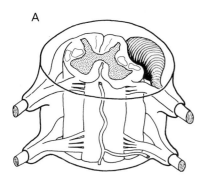

A neurofibroma on the left D.9. dorsal root is shown

The root is irritated causing root pain at D9

B
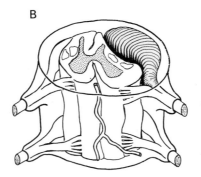

The cord is now seriously distorted and definite sensory loss occurs in the root zone and in the opposite spinothalamic distribution

C
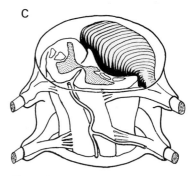

The terminal stage of cord compression has been reached. Total paralysis of the legs with rapidly ascending sensory loss occurs

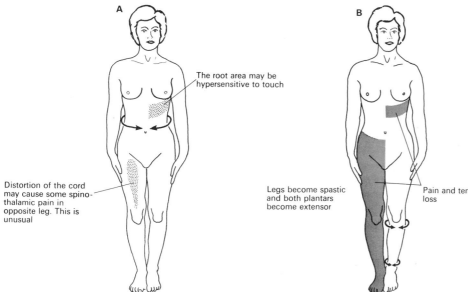

A

The root area may be hypersensitive to touch

Distortion of the cord may cause some spino-thalamic pain in opposite leg. This is unusual

Root pain may be worse on coughing
Tight band or cold bands around abdomen noticed
May be some deep pain in opposite limb
No sensory loss may be detected
Leg reflexes may be brisk
Plantar may be extensor
May be urinary urgency

B
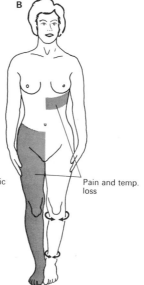

Legs become spastic and both plantars become extensor

Pain and temp. loss

Root area now numb
Band sensations in legs occur
Opposite leg may feel "different"
Partial Brown-Séquard lesion
Radicular loss of sensation
Pain and temp. loss in opposite leg
(May be some joint position sense loss on same side)
Legs now spastic and weak
Reflexes brisk. Plantars extensor
May be marked sphincter upset

C
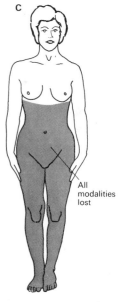

All modalities lost

Final stage—may be acute after long stage A and B or can go from A—C over a matter of hours
Sensory level to *all* modalities to level of lesion
Flaccid, areflexic paralysis in spinal shock phase.
Reflexes often *increased* above the level of transection

Figure 14.7. Development of a Central Cord Lesion

This picture would be seen in syringomyelia, ependymoma, and intrinsic glioma
or astrocytoma. The progress of the signs
relates directly to degree of involvement
shown in the cord sections

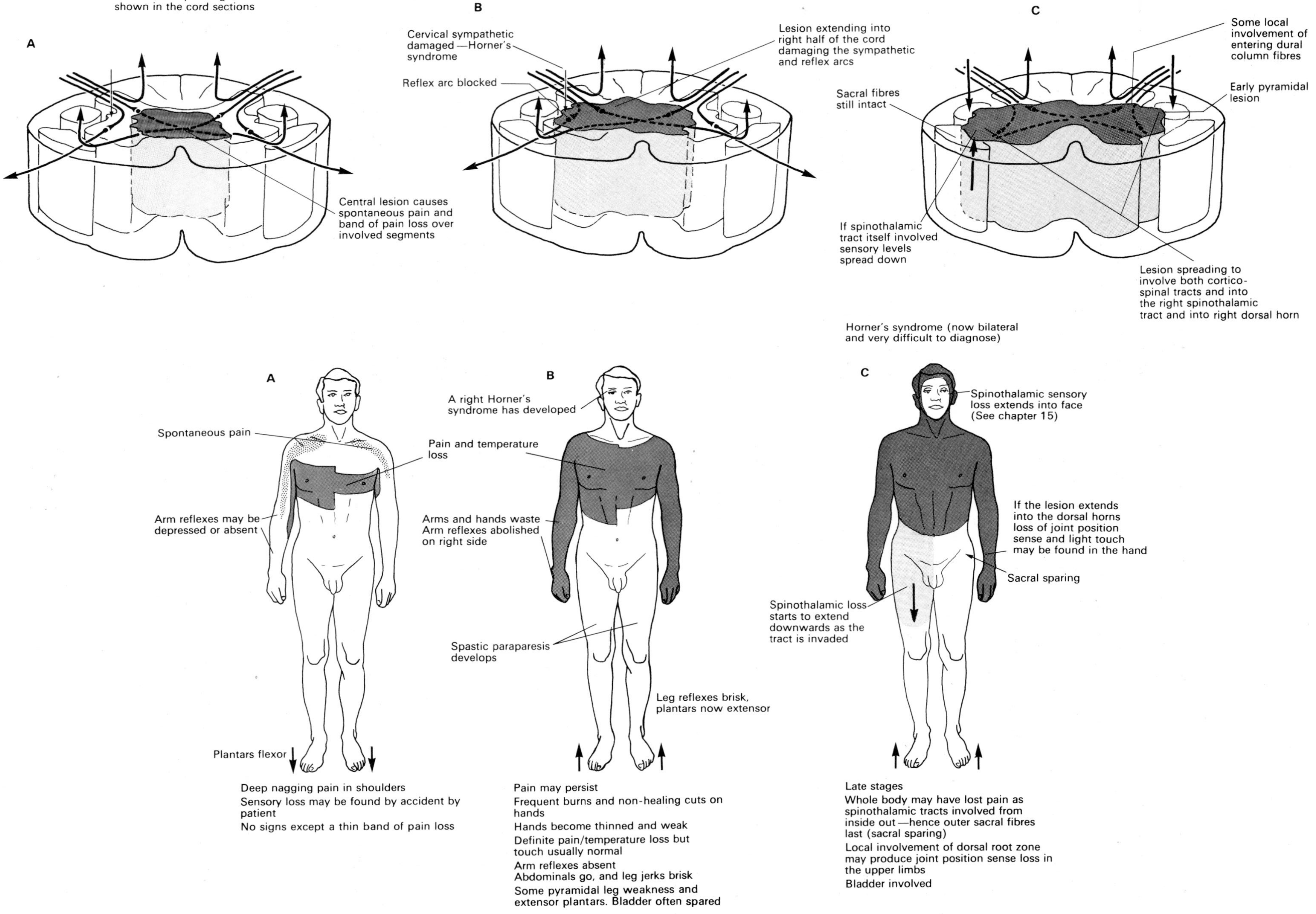

A

Some local
involvement of
entering dural
column fibres

Early pyramidal
lesion

Lesion extending into
right half of the cord
damaging the sympathetic
and reflex arcs

Cervical sympathetic
damaged—Horner's
syndrome

Reflex arc blocked

Central lesion causes
spontaneous pain and
band of pain loss over
involved segments

B

Lesion spreading to
involve both cortico-
spinal tracts and into
the right spinothalamic
tract and into right dorsal horn

Sacral fibres
still intact

If spinothalamic
tract itself involved
sensory levels
spread down

C

Horner's syndrome (now bilateral
and very difficult to diagnose)

Spinothalamic sensory
loss extends into face
(See chapter 15)

If the lesion extends
into the dorsal horns
loss of joint position
sense and light touch
may be found in the hand

Sacral sparing

Spinothalamic loss
starts to extend
downwards as the
tract is invaded

Late stages
Whole body may have lost pain as
spinothalamic tracts involved from
inside out—hence outer sacral fibres
last (sacral sparing)
Local involvement of dorsal root zone
may produce joint position sense loss in
the upper limbs
Bladder involved

A

Spontaneous pain

Deep nagging pain in shoulders
Sensory loss may be found by accident by
patient
No signs except a thin band of pain loss

Arm reflexes may be
depressed or absent

Plantars flexor

B

A right Horner's
syndrome has developed

Pain and temperature
loss

Arms and hands waste
Arm reflexes abolished
on right side

Spastic paraparesis
develops

Leg reflexes brisk,
plantars now extensor

Pain may persist
Frequent burns and non-healing cuts on
hands
Hands become thinned and weak
Definite pain/temperature loss but
touch usually normal
Arm reflexes absent
Abdominals go, and leg jerks brisk
Some pyramidal leg weakness and
extensor plantars. Bladder often spared

spino-thalamic symptoms should be carefully checked for loss of reflexes. Reflex loss applies only to lesions affecting the standard reflex arcs in the arms and the legs. In the cervical cord the sympathetic will be affected at this stage producing a unilateral or bilateral Horner's syndrome. If the lesion extends into the anterior horn cells focal wasting and weakness may appear, typically affecting the small muscles of the hand. The location of these new signs will depend on the site of the lesion. If the lesion is in the mid-thoracic cord, it is very unlikely that the patient will notice wasting and weakness of individual intercostal muscles, although this should certainly be looked for in a patient with spino-thalamic symptoms in the thoracic region. It is only when the cord becomes expanded that the long tracts become involved. This may take several years. Bilateral pyramidal signs then appear with brisk reflexes in the legs and extensor plantar responses. The inner part of the spino-thalamic tract may be damaged causing descending spino-thalamic sensory loss. In the final stages of the process only the peripheral fibres carrying sensation from the sacral area will survive and the patient develops what is known as sacral sparing, a rare but diagnostic feature of an intrinsic lesion of the spinal cord. The dorsal columns seem very resistant to infiltration by tumours and in general dorsal column signs are a late feature of intrinsic lesions. The sequence and anatomical correlation of the signs at various stages are illustrated in Figure 14.7.

THE BLOOD SUPPLY OF THE SPINAL CORD
(Figure 14.8)

The spinal cord is not supplied by segmental arteries or by a continuous vessel running down its length. There is a fairly constant territorial distribution of blood supply in the transverse plane. The central area is supplied by the sulcal arteries which are given off alternately from each side of the anterior spinal artery which lies in the ventral sulcus of the cord. The anterior spinal artery also gives off circumferential arteries which lie on the surface of the cord forming a surface plexus by anastomosing with branches of the posterior spinal arteries and supplying the periphery of the cord. The paired posterior spinal arteries form a plexus over the dorsal columns, which they supply. The posterior spinal arteries are less defined than the anterior spinal artery, although even this vessel may be incomplete and often peters out at lower dorsal cord levels and starts again below as a new vessel.

Although these small vessels are affected by disease processes such as syphilis, diabetes, arteritis and arteriosclerosis clinical disorders of the cord circulation are usually due to disease in the feeder vessels which replenish the artery at various points along its course.

The anterior spinal artery arises from the vertebral arteries in the foramen magnum as two vessels that join to become a single vessel opposite the odontoid peg. It is replenished by a fairly constant vessel which enters the canal on the C3 or C4 root and comes from the thyrocervical trunk which may be damaged in surgical procedures in the neck. This upper part of the vessel supplies the cord down to about D4.

The dorsal spinal cord segment of the artery is supplied by a variable branch from one of the intercostal arteries but the main feeder vessel is the arteria magna of Adamkewicz. This arises from the D10, D11 or D12 intercostal artery in seventy-five per cent of patients. It is easily damaged during thoracic operations, sympathectomy, nephrectomy, adrenal exploration, lumbar aortography and intercostal nerve blocks. In any of these procedures damage to the vessel may cause infarction of the entire lumbar enlargement and the thoracic cord up to mid-dorsal level.

The terminal spinal cord and the nerve roots of the cauda equina are supplied by a variable vessel entering the canal on one of the upper lumbar roots.

Vascular Syndromes

The surgical causes of vascular cord disease have been listed above.

Medical causes are dominated by atheromatous changes in the vessels and in particular disease of the vertebral arteries occluding the origin of the anterior spinal artery, which causes infarction of the central medulla (see Chapter 11).

At any cord level diabetes mellitus, syphilis, any coagulopathy, embolic phenomena (subacute bacterial endocarditis, atrial fibrillation, myocardial infarction), dissecting aneurysm of the aorta, intravascular air bubbles in decompression sickness, and sickle cell disease are notable causes of feeder vessel occlusion.

When the arteria magna is occluded by any of these processes the level of the lesion is usually found between D4 and D6. The entire anterior half of the cord is infarcted so that the picture is that of an acute flaccid paraplegia, with retention of urine, spinothalamic sensory loss to the level of the lesion but with complete preservation of joint position sense and touch. The onset is often accompanied by local pain in the back.

The lumbar feeder vessel may be involved in disc lesions in patients with congenitally narrowed lumbar canals causing the syndrome of "intermittent claudication of the cauda equina". In this condition root pain and weakness appear during exercise and rapidly pass off when the patient rests. Decompressive laminectomy usually relieves this condition.

Figure 14.8. Diagram to Show the Blood Supply of the Spinal Cord

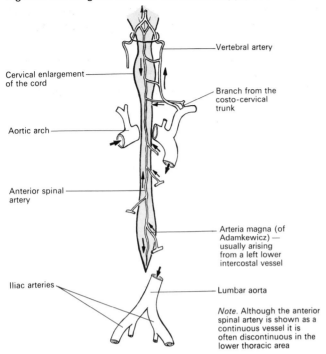

Vertebral artery

Cervical enlargement of the cord

Branch from the costo-cervical trunk

Aortic arch

Anterior spinal artery

Arteria magna (of Adamkewicz) — usually arising from a left lower intercostal vessel

Iliac arteries

Lumbar aorta

Note. Although the anterior spinal artery is shown as a continuous vessel it is often discontinuous in the lower thoracic area

Posterior spinal artery occlusion is less likely to produce classical signs as the vessel is part of a plexus and does not have a constant territory to supply.

There is no doubt that the effects of spinal cord compression are initially due to vascular factors and it seems likely that impaired venous drainage leads to back pressure and capillary stasis. This will be maximal in the watershed areas and the central cord indicated in Figure 14.9. This would also account for the fact that evidence of cortico-spinal tract damage dominates the early clinical picture in cord compression.

There are some other rare, but interesting vascular lesions that may affect the spinal cord.

1. Spinal cord angiomas, usually found in the lower mid dorsal segment of the cord may cause repeated attacks of paraparesis with severe back pain. An associated angioma in the skin of the back may be found on careful examination.

2. Telangiectasia of the spinal cord may cause spontaneous haemorrhage into the substance of the spinal cord or spinal subarachnoid haemorrhage with cord compression.

Figure 14.9. Diagram to show the Segmental Blood Supply of the Spinal Cord

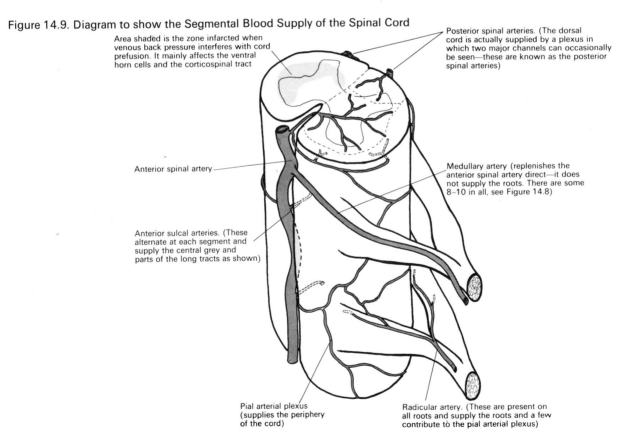

Area shaded is the zone infarcted when venous back pressure interferes with cord prefusion. It mainly affects the ventral horn cells and the corticospinal tract

Posterior spinal arteries. (The dorsal cord is actually supplied by a plexus in which two major channels can occasionally be seen—these are known as the posterior spinal arteries)

Anterior spinal artery

Medullary artery (replenishes the anterior spinal artery direct—it does not supply the roots. There are some 8–10 in all, see Figure 14.8)

Anterior sulcal arteries. (These alternate at each segment and supply the central grey and parts of the long tracts as shown)

Pial arterial plexus (supplies the periphery of the cord)

Radicular artery. (These are present on all roots and supply the roots and a few contribute to the pial arterial plexus)

154

3. Coarctation of the aorta is sometimes associated with massive enlargement of the mid-thoracic feeder vessel which may be large enough to compress the spinal cord.

4. Haemangioblastomas of the cord are dense vascular tumours usually found in the upper dorsal cord, often continuous with a syringomyelic cavity. They are usually found in patients with retinal and cerebellar haemangioblastomas (Hippel—Von Lindau disease).

5. Vertebral haemangiomas are vascular malformations of the vertebral body or arch. They may cause vertebral collapse or produce an extradural mass due to gross thickening of the vertebral arch.

The differential diagnosis is metastatic malignant disease because these malformations usually cause symptoms in adulthood; and the x-ray appearances may suggest osteolytic or osteosclerotic metastases.

Chapter 15

THE SPINAL CORD IN RELATION TO THE VERTEBRAL COLUMN

DEVELOPMENTAL ANATOMY OF THE NERVOUS SYSTEM

In the early stages of development of the embryo the oval disc lying on the yolk sac is differentiated into a superficial ectodermal layer and a deeper entodermal layer derived from the yolk sac. The former becomes thickened along the midline to form the neural plate and the latter gives origin to the underlying notochord (Figure 15.1). Abnormalities in the development of the notochord may be responsible for some of the conditions in which vertebrae are absent, fused or malformed. The only residual notochord in the adult is the nucleus pulposus of the intervertebral discs. In the embryo, the notochord extends from the region of the pituitary fossa to the sacrum. Notochord remnants persisting at either side may give rise to malignant chordomas, tumours found only in the basilar part of the occipital bone or in the sacrum.

The neural plate heaps up on either side of the midline forming the neural folds. The neural crest, at the tip of each fold, is the tissue that migrates laterally to form the spinal ganglia and the autonomic nervous system. Residual tissue of this type may give rise to extradural malignant ganglio-neuromas in children. By the third week of embryonic life the somites, developing segments of mesoderm, appear alongside the invaginating neural groove. As invagination is completed, the ectoderm begins to close over the neural tube along the midline (Figures 15.1b and 15.1c). This process begins in the cervical region and is first completed at the head end. The lower end closes later at the posterior neuropore. Any teratogenic factor operating at this stage of development may lead to defects in neural tube closure, the most typical being spina bifida. There will also be a high probability that tube closure at the head end is simultaneously affected, and this accounts for the frequent association of spina bifida with hydrocephalus, caused by developmental anomalies in the posterior fossa.

When the neural tube is completely closed the vertebral bodies begin to form around the notochord (Figure 15.1d). If neural development is incomplete the vertebrae cannot develop normally and the vertebral arches overlying closure defects are usually absent. However, bony defects without neurological problems can occur as in spina bifida occulta which occurs in about five per cent of the population. In normal development the arches of S4, 5 and coccygeal 1 are never completed. Conversely, soft tissue abnormalities in the spinal cord can occur in the absence of detectable bony abnormality.

In the development of the brain a critical stage occurs as neural tube closure is completed. This is the development of the pons and the fourth ventricle. The primitive brain is a tube divided into two areas, the forebrain and the hindbrain, demarcated by the mesencephalic and cervical flexures respectively. In the next stage of development a transverse flexure develops on the dorsum of the hindbrain. This has a similar effect to the flexing of a thick rubber tube: the hindbrain flattens and widens producing a rhomboid shape enclosing what will become the fourth ventricle (Figures 15.1e and 15.1f). The area is roofed over by a thin membrane that perforates in the seventh week to establish the normal pathway of C.S.F. flow. If the membrane remains intact a condition known as the Dandy–Walker syndrome occurs in which the posterior fossa is occupied by a giant cystic fourth ventricle. If the pontine flexure fails to develop (and remember that it does so at the same time as the final closure of the neural tube) the pons remains long and thin. Furthermore, the cerebellum which develops from the anterior lip of the pontine flexure will also develop abnormally. As a result, when the cerebral hemispheres rapidly expand during the eighth to twelfth weeks of foetal life they can easily push the maldeveloped pons, medulla and cerebellum into the cervical canal. The displaced fourth ventricle becomes kinked and the resulting C.S.F. block produces hydrocephalus, further aggravating the situation. This condition is known as the Arnold–Chiari syndrome and is almost always associated with severe spina bifida suggesting a common aetiological factor operative in the fourth week of development. The affected child usually dies within the first few months of life.

If development is proceeding normally at this stage the spinal cord is still a thin-walled tube. As soon as the fourth ventricle opens, the C.S.F. pressure in the lumen falls and the spinal cord develops by a combination of glial migration and tract enlargement until, in the adult, the central canal is barely visible. If normal C.S.F. flow is *not* established, together with the gross developmental anomalies already described, the child almost invariably has a large syringomyelic cavity in the cervical cord. It has recently been

Figure 15.1. Embryology of the CNS

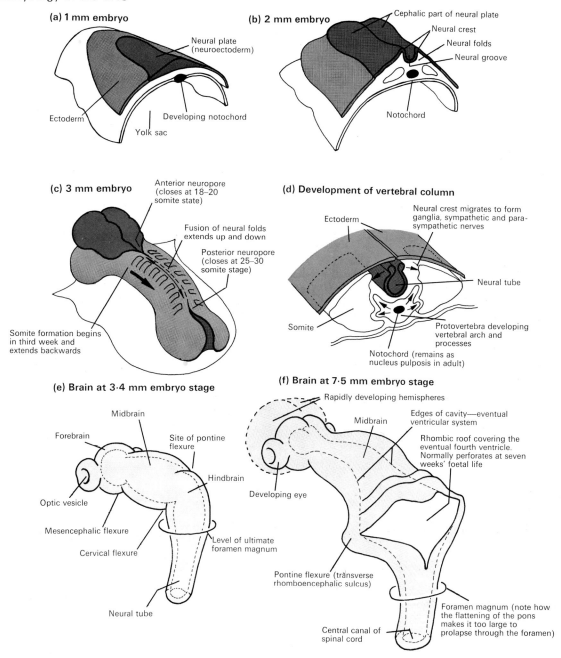

(a) 1 mm embryo

Neural plate (neuroectoderm)

Ectoderm

Developing notochord

Yolk sac

(b) 2 mm embryo

Cephalic part of neural plate

Neural crest

Neural folds

Neural groove

Notochord

(c) 3 mm embryo

Anterior neuropore (closes at 18–20 somite state)

Fusion of neural folds extends up and down

Posterior neuropore (closes at 25–30 somite stage)

Somite formation begins in third week and extends backwards

(d) Development of vertebral column

Neural crest migrates to form ganglia, sympathetic and para-sympathetic nerves

Ectoderm

Neural tube

Somite

Protovertebra developing vertebral arch and processes

Notochord (remains as nucleus pulposis in adult)

(e) Brain at 3·4 mm embryo stage

Midbrain

Forebrain

Site of pontine flexure

Hindbrain

Optic vesicle

Mesencephalic flexure

Cervical flexure

Level of ultimate foramen magnum

Neural tube

(f) Brain at 7·5 mm embryo stage

Rapidly developing hemispheres

Midbrain

Edges of cavity—eventual ventricular system

Rhombic roof covering the eventual fourth ventricle. Normally perforates at seven weeks' foetal life

Developing eye

Pontine flexure (transverse rhomboencephalic sulcus)

Central canal of spinal cord

Foramen magnum (note how the flattening of the pons makes it too large to prolapse through the foramen)

established that many patients who first show evidence of syringomyelia in adulthood have a very mild degree of the Chiari malformation which, over many years, leads to ballooning of the central canal with C.S.F. Surgical decompression often arrests and may even reverse the condition. This is one of the most important advances in neurology in recent years.

The other feature of C.N.S. development that may lead to delayed neurological problems concerns the length of the spinal cord. Initially the cord is the same length as the spinal canal, but as the foetus develops the rapid lengthening of the vertebral column out-strips cord growth and by birth the end of the cord has been pulled up to the level of L3 vertebra. The lumbar and sacral roots are pulled into the spinal canal to

Figure 15.2. Some Common Foramen Magnum Anomalies

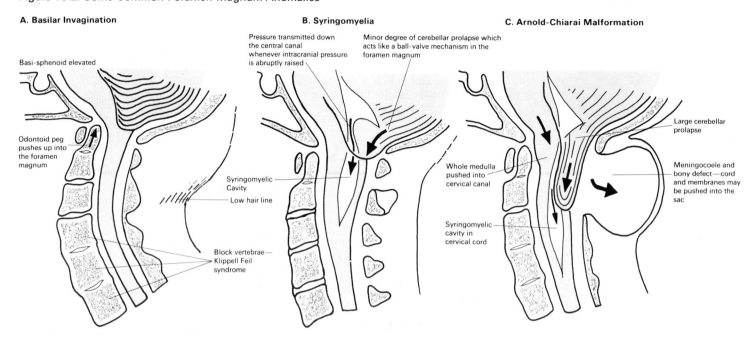

A. Basilar Invagination

Basi-sphenoid elevated

Odontoid peg pushes up into the foramen magnum

Block vertebrae— Klippell Feil syndrome

B. Syringomyelia

Pressure transmitted down the central canal whenever intracranial pressure is abruptly raised

Minor degree of cerebellar prolapse which acts like a ball-valve mechanism in the foramen magnum

Syringomyelic Cavity

Low hair line

Block vertebrae— Klippell Feil syndrome

C. Arnold-Chiarai Malformation

Large cerebellar prolapse

Whole medulla pushed into cervical canal

Meningocoele and bony defect—cord and membranes may be pushed into the sac

Syringomyelic cavity in cervical cord

form the cauda equina. During childhood the cord pulls up further to reach the lower border of L1 by eight years of age. Any developmental abnormality of the bony or fibrous structures in the lumbar canal may tether the cord and prevent it rising, causing a progressive cauda equina syndrome. This may occur in the absence of x-ray evidence of abnormality and exploration may be required completely to exclude cord tethering in a child with a progressive cauda equina syndrome.

Although these malformations are relatively rare, they cause considerable clinical and ethical problems. Abnormalities in the lumbar area may range from simple cutaneous lesions, such as a hairy mole, a pilonidal sinus, a dermal sinus, telangiectasia or a subcutaneous lipoma to severe defects such as a double spinal cord, separated by a bony spur, a tethered conus, an intradural lipoma or dermoid or a full-blown spina bifida. Vertebral defects alone may be of little consequence but an underlying soft tissue defect should always be suspected if neurological problems occur. In the cervical region the more serious defects are usually fatal. Fused cervical vertebrae (the Klippel–Feil syndrome) are usually associated with a family history of a short neck and low hairline, and lead to severe early degenerative cervical spine disease. A dermal sinus in the hairline may lead to recurrent attacks of meningitis. At the foramen magnum maldevelopment of the first cervical vertebra and the skull base, leading to basilar invagination may cause pressure on the medulla or hindbrain circulation leading to a clinical

picture simulating a posterior fossa tumour, a high cervical tumour or transient brain stem ischaemic attacks. Careful x-rays of the foramen magnum are indicated in any of these clinical situations.

It is very important to recognise that although many of these abnormalities are congenital, symptoms may not occur until late middle age in many instances. Perhaps the best example is syringomyelia.

SYRINGOMYELIA

We have already mentioned this condition in Chapter 13 in relation to the clinical signs of an expanding lesion in the cervical cord. In a previous paragraph the recent recognition that the ballooning of the central cavity of the cord is associated in a majority of cases with a congenital abnormality at the foramen magnum was mentioned. This usually consists of a mild degree of Arnold–Chiari malformation with the cerebellar tonsils lying in the posterior foramen magnum (see Figure 15.2B). Throughout life sudden pressure rises during coughing or straining impact the cerebellar tonsils in the foramen magnum and transmit the increased C.S.F. pressure into the central canal instead of it being dissipated into the spinal C.S.F. Occasionally patients develop acute syringomyelia during a cough or a sneeze. Operations to decompress the posterior foramen magnum may relieve the situation *and* improve the patient's clinical

Figure 15.3. The Anatomy of the Sensory Deficit in Syringomyelia

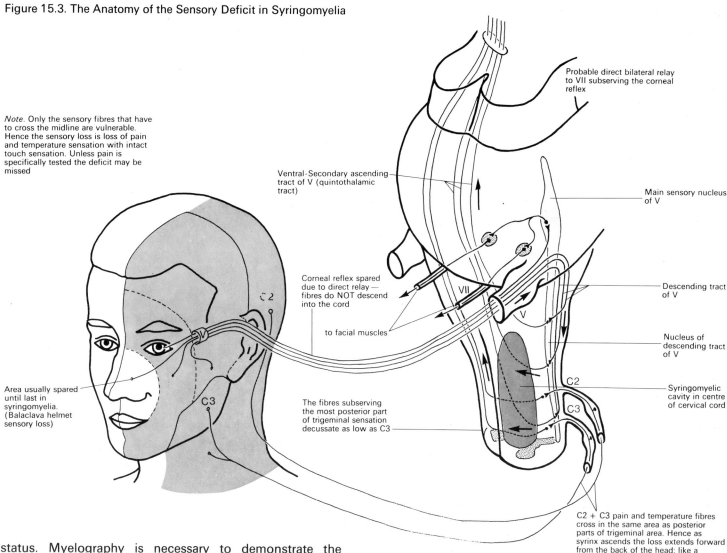

Note. Only the sensory fibres that have to cross the midline are vulnerable. Hence the sensory loss is loss of pain and temperature sensation with intact touch sensation. Unless pain is specifically tested the deficit may be missed

Probable direct bilateral relay to VII subserving the corneal reflex

Ventral-Secondary ascending tract of V (quintothalamic tract)

Main sensory nucleus of V

Corneal reflex spared due to direct relay — fibres do NOT descend into the cord

Descending tract of V

to facial muscles

VII

V

Nucleus of descending tract of V

Area usually spared until last in syringomyelia. (Balaclava helmet sensory loss)

The fibres subserving the most posterior part of trigeminal sensation decussate as low as C3

C2

Syringomyelic cavity in centre of cervical cord

C3

C2 + C3 pain and temperature fibres cross in the same area as posterior parts of trigeminal area. Hence as syrinx ascends the loss extends forward from the back of the head; like a balaclava helmet

status. Myelography is necessary to demonstrate the lesion as bony abnormalities are not always present. In addition to the symmetrical dilation of the central canal, slit-like cavities adjacent to but in continuity with the central canal can produce asymmetry of the physical signs. Why the cavitation begins at C7-D1 level is not clear. The cord may expand with greater ease in the cervical enlargement. The mechanism may be compared to the way a balloon, made with expanded sections, inflates to a series of bulges. As the lesion expands upwards into the region of the fourth ventricle the condition known as syringobulbia develops. Progressively higher sensory loss occurs and as the decussating pain fibres from the descending tract of the fifth nerve are affected the sensory loss spreads from C3→C2 and then forward on to the face like a balaclava helmet. This is shown in detail in Figure 15.3. The earliest cranial nerve

nuclei to be affected are the hypoglossal nuclei in the floor of the canal under the obex. This causes bilateral wasting and weakness of the tongue. There is also disruption of vestibular afferents from the neck muscles and nystagmus is usually present by the time the sensory loss extends onto the face.

Although this is a classical neurological disorder it is often completely misdiagnosed. The main reason is the failure to realise that cutaneous sensation is *normal* and unless pain sensation is specifically and carefully tested over the arms, upper thorax, back of head and face no sensory loss will be documented. Multiple sclerosis, motor neurone disease and cervical spondylosis are the alternative diagnoses that are usually suspected.

THE CERVICAL SPINE AND CERVICAL SPONDYLOSIS

In the cervical region vertebral disease may affect both the spinal cord and the nerve roots. There are many features of the anatomy of this area that must be appreciated to understand the pathogenesis and neurological syndromes caused by cervical spondylosis (Figures 15.4 and 15.5).

1. The cervical spinal cord is slightly expanded and the canal is narrow. The usual variation in sagittal diameter ranges from 15–20 mm. Patients with a diameter of less than 13 mm. may develop cord compression with quite mild degrees of spondylosis.

2. The C1 root emerges *over* the top of the first cervical vertebra. Therefore the other roots emerge above their respective vertebra, that is the C6 root emerges in the C5/6 interspace (compare with the lumbar roots).

3. Cervical spondylosis is caused by disc degeneration and protrusion with bony overgrowth of the adjacent vertebrae. These bony ridges plus the extruded disc material constitute the spondylotic bar that may compress the cord.

4. These changes are maximal at C5/6, C6/7 and C4/5 spaces respectively. These are the joints at which most movement occurs. The atlanto-occipital joint allows only nodding movements and C7/D1 is immobilised by the thoracic cage.

5. The mobility of the neck makes great demands on the cervical cord. In forward flexion the length of the canal is increased by 2 cm. and the cord must stretch. This stretching of the cord probably accounts for the transient cord symptoms known as Lhermitte's sign (or in the U.S.A. as the barber's chair sign). This consists of tingling in all four limbs or electric shock-like feelings down the back produced on flexing the neck if the cervical cord is damaged by multiple sclerosis, cervical spondylosis or any other condition. In hyperextension of the neck the canal shortens and the cord buckles. In this position it may be squeezed between the spondylotic bar and the buckled ligamentum flavum (Figure 15.5).

6. The cord is not free to ride these blows as it is held forwards by the anteriorly directed nerve roots and prevented from riding backwards by the ligamentum denticulatum at each side.

Figure 15.4. Lateral View of Cervical Spine

Vertebral arch cut away at C5 and C6 to
show the cord being compressed by a
spondylotic bar

Left Anterior Oblique View of the Cervical Spine

The transverse process of C5 is cut away to
show the emerging C6 root damaged by
the osteophytes in the exit foraminae

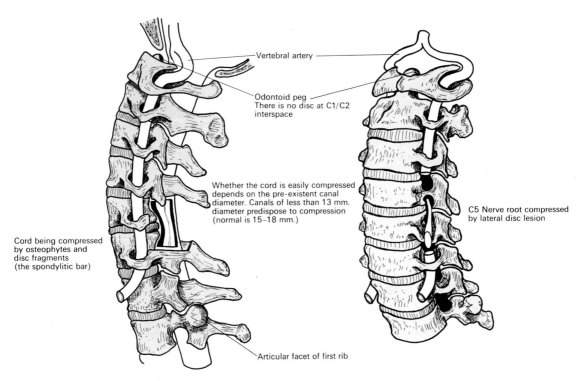

Vertebral artery

Odontoid peg
There is no disc at C1/C2
interspace

Whether the cord is easily compressed
depends on the pre-existent canal
diameter. Canals of less than 13 mm.
diameter predispose to compression
(normal is 15–18 mm.)

Cord being compressed
by osteophytes and
disc fragments
(the spondylitic bar)

C5 Nerve root compressed
by lateral disc lesion

Articular facet of first rib

Figure 15.5. Lateral View of the
Cervical Spine in Forward Flexion

Lateral View of the Cervical
Spine in Hyperextension

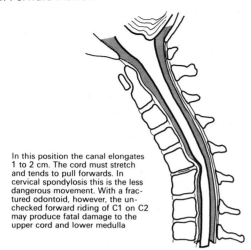

In this position the canal elongates 1 to 2 cm. The cord must stretch and tends to pull forwards. In cervical spondylosis this is the less dangerous movement. With a fractured odontoid, however, the unchecked forward riding of C1 on C2 may produce fatal damage to the upper cord and lower medulla

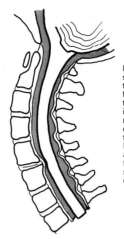

In this movement the cord shortens and would appear to be able to 'flop back' from the bars. But it is by far the most dangerous movement in cervical spondylosis. The roots (see above) the denticulate ligaments, and the forward bulging of the buckled ligamentum flavum all tend to hold the cord forwards. Which is the most significant in causing damage is much disputed

Clinical Features of Cervical Spondylosis (Figure 15.6)

There are two clinical syndromes which may co-exist in some patients; these are the root syndromes and compressive cervical myelopathy.

The Cervical Root Syndromes

The roots most often affected are in order C6, C7 and C5. C3, C4 and D1 are affected infrequently so that other possible causes should be carefully excluded before accepting that damage to any of these roots is caused by spondylosis. The clinical details of the individual root lesions are fully described in Chapter 16. At this stage it is sufficient to note that the pain in the affected root territory is usually related to neck movement, is generally worse on waking, and often originally provoked by unusual exercise such as painting a ceiling. Efforts to prevent the damaged root being pulled in and out of the intervertebral foramen should be made. This is best achieved by a soft collar. This should serve to remind the patient not to move his neck and as a mild physical restraint. The symptoms usually subside in a few weeks and may not recur for years if the provoking activity is avoided.

Compressive Cervical Myelopathy

Fortunately this condition occurs less frequently than the root syndromes. The patient probably has to be predisposed to compression by a congenitally narrow canal, and will usually present with a progressive spastic paraparesis.

Although root symptoms may not be a feature of the history, quite often the exminer will find that the biceps and

Figure 15.6. To Show the Dual Effects of Cervical Spondylosis on the Spinal Cord and the Cervical Roots

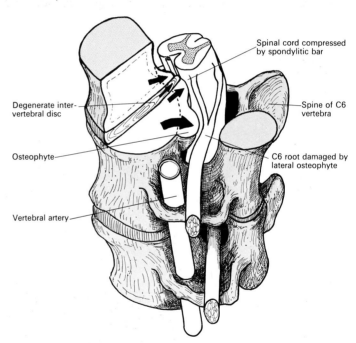

Spinal cord compressed by spondylitic bar

Degenerate intervertebral disc

Osteophyte

Vertebral artery

Spine of C6 vertebra

C6 root damaged by lateral osteophyte

supinator reflexes (C5 and C6) are absent, and that the triceps reflex (C7) is brisk. This indicates that the cord and roots are being compressed at the C5/6 interspace and this combination is almost pathognomonic of cervical spondylosis with cord compression. Myelography is always indicated, and surgical efforts to decompress the cord, although carrying some risk and no guarantee of improvement, are usually indicated. A collar is often advised but this rarely

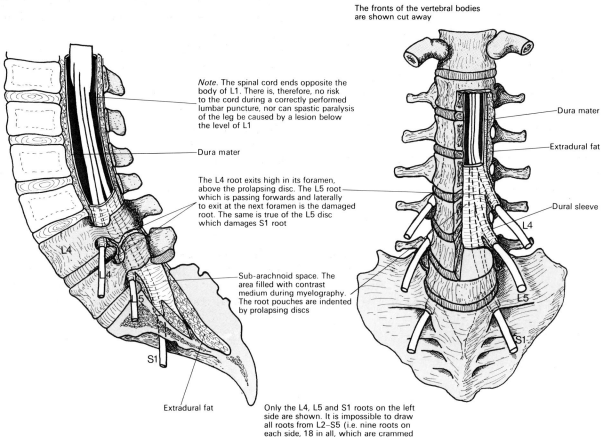

Figure 15.7. The Lumbar Spine and Cauda Equina
(lateral view)

(anterior view)

The fronts of the vertebral bodies
are shown cut away

Note. The spinal cord ends opposite the
body of L1. There is, therefore, no risk
to the cord during a correctly performed
lumbar puncture, nor can spastic paralysis
of the leg be caused by a lesion below
the level of L1

Dura mater

The L4 root exits high in its foramen,
above the prolapsing disc. The L5 root
which is passing forwards and laterally
to exit at the next foramen is the damaged
root. The same is true of the L5 disc
which damages S1 root

Sub-arachnoid space. The
area filled with contrast
medium during myelography.
The root pouches are indented
by prolapsing discs

Extradural fat

Only the L4, L5 and S1 roots on the left
side are shown. It is impossible to draw
all roots from L2–S5 (i.e. nine roots on
each side, 18 in all, which are crammed
into the cauda equina)

Dura mater

Extradural fat

Dural sleeve

seems to have any effect on the condition, although it may relieve any co-existent root pain.

Unfortunately so many middle-aged patients have some degree of cervical spondylosis on plain x-rays that its presence cannot be regarded as confirming that the patient's illness is due to the condition. Subsequent myelography may show no evidence of compression and the diagnosis then often turns out to be multiple sclerosis or motor neurone disease. On the other hand, an unexpected neurofibroma or meningioma is occasionally discovered. As discussed previously it is wise to keep the diagnosis of cervical spondylosis with neurological complications under continual review.

THE LUMBAR SPINE AND LUMBAR DISC LESIONS

The most important anatomical difference between the cervical and lumbar spine is that the spinal cord ends opposite the lower border of L1 vertebra. Therefore, lumbar disc lesions can only cause root syndromes. Any lesion below L1 vertebral level *cannot* cause a spastic paraparesis. As there are eight cervical roots and only seven cervical vertebra the relationship of the root to the interspace alters below D1. Therefore, the lumbar roots emerge *below* their respective vertebrae, that is, the L4 root emerges at the L4/5 interspace. It also follows that a disc lesion may damage a root anywhere between its origin from the cord and its exit foramen (the S1 root, for example, could be damaged anywhere along its six-inch intraspinal course). Fortunately, disc lesions produce anatomically accurate root damage in the majority of cases.

Individual roots are most vulnerable just above their exit foramina, as they are then the most anterior and most lateral root in the canal and lie in the immediate path of a lateral disc prolapse (Figure 15.7 and 15.8). The root exits very high in its foramen, usually *above* a disc that is prolapsing into its own interspace. The disc, therefore, damages the root that is passing to the interspace below. Thus, a disc lesion at L4/5 will damage the L5 root and a disc at L5/S1 will damage the S1 root.

These anatomical features require very careful consideration when one is investigating a patient with lumbar or sacral root lesions. False negative myelograms occur, especially with disc lesions at the L5/S1 interspace. False positive myelograms are usually the result of over-interpretation of a bulging disc. The most important point to remember is that if no lesion is seen at L5/S1 in a patient with S1 root symptoms the myodil must be run up to at least D10 level before it can be stated that there is *no* lesion involving the root. A neurofibroma on the L2 root, for example, can easily present as an S1 root lesion because of the peculiar anatomy of the cauda equina.

The other consideration depends on the frequency of disc lesions at various sites. Lesions affecting L5 and S1 roots account for ninety-five per cent of disc lesions. Lesions affecting L2, L3 and L4 account for only five per cent and the majority of these are at the L4 level. It follows that L2 and L3 root lesions are very unlikely to be a result of uncomplicated disc disease, and urgent investigation is indicated. There are four syndromes produced by upper lumbar root lesions that may prove to be due to disc lesions.

Anterior Thigh Pain

Pain in the anterior thigh, with wasting of the quadriceps and an absent knee jerk, is produced by lesions affecting the L3 or L4 roots. Disc lesions are an *unusual* cause of this picture. Metastatic carcinoma of the prostate gland and diabetic amyotrophy are the main conditions to be excluded.

Low Back Pain without Radicular Symptoms

One relies so much on radicular symptoms in the leg that if these are absent the question of a disc lesion is not raised. Occasionally, lesions at the L3/4 level may produce severe local back pain without radicular pain. The most ominous historical feature is rest pain. If the back pain is worse at night or in a lying position the chance of finding a serious underlying cause is very high.

Sciatic Syndrome

We have already pointed out this situation in relation to a neurofibroma. A disc lesion as high as L2/3 interspace may fail to damage the appropriate roots and present as pain in the L5 or S1 distribution. This adds further emphasis to the need for a complete myelographic examination of the area, up to and including the lower cord.

Figure 15.8. Diagram to show the effect of a Central Disc Prolapse

Diagram to show the effect of a Lateral Disc Prolapse

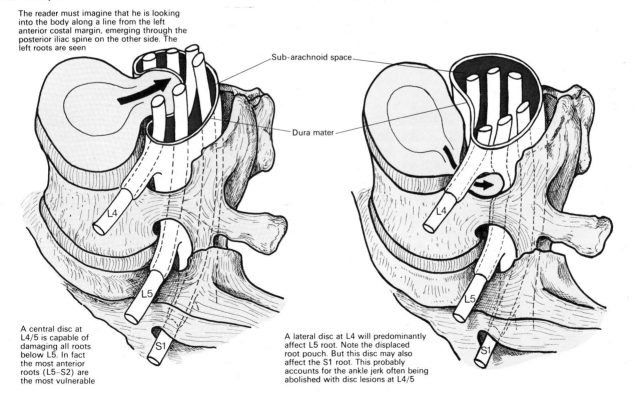

The reader must imagine that he is looking into the body along a line from the left anterior costal margin, emerging through the posterior iliac spine on the other side. The left roots are seen

Sub-arachnoid space

Dura mater

L4

L5

S1

A central disc at L4/5 is capable of damaging all roots below L5. In fact the most anterior roots (L5–S2) are the most vulnerable

L4

L5

S1

A lateral disc at L4 will predominantly affect L5 root. Note the displaced root pouch. But this disc may also affect the S1 root. This probably accounts for the ankle jerk often being abolished with disc lesions at L4/5

Acute Cauda Equina Syndrome

An acute disc prolapse at the L2/3 level may cause bilateral multiple root lesions. The patient complains of severe bilateral leg pain, flaccid paralysis of both legs and retention of urine. This is a surgical emergency; and immediate exploration of the cauda equina is indicated.

One other rarity worth including is the condition known as "claudication of the cauda equina". The patient complains that while walking he develops root pain and leg weakness, usually a foot drop. This rapidly recovers on resting. This is usually due to a combination of a disc lesion and a congenitally narrowed lumbar theca which interferes with the blood supply of the spinal cord during activity. The situation is rather similar to the narrow cervical canal that predisposes to cord compression in cervical spondylosis.

CAUDA EQUINA LESIONS

A lesion in the spinal canal at any level below the D10 vertebra can cause a cauda equina syndrome. There is often a tendency to think of the cauda equina as comprising only the nerve roots lying in the sacrum. It includes the terminal spinal cord, all the spinal roots from D12 to S5 and the filum terminale—the fibrous band that extends from the tip of the cord to attach to the sacrum (see Figure 15.7).

Cauda Equina Lesions in Childhood

The embryology of the vertebral column has already been described and the variety of developmental defects that may occur in the lumbar-sacral region mentioned. It is important to remember that *disc* lesions are exceedingly rare before 15 years of age.

1. Symptoms present since birth

Spina Bifida Occulta

Many patients with spina bifida occulta remain asymptomatic throughout life but associated developmental abnormalities may cause problems. Progressive wasting and weakness affecting particularly L4, L5 and S1 are found. Absent ankle jerks and trophic changes in the feet often first manifest as recurrent chilblains may be found. The picture may remain static but close follow-up until seven years of age is necessary to exclude any progression.

Spina Bifida Cystica

Severe defects in the vertebral column are associated with variable degrees of neural abnormality. These include bulging meninges (meningocoele), a sac containing parts of the terminal cord and nerve roots (myelomeningocoele), and a lump of malformed neural tissue lying free on the surface (myelocoele). Both latter varieties are often associated with Arnold—Chiari malformation and initial surgical enthusiasm for active treatment is now being tempered by the ethical dilemma presented as the grossly disabled survivors reach adulthood. Further discussion of this tragic and emotive subject is beyond the scope of the present text.

2. Symptoms occurring in later childhood

Mild developmental abnormalities may not produce any disability at birth but the ascent of the spinal cord in the first five years of life may cause problems due to cord stretching. Occasionally symptoms or signs may not occur until adulthood. The development of any weakness, numbness, trophic change or disparity in the size or shape of the feet should prompt careful investigation. Progressive symptoms may require surgery even in the absence of myelographic abnormalities as a tethered cord may not produce myelographic signs.

Pain is an unusual feature in the developmental cauda equina syndromes of childhood. Pain should prompt an urgent search for evidence of primary malignant disease in the vertebral column or sacrum, retro-peritoneal malignancy and the possibility of seeding of the lumbar theca by a medulloblastoma should be considered.

CASE REPORT

A 16-year-old boy went camping at Easter. The weather was extremely bad and he developed a "chill". He came home early looking very pale, had a low-grade fever, severe low backache and pain in the left thigh. Over the next three weeks he lost weight and the main symptoms continued. On examination he looked very ill, but there was no hepatosplenomegaly or lymphadenopathy. The left knee jerk was absent. He was investigated for malignant disease and found to be suffering from acute lymphatic leukaemia. His symptoms remitted with appropriate chemotherapy.

Cauda Equina Lesions in the Adult

There are three main clinical pictures.

a. *The Lateral Cauda Equina Syndrome* (Figure 15.9)

The most frequent cause of the lateral cauda equina syndrome is a neurofibroma. Rarely, a high disc lesion may be responsible. The symptoms include anterior thigh pain, quadriceps wasting, weakness of inversion of the foot (L4 root lesion) and an absent knee jerk. If the lesion is very high and lies lateral to the terminal spinal cord there may even be pyramidal signs *below* the lesion, in which case the ankle jerks may be very brisk with ankle clonus and an extensor plantar response. In this situation sphincter disturbance is likely to be due to cord compression.

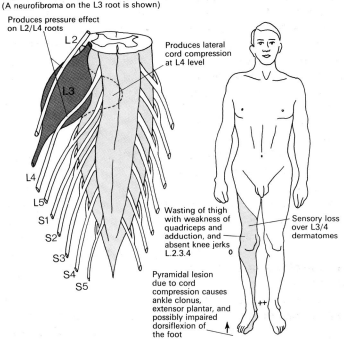

Figure 15.9. High lateral Cauda Equina lesion
(A neurofibroma on the L3 root is shown)

Produces pressure effect on L2/L4 roots

L2

L3

Produces lateral cord compression at L4 level

L4

L5

S1

S2

S3

S4

S5

Wasting of thigh with weakness of quadriceps and adduction, and absent knee jerks L.2.3.4

Sensory loss over L3/4 dermatomes

Pyramidal lesion due to cord compression causes ankle clonus, extensor plantar, and possibly impaired dorsiflexion of the foot

Figure 15.10. Midline (conus lesion) of the Cauda Equina
(Usually an ependymoma) Affects S5-4-3 roots bilaterally

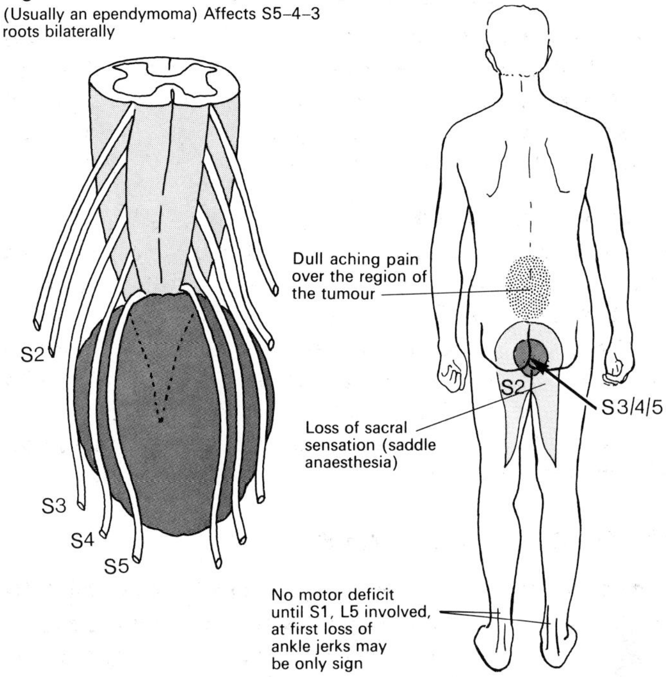

S2

S3

S4

S5

Dull aching pain over the region of the tumour

Loss of sacral sensation (saddle anaesthesia)

S2

S3/4/5

No motor deficit until S1, L5 involved, at first loss of ankle jerks may be only sign

b. *Midline Cauda Equina Lesions from Within* (Figure 15.10)

This is also known as a "conus lesion". The usual causes are an ependymoma, a dermoid tumour or a lipoma of the terminal cord. The roots are damaged from the inside i.e. S5→S4→S3 and so on. The initial symptoms include rectal pain, genital pain, micturition disturbances and loss of potency with no definite physical signs *unless* the perianal sensation and anal reflex are carefully tested. Later loss of the ankle jerks and weakness of the L5 and S1 muscle groups occurs. In the case of an ependymoma the patient may have a five-year history of dull backache *before* any other symptoms or signs appear.

An important benign cause of rectal pain that must be considered is the benign, but excruciating pain syndrome known as Proctalgia fugax. This can occur in either sex at any age, but seems to be more frequent in men. Attacks are mainly nocturnal and may accompany erection or ejaculation. The pain is an intense gripping sensation around the rectum about 2" inside the anal ring. Attacks typically last 15–20 minutes and then subside. Bearing down may relieve the pain slightly. It is thought to be due to cramp in the Levator ani muscles.

c. *Midline Cauda Equina Lesions from Outside*

The hallmark of this situation is bilateral lumbar and sacral root lesions. Root pain in unusual dermatomes (L2 or 3) (or S2 or 3) should be regarded with great suspicion, but pain in L4, L5 or S1 may be readily and not unreasonably ascribed to simple disc disease. Severe pain not relieved by appropriate measures, and the detection of neurological signs indicates the need for myelography, not just to confirm a disc lesion but to exclude alternative pathology. In the adult the alternatives are extremely unpleasant and include primary sacral bone tumours (chordomas) metastatic disease (especially prostatic disease), reticulosis, leukaemia or direct seeding from malignant tumours in the C.N.S. notably medulloblastomas, ependymomas or pinealomas.

CASE REPORT

A 20-year-old female was admitted as an emergency with severe headaches of one month's duration and papilloedema. She gave a five-year history of left S1 root pain ascribed to a disc lesion. On physical examination there was papilloedema, neck stiffness, a positive Kernig test and absence of the left ankle jerk. An ependymoma with a spinal subarachnoid haemorrhage was suspected but at operation a piloid astrocytoma was found, with evidence of recent haemorrhage. This case emphasises the danger of diagnosing a disc lesion in a 15-year-old and the surprisingly slow clinical course of lesions in this situation.

Although low backache and various aches and pains in the legs are one of the most frequent reasons for hospital referral the importance of detecting *unusual* features in the history and a *careful* neurological examination in all cases cannot be over-emphasised.

TUMOURS AND THE SPINAL CORD

Now that the anatomy of the spinal cord in relation to the vertebra has been fully described it is appropriate to consider tumours and the spinal cord. This subject has been deferred until this stage because from an investigational and pathological point of view the relationship of the tumour to the vertebral column is of great importance. Furthermore, the relationship of the tumour to the cord and its coverings often provides a pre-operative clue to the pathology and to some extent governs the surgical approach.

As so often in neurological disease, we have to consider cord tumours in children and adults separately as there is a dramatic difference in the pathological possibilities in different age groups, and for certain tumours a marked difference in the sex incidence. As was the case in regard to cerebral tumours there is also a significant risk of a spinal tumour being due to a metastasis from malignant disease elsewhere. In children fifty per cent of spinal tumours are metastatic usually by direct spread from retroperitoneal neuroblastomas, ganglioneuromas and sarcomas. In adults some twenty to thirty per cent of all spinal tumours are metastatic. Metastases from carcinoma of the breast in the female (68 per cent) and prostate in the male (40 per cent) account for the majority. Lung (25 per cent), thyroid (15 per cent), uterus and cervix (10 per cent) and direct spread of Hodgkin's Disease and Multiple myeloma are the other major causes. In all these instances plain films will often show evidence of either the primary lesion or of the bone involvement and often the site of the primary can be guessed from the plain film changes.

Tumours in both groups are defined as extradural, intradural/extramedullary and intramedullary if actually in the substance of the cord.

The striking difference between childhood and adulthood is best seen in the following classification:

When a patient presents with symptoms and signs suggesting a cord lesion (see Chapter 13) the initial clinical evaluation should enable a distinction to be made between an intrinsic (intramedullary) lesion of the cord and a compressive (extradural or intradural) lesion. Considering the age, sex and site of the damage the probable nature of the lesion can be deduced but operative diagnosis and histology is always required.

The following brief profiles of different tumours may be used as a guide:

Neurofibromas: Sex incidence equal, 30–50 years age, 60 per cent above L1 causing spastic paraparesis, 30 per cent below L1 causing root pain and mimicking a disc lesion (16 per cent are sarcomas).

Meningiomas: Female/male ratio 9:1, nearly all mid-dorsal (D3–D6). Few in foramen magnum; female/male ratio 2:1 at this site.

Ependymomas: Male/female ratio 2:1, average age 30 years, either intrinsic in cord at C6–D2 (mimics syringomyelia) or on filum terminale (central cauda equina syndrome). Very high incidence of associated syringomyelic cavity, making the lesion seem much more extensive than its actual size.

Gliomas: Sex incidence equal, average age 35–45, nearly all in cervical cord.

Dermoids: All sacrococcygeal, usually associated with spina bifida; present at 15–20 years of age.

Chordomas: Slight male predominance, 80 per cent sacrococcygeal, 12 per cent in sphenoid. Considerable bone destruction and pain are features.

Vascular tumours affecting the cord are discussed in Chapter 14.

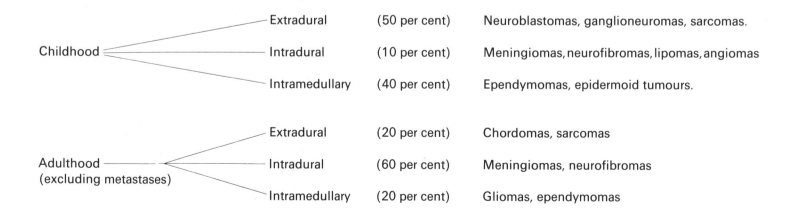

Childhood	Extradural	(50 per cent)	Neuroblastomas, ganglioneuromas, sarcomas.
	Intradural	(10 per cent)	Meningiomas, neurofibromas, lipomas, angiomas
	Intramedullary	(40 per cent)	Ependymomas, epidermoid tumours.
Adulthood (excluding metastases)	Extradural	(20 per cent)	Chordomas, sarcomas
	Intradural	(60 per cent)	Meningiomas, neurofibromas
	Intramedullary	(20 per cent)	Gliomas, ependymomas

Figure 15.11. Plain Film X-ray Appearances of
Intra-Spinal Tumours

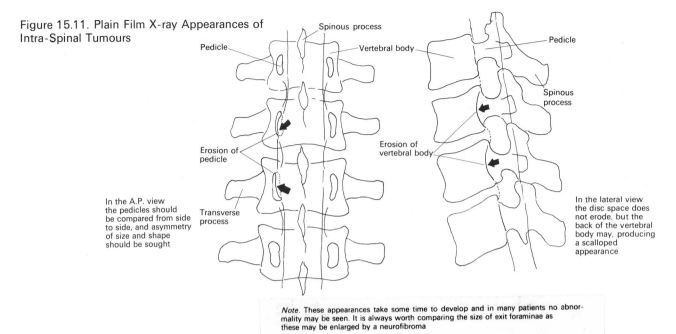

Spinous process

Pedicle

Vertebral body

Pedicle

Spinous
process

Erosion of
pedicle

Erosion of
vertebral body

In the A.P. view
the pedicles should
be compared from side
to side, and asymmetry
of size and shape
should be sought

Transverse
process

In the lateral view
the disc space does
not erode, but the
back of the vertebral
body may, producing
a scalloped
appearance

Note. These appearances take some time to develop and in many patients no abnormality may be seen. It is always worth comparing the size of exit foraminae as these may be enlarged by a neurofibroma

The Investigation of Spinal Tumours

Routine physical examination and chest x-ray to exclude a primary neoplasm is essential. A rectal examination is particularly important in the male to detect carcinoma of the prostate. In the absence of any focal signs or symptoms to indicate the level of the tumour the cervical spine, including the foramen magnum and thoracic spine, including L1, should be x-rayed *if* the clinical picture is that of a spastic paraparesis.

If the picture is one of low backache, lumbar root pain and mixed upper and lower motor neurone signs in the legs the region D10–L3 is the most important from a radiological point of view.

If the symptoms started with rectal or genital pain the sacrum should be included in the x-rays but the importance of including the spinal column up to D10 must be stressed.

The correct investigation is a myelogram and this can be easily performed in most hospitals. However, the temptation to use this facility should be resisted *unless* neurosurgical help is available and under *no* circumstances should a simple lumbar puncture be performed. The reason for this advice is that often a highly delicate haemodynamic situation exists by the time cord compression is evident. Myelography or an L.P. by upsetting these dynamics, particularly if Queckenstedt's test is performed, may lead to acute worsening of the situation, requiring immediate neurosurgery. Furthermore, a simple L.P. may make it impossible to perform myelography for several days as well as worsening the clinical situation. In some patients myodil must also be put in through a cisternal puncture to demonstrate the upper limit of a tumour that is completely blocking the canal. This investigation should be performed only in a neurosurgical unit immediately prior to operation.

The plain film and myelographic appearances of the different types of tumour are shown in Figures 15.11 and 15.12.

Figure 15.12. Diagram to Show Myelographic
Appearances of Intraspinal Tumours

A. Extradural tumour

B. Intradural tumour

C. Intramedullary tumour

Ghost of spinal cord

The tumour lifts the
dura away from the
vertebrae producing a
smooth sloping effect

The tumour sits in the
myodil column and
produces a meniscus-
shaped defect

The expanded cord
occupies the canal and
attenuates the myodil
column on either side

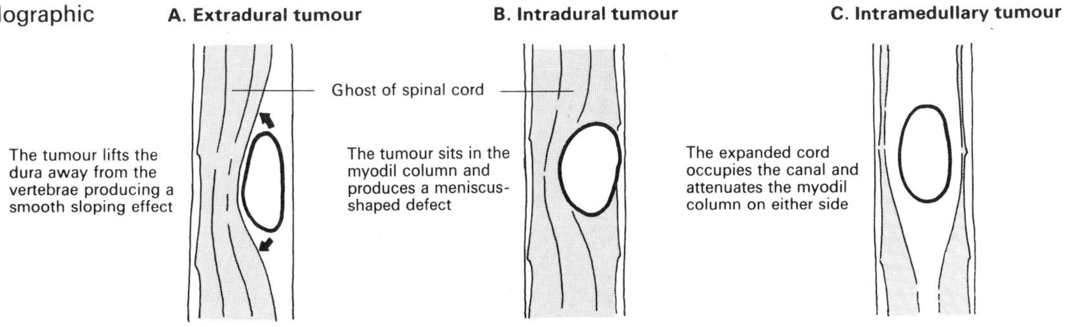

MICTURITION AND NEUROLOGICAL DISEASE
(Figure 15.13)

Micturition disturbances are a common feature of spinal cord disease and cauda equina lesions and it is therefore most appropriate to discuss micturition disturbances at this point.

The normal anatomy and physiology of micturition are not well understood and hence the mechanisms of micturition disturbance in disease remain rather speculative. Males have a very considerable advantage over the females in both the length of urethra and additional sphincter mechanisms designed to isolate the bladder and contract the urethra

Figure 15.13. Schematic diagram of the Neural Control of Micturition

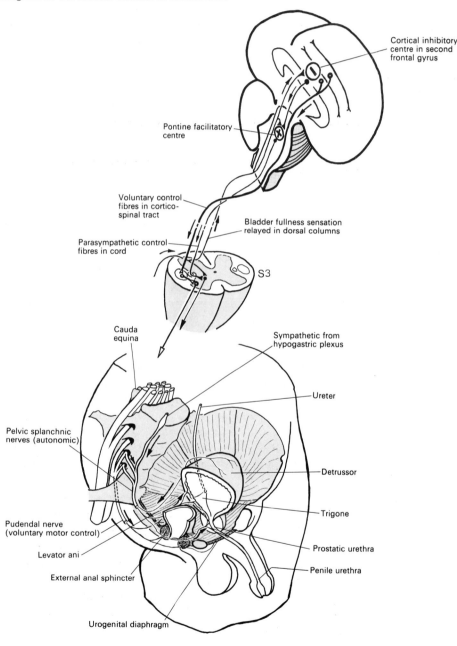

during erection and ejaculation. In neither sex is there a true internal sphincter mechanism; there are arrangements of smooth muscle that produce a "sphincteric" action complete with a condensation of elastic tissue that keeps the urethra in a collapsed state. The angle the bladder makes with the urethra is important and in both sexes collapse of the pelvic floor, allowing the bladder to flop back or gross faecal impaction, by tilting the bladder forward, may have some effect on bladder function for purely mechanical reasons. These possibilities should always be explored. There is a true external sphincter muscle under voluntary control at the uro-genital diaphragm. It is not capable of completely controlling continence—a fact well known to examination candidates!

The anatomy of the bladder and pelvis is shown schematically in Figure 15.13. It is important to notice that part of the urethra lies *in* the abdomen and is subject to the same external pressure alterations as the bladder itself, so that a high pressure differential is not created by coughing or sneezing.

The neural control of the bladder is extremely complicated.

The following details are essential to an understanding of pathological bladder function:

1. The bladder is basically a hollow bag of smooth muscle containing stretch receptors and contracting under the influence of parasympathetic nerves. This constitutes an autonomic stretch reflex.

2. The parasympathetic reflex is based on the S3 roots and S3 segment of the cord. The sympathetic supply descends into the pelvis from the hypogastric plexus but has no certain role in micturition although sympathetic endings on both the detrussor and urethra have been demonstrated and pharmacological evidence suggests that at urethral level the sympathetic may have a major role in the urethral sphincter mechanisms.

3. The stretch receptors fire impulses proportional to the stretch and weight of urine in the bladder. Therefore, there is less afferent activity lying down than standing, hence the instant desire to pass urine on getting up in the morning. Any infection or inflammation of the bladder wall will heighten the sensitivity of the stretch receptors. Stimulation of the perineum and anal canal inhibits the discharge.

4. The basic sacral reflex arc controls micturition in infancy, senility, unconsciousness and following various lesions to the nervous system.

5. The voluntary mechanisms involve both inhibition of the conditioned reflex, volitional control over the hy-pothalamic and pontine facilitating centres and direct physical control over the rather weak external sphincter and pelvic floor. This is all controlled by an area in the second frontal gyrus and the main descending pathways lie in or adjacent to the cortico-spinal tracts. This accounts for the early disturbance of micturition control in patients with spinal cord compression.

Micturition involves complete relaxation of volitional control; the external sphincter and pelvic floor relax and the local reflex is allowed to take over. As the detrusor contracts the bladder neck is pulled open and this combined with inhibition of the weak internal sphincter allows urine to flow by a combination of rising intravesical pressure and gravity. If there is any mechanical obstruction to flow an additional voluntary increase in intra-abdominal pressure by a combination of the Valsava manœuvre and contraction of the abdominal muscles can be used. This is the main cause of the condition known as micturition syncope (see Chapter 22).

Neurological Disorders

There are four main types of neurological bladder:

1. *The Uninhibited Bladder*

This condition is due to a lesion affecting the second frontal gyrus. These include local lesions such as frontal lobe tumours, parasagittal meningiomas and anterior communicating artery aneurysms. It is also a feature of dementia and as stressed before, if dementia *starts* with a micturition upset a focal frontal lesion should be carefully excluded.

The features are:

Urgency at low bladder volumes.
Sudden uncontrolled evacuation.
No residual urine.
If intellectual deterioration occurs urine may be passed anywhere without concern.

2. *The Spinal Bladder*

This condition results from damage to the spinal cord by trauma, cord tumour or multiple sclerosis.

The features are:

Bladder fullness is not appreciated, but may cause sweating pallor, flexor spasms and rises in the blood pressure to very high levels.
The bladder empties suddenly and reflexly.
Evacuation may be incomplete but with training can be complete and at will if the bladder is massaged by suprapubic pressure.
The bladder is spastic and only holds a small volume (less than 250 mls.).

3. The Autonomous Bladder

An autonomous bladder results from damage to the motor and sensory components in the cauda equina or pelvis. It is a feature of cauda equina lesions, pelvic surgery, pelvic malignant disease, spina bifida and high lumbar disc lesions.

The features are:

Continual dribbling incontinence.
Considerable residual urine with high infection risk.
No sensation of bladder fullness.
Associated with perineal numbness and loss of sexual function.

4. The Sensory Bladder

Although the features are similar to an autonomous bladder the anatomical explanation is hard to understand. It is a consequence of several disorders—tabes dorsalis, subacute combined degeneration of the cord, multiple sclerosis and diabetes mellitus. The striking feature is loss of awareness of bladder fullness combined with loss of the spinal reflex. This leads to massive retention of urine.

The features are:

Dribbling incontinence of quite large volumes.
Residual urine measured in litres with high infection risk.
Can be voided by considerable straining, but evacuation incomplete.

During history-taking the main questions to ask a patient with possible neurological bladder dysfunction are:

Is there any sense of bladder filling?
Can the patient feel the urine passing?
Can the patient stop urine passing in midstream at will?
Does the bladder leak continually or suddenly pass large volumes?
Is there any associated rectal disorder?
Is there any disorder of potency in the male?
Is there any numbness in the perineum?

Based on the type of dysfunction further history and examination must be directed to the exclusion of the neurological disorders potentially responsible for the disorder described.

Neurological bladder dysfunction is very difficult to treat. Incontinence may be helped by anti-cholinergic drugs such as emepronium bromide or imipramine. If drugs fail various pelvic nerve sections, urinary diversion or the creation of an artificial bladder may be considered. The most obvious solution, permanent catheterisation, although effective in many instances has the serious and potentially fatal risk of infection. In some females the urethra may become so enlarged that the catheter is ineffective in preventing leakage of urine. The seriousness and misery of bladder dysfunction in neurological disease is a major and often insoluble problem in neurological management.

DISORDERS OF POTENCY

Although the impact of perineal sensory loss or urinary incontinence is the same in both sexes the associated disorder of potency in the male is a source of great frustration and anxiety and often leads to divorce in patients with chronic neurological disease.

There are two components to sexual function in the male; erection and ejaculation. Both functions are basically autonomic reflexes and yet the importance of psychic influences, descending cord pathways and the endocrine status greatly complicate the issue and lead to a wide range of causes of impotence that are not always easy to explain.

1. Erection requires a suitable psychic state and an intact parasympathetic reflex arc at S2/3. The sympathetic plays a minor role at this stage. However the initiation and maintenance of erection requires a strong sensory input from the glans penis and adjacent skin and as this is mainly through the S2 dermatome sensory loss in this region is usually accompanied by damage to the reflex arc itself.

Malignant infiltration of the S2/3 roots, usually due to malignant lymphomas or leukaemia may cause a constant painful erection, a condition known as priapism.

2. Ejaculation is primarily controlled by the sympathetic through the L1 root and the hypogastric plexus which lies in front of the body of the first lumbar vertebra. Voluntary inhibition of ejaculation and to some extent voluntary ejaculation is possible in the final stages. The initial reflex, under sympathetic control, moves semen from the seminal vesicles into the prostatic urethra and contracts the bladder neck to prevent reflux. Then clonic contractions of the bulbo-cavernosus and ischio-cavernosus muscles milk semen along the length of the urethra. This final phase is under some degree of voluntary control.

Causes of loss of potency

1. Psychic disorders

Anxiety states, depression and psychoses may all cause impotence. In recent years it has also been recognised that impotence may be an early symptom of a temporal lobe tumour, and as such tumours may also be associated with personality changes there is a real risk of serious misdiagnosis. A useful clue to intact reflex mechanisms is the history that the patient still has normal morning erections or that successful intercourse outside the marital situation has been achieved.

2. *Spinal Cord Lesions*

Spinal cord compression, transection, multiple sclerosis, tabes dorsalis and sub-acute combined degeneration of the cord all cause impotence. In many instances the exact cause of the difficulty cannot be stated with certainty. Following spinal cord transection reflex erection can easily be produced even though there is no sensory appreciation at cortical level and no descending influences. Ejaculation does not occur in this situation.

3. *Cauda Equina Lesions*

Cauda equina lesions tend to affect erection by a combination of penile sensory loss and direct damage to the reflex arc. In this situation dribbling emission of semen may occur. Causes of cauda equina lesions are discussed earlier in this chapter.

4. *Autonomic Nerve Lesions*

Autonomic neuropathy occurs in diabetes mellitus, chronic polyneuropathy due to any cause (see Chapter 17) and as an important part of the Shy–Drager syndrome (see Chapter 12). Impotence in these cases is usually associated with micturition disturbance and postural hypotension.

The sympathetic nerve supply itself may be injured by crush fractures of the L1 vertebra or deliberate surgical extirpation for peripheral vascular disease. In both cases normal erection may occur but ejaculation is impossible or incomplete. Ganglion blocking agents block both erection and ejaculation but modern anti-hypertensive agents which confine their action to adrenergic nerve endings may cause loss of ejaculation without affecting erection.

5. *Endocrine Disorders*

Potency is affected in many endocrine diseases in which the clinical signs are usually obvious. From a neurological point of view the most important consideration is the possibility of pan-hypopituitarism due to a pituitary tumour. In the male the first symptom is invariably declining sexual function, often occurring several years before field defects or headaches appear (see Chapter 3). The patient himself rarely mentions this symptom unless specifically asked. Usually the wife refers to the problem colloquially as "he hasn't been himself". Body hair, skin texture and testicular size should be carefully assessed, the visual fields examined, and careful x-rays of the pituitary fossa obtained in these patients.

Most endocrinological departments can provide full screening to exclude sub-clinical endocrine dysfunction and this is recommended in those patients who are impotent and are not thought to have psychological problems or neurological disease.

Chapter 16

PERIPHERAL NEUROPATHY AND DISEASES OF THE LOWER MOTOR NEURONE

The classical signs of a lower motor neurone lesion are wasting and weakness of muscles and loss of reflexes. These signs may be associated with other phenomena such as muscle cramps, muscle pain on exercise, easy fatigue and fasciculation. These additional features may indicate specific entities such as motor neurone disease or myasthenia gravis. Unfortunately all or any of these symptoms and signs can be found in *any* condition that affects the lower motor neurone anywhere on its course from the ventral horn cell to the muscle end plate.

The symptoms and signs of a neuropathy vary widely depending on the disease responsible. Sometimes sensory symptoms dominate the picture, varying from mild para-esthesiae to severe pain. Actual sensory impairment may range from slight numbness with hypersensitivity to painful stimuli to gross loss of pain perception. In others the picture is essentially a motor one almost to the exclusion of sensory phenomena. The only constant physical finding is depression or absence of reflexes. As a broad generalisation, if a patient has normal reflexes it is unlikely that he is suffering from a peripheral neuropathy.

These symptoms and signs must be very critically evaluated in every case and it is essential to remember that it may be quite impossible to distinguish between nerve and muscle disease on clinical grounds alone.

THE PHENOMENA OF PERIPHERAL NERVOUS SYSTEM DISEASE

Muscle Wasting

Muscle atrophy is a feature of all lower motor neurone disorders and muscle diseases with the exception of pseudohypertrophy and hypertrophy secondary to myotonia (see Chapter 19).

Muscles normally thin with age and as part of any generalised weight loss. In both situations muscle stamina may decrease but strength is *not* affected. Even very frail patients should be able to produce one full-strength effort in each muscle. If they can do so it is unlikely that they have peripheral nerve or muscle disease. If called upon to make repeated efforts with the same muscle, fatigue may rapidly

occur and raise the suspicion of myasthenia gravis, but the absence of ocular or bulbar muscle weakness excludes this diagnosis in most cases.

Certain muscles waste rapidly with disuse, the best example being the quadriceps which often show appreciable wasting within days of a patient being confined to bed. In this situation the muscle is not weak. The important point is that wasting is *not* necessarily associated with weakness and disuse atrophy in particular affects stamina and not strength.

Muscle Weakness

Patients in pain have difficulty in co-operating with muscle testing. It is essential that they do so and the majority of patients are prepared to bear the pain for one maximal effort. Patients who absolutely refuse to do so are often suffering from a non-organic pain syndrome. Weakness in the legs secondary to unbearable back pain is a common feature in depressive low back pain syndromes and the weakness affects *all* muscle groups. In patients with organic disc disease if weakness *is* present, it will be confined to muscles innervated by one root (i.e. L5 or S1).

Non-organic weakness is usually described as "give-away" weakness. This is a bad term as all weakness leads to the muscle giving way. But in non-organic weakness there is a typical variable weakness proportional to the amount of resistance offered by the examiner. If the examiner suddenly exerts less effort after a brief lag the patient stops trying and "gives-way". Often the patients' performance on testing is grossly at variance with their ability to walk into the clinic, undress and climb on to a couch. Occasionally when total weakness of a muscle is present on a non-organic basis, if the antagonist muscles are palpated at the same time they will be felt to contract every time the patient tries to use the "weak" muscle. There is an enormous amount of grunting and groaning, facial grimacing and stiffening of the entire body in such cases, quite different to the quiet but ineffectual efforts made by the organically paralysed patient.

Loss of Reflexes

Many normal people have depressed or absent reflexes. Such patients often recollect being asked to perform the reflex reinforcement manœuvres at previous physical examinations or recall being told that their reflexes were absent. Recent loss of previously intact reflexes is a very important physical sign. Total loss of reflexes is a feature of peripheral neuropathy and often occurs in patients with muscle disease. Loss of isolated reflexes indicates disease affecting the nerve root or peripheral nerve conveying that reflex (see Chapters 16 and 17).

Muscle Cramps

Muscle cramps are a common experience. They usually occur when a muscle contracts when already shortened, i.e. the small foot muscles when the foot is already flexed by the weight of bedclothes. Salt depletion or a low serum calcium may predispose to cramping but usually in obvious climatic situations or associated with disease. The majority of patients with cramps do *not* have an electrolyte disturbance or any physical disease; it is a physiological phenomenon. Although muscle cramps are a common feature in motor neurone disease unless other definite signs are present this diagnosis should not be entertained.

Muscle Pain on Exercise

Muscle pain during or following exercise is invariably the result of unusual activity. The whole basis of training for any form of sport or activity is to reduce muscle pain or delay its onset. Probably the commonest type is known as "shin-splints". This consists of severe pain in the tibialis anterior muscle following unaccustomed activity. Occasionally the swelling of the muscle within its confined compartment may lead to ischaemic damage and surgical decompression may be required.

Fasciculation

Visible spontaneous contractions of groups of muscle fibres are known as fasciculation. This is usually a physiological phenomenon, often following exertion. It is particularly common in previously athletic patients who have reduced their participation in sports. It is most striking in relaxed dependent muscles such as the calves. Although it does occur in motor neurone disease it is *not* specific for this condition and may occur in any disease of the lower motor neurone. In the absence of any other signs such as wasting or weakness of the fasciculating muscle it is unlikely to be of any significance. Doctors who notice fasciculation in their own muscles usually require very considerable reassurance before they will accept that they do *not* have motor neurone disease.

Sensory Symptoms

In the context of peripheral nervous system disease we are concerned with symmetrical sensory symptoms. These usually begin in the legs and rarely affect the hands until the symptoms in the leg reach knee level. They consist of *non-stop* fine tingling paraesthesiae, coupled with subjective numbness although it is often difficult to detect any actual sensory loss. These sensations may be more severe in a warm bed or while standing but do not remit completely. Patients with *intermittent* peripheral paraesthesiae are almost invariably suffering from an anxiety state with hyperventilation (see Chapter 23). Similar *non-stop* symptoms occur in multiple sclerosis and the distinction is best made by the state of the reflexes. If the reflexes are present or brisk multiple sclerosis is the likely diagnosis; if absent or depressed a peripheral neuropathy may be the cause. As the tingling extends centrally numbness follows in its wake in a "glove and stocking" distribution. This is another expression that is subject to serious misinterpretation as it is often used to describe non-organic sensory deficits, ignoring the fact that organic sensory loss produces the *same* type of loss. In organic sensory loss the sensation gradually becomes normal over a few inches with an intermediate zone of altered sensation. In non-organic loss there is usually a sharp transition from total sensory loss to intact sensation. Furthermore, in organic sensory loss it is unusual for all modalities to be equally affected and relative preservation of some modalities is often found. In non-organic situations *complete* sensory loss to all modalities is claimed.

Further discussion will be divided into two major groups of diseases, those affecting the ventral horn cells and those affecting both the motor and sensory peripheral nerve fibres.

VENTRAL HORN CELL DISEASE

These are a group of disorders due to a variety of genetic, infective or toxic causes, many of which have a lethal prognosis.

1. Inherited Ventral Horn Cell Disease

This category includes three or possibly four conditions if we include the fact that five per cent of patients with motor neurone disease have a family history of this disorder.

a. *Werdnig–Hoffman Disease*

This lethal disease is inherited as an autosomal recessive. The disease may begin in utero and death within the first year of life is the usual outcome. The child is hypotonic from birth and may have difficulty feeding. Motor development is poor and the child is unable to lift its head and the upper limbs tend to flop to the sides. It can be very difficult to detect muscle wasting and fasciculation due to the amount of subcutaneous fat, but fasciculation may be evidenced by sudden twitches of the fingers or toes, as they are pulled by the fasciculating muscle. The facial and tongue muscles are often spared but respiratory muscle paralysis occurs early and is responsible for death in most instances. This is often detectable as indrawing of the intercostal spaces as the child breathes in.

b. *Intermediate Form of Werdnig—Hoffman Disease*

In this variety the child may develop normally in the first year of life until weakness of the legs becomes apparent when the child should start walking. The arms may be mildly affected and unlike the classical disease tongue wasting and fasciculation are prominent. The disease appears to arrest and if respiratory involvement does not occur the child may survive. Whether this represents variable expression of the Werdnig—Hoffman gene or is a separate disease is unknown.

c. *Kugelberg—Welander Syndrome*

This is the mildest of the inherited motor neurone diseases, the onset often being delayed into adulthood. The weakness is most pronounced in the pelvic girdle and the disease is often misdiagnosed as a girdle myopathy. The prognosis is relatively good with some gait disability and later some shoulder girdle weakness but rarely any bulbar muscle involvement. Whether this is a separate genetic disorder or a benign form of Werdnig—Hoffman disease is uncertain.

d. *Motor Neurone Disease (Progressive Muscle Atrophy Type)*

Motor neurone disease in the classical form with combined cortico-spinal and ventral horn cell damage has been discussed in Chapter 14. In this section we are mainly concerned with the variety that primarily affects the ventral horn cells—producing progressive wasting and weakness without long tract signs and running a slower but ultimately fatal course. This type often begins in the legs, particularly affecting the anterior compartments and may be misdiagnosed initially as a peroneal nerve palsy. The reflexes usually remain intact which excludes peripheral nerve disease. Five per cent of cases are on a familial basis and it has been argued that these patients have a less malignant course.

2. Infective Ventral Horn Cell Disease (Acute Anterior Poliomyelitis)

Anterior poliomyelitis has become a rare disease since immunisation was developed in the 1950's. Prior to this yearly epidemics occurred usually causing an aseptic meningitis, which in one per cent of cases went on to paralytic and potentially fatal poliomyelitis. The disease was also known as "infantile paralysis", an expression which belied the fact that a great many adults were also affected and more likely to die.

This may also account for a personal impression that in the past *any* form of paralysis in childhood was likely to be called "polio". A large number of patients have been seen by the author with conditions ranging from cerebral palsy and spina bifida to Friedreich's ataxia whose families had been told they had had "polio". It would seem a wise precaution to carefully review the physical signs in any patient who gives such a history. "Old polio" typically produces a group of severely atrophied and weak muscles with loss of reflexes. Often vasomotor changes in the affected limb produce a violaceous swollen, sweaty extremity. If there is ataxia, sensory loss *or* the reflexes are intact the diagnosis is *not* "old polio"!

The illness still occurs in the non-immune and remains a major risk to travellers in the tropics and less sanitary areas who have *not* been immunised. It is ushered in by an "influenzal" illness with a mild gut upset; this may progress to meningism with headache and a stiff neck. If the paralytic stage is reached the affected muscles become extremely painful and then rapidly waste with severe weakness and loss of the local reflex. The C.S.F. shows a mild pleocytosis.. Facilities for respiratory assistance should be available. Following even severe generalised weakness there is often considerable recovery. There is thought to be a higher risk of a motor neurone disease-like illness developing in survivors of poliomyelitis although this concept has always been disputed. Fortunately with the demise of the disease this consideration is becoming academic.

3. Toxic Ventral Horn Cell Disease

Fortunately there are no drugs that are known to damage the ventral horn cell but at least one chemical, tri-ortho-cresyl-phosphate does and this has twice caused tragic outbreaks of disease in the last fifty years. The first was its use as "Jamaica-ginger", an abortifacient used in the U.S.A. in the 1920's. The second occurred fairly recently when aviation oil containing the chemical was sold as cooking oil in Morocco. An epidemic of poisoning occurred with many severely disabled survivors.

The second "toxic" cause of ventral horn cell damage, or at least a "polio-like" illness is tick paralysis. This is due to a toxin released from a tick embedded in the skin, usually in the scalp or neck. The particular species involved are found in the Rocky Mountains of Canada and the U.S.A. and also occur in South Africa, Australia and South-East Europe, including the Balkan states. Within days of the entry of the tick, fever, delusions, facial paraesthesiae and difficulty in swallowing occur. This is rapidly followed by ascending paralysis, which may prove fatal if the tick is not found and removed.

4. Electric Shock and Ventral Horn Cell Disease

In recent years it has been recognised that survivors of severe electric shock may develop acute spinal cord damage in the affected area of the spinal cord. As the shock often enters through the arm and goes to earth through the opposite arm or leg the cord at C5, C6 or C7 is maximally affected. Within months progressive wasting and weakness in these motor units occurs, producing symptoms and signs indistinguishable from motor neurone disease. The condition usually arrests but the damage is permanent.

PERIPHERAL NEUROPATHY

Lesions affecting individual nerve roots and peripheral nerves are discussed in Chapters 16 and 17. In this section we are concerned with inherited, infective, metabolic, toxic and obscure disorders in which the peripheral nerves are diffusely damaged.

In infancy and childhood peripheral neuropathy may cause failure to achieve normal motor milestones, clumsiness or abnormal gait. Rarely does the child complain of peripheral paraesthesiae, the classical symptom of a neuropathy. Because of the absence of subjective symptoms children with peripheral nerve damage are often thought to have muscular dystrophy.

In the adult the typical symptoms of peripheral paraesthesiae, sensory loss and clumsiness usually due to a mixture of slight loss of dexterity and sensory impairment make the diagnosis more obvious even though the aetiology often remains obscure.

In all age groups a very detailed family history is vital. Sometimes several members of a family are found to have the same disease, masquerading under several different diagnostic labels. If there is any doubt it is worth examining other family members to establish whether or not an inherited disorder is present. A detailed history of all drugs used within the previous two years and any possible chemical exposure, dietary habits, previous surgical procedures and alcohol intake should be included.

1. Inherited Peripheral Neuropathies

Peroneal Muscular Atrophy (Charcot-Marie-Tooth Disease)

This condition may be inherited as a dominant or recessive gene and may produce physical signs at any age. Typically the illness starts with wasting and weakness of the peroneal muscles producing a foot drop and pes cavus. Later the calf muscles and the distal third of the thigh atrophy producing a leg shaped like a "stork leg" or a "champagne glass". Vibration sense is impaired and later some joint position sense loss may occur. The motor disabilities are always much more in evidence than sensory deficit. In a very florid case the distal forearms and small hand muscles may also waste. Reflexes are absent and some thickening of the peripheral nerves is detectable in about 25 per cent of cases.

Hypertrophic Peripheral Neuropathy (Dejerine–Sottas Disease)

This form of peripheral neuropathy usually causes symptoms in adolescence or adulthood. A diffuse peripheral neuropathy eventually results including the cranial nerves. Marked thickening of the involved nerves is the striking feature of the disorder and is often first detected in the supraclavicular nerves or in the cutaneous nerves over the dorsum of the foot. Ultimately all the peripheral nerves become thickened up to twice their usual size. Rarely the nerve roots in the spinal canal become so large that they compress the spinal cord. The C.S.F. protein is usually very elevated in this condition.

Friedreich's Ataxia

This hereditary disease has already been described in Chapter 14 as it mainly affects spinal cord pathways. However, a diffuse peripheral neuropathy manifest as areflexia is a constant feature of the illness, which appears to be part of a spectrum of inherited disorders, including those discussed above.

In all the inherited neuropathies discussed above both affected and non-affected family members may have had "pes cavus" from childhood with difficulty in obtaining shoes that fit.

Hereditary Sensory Neuropathy

This familial disorder almost specifically affects pain sensation and to a lesser extent other modalities particularly in the legs. The underlying lesion appears to be a degenerative process in the dorsal root ganglia and the disorder is very slowly progressive. The main problems are due to recurrent painless trauma and ulceration of the feet, later progressing to a severe destructive arthropathy of the ankle joints (Charcot's joint).

Hereditary Ataxic Neuropathy (Refsum's syndrome)

This is a rare disorder and consists of a combination of cerebellar damage, peripheral neuropathy, deafness and retinitis pigmentosa. The serum phytanic acid (hexadec-anoic acid) is markedly elevated but as in so many metabolic disorders the relationship of this chemical abnormality to the disease is not clear.

Amyloid Neuropathy

There are three varieties of amyloid neuropathy. The first type to be reported is almost exclusively confined to patients of Portuguese extraction. This produces a very unpleasant, relentlessly progressive and ultimately fatal neuropathy that starts in the legs in the third decade and runs its course over some ten years. The second variety has been reported in Swiss families and is a milder disorder usually starting in the arms with a carpal-tunnel like syndrome. Vitreous opacities are common in this variety. The third variety is not determined on an ethnic or familial basis but occurs in a sporadic form and has been increasingly recognised since peripheral nerve biopsies became a routine investigation.

Lipoprotein Neuropathies

Two neuropathies associated with disorders of lipoprotein metabolism have been reported. These are Tangier Disease and Bassen–Kornzweig syndrome. In both the serum cholesterol is very low (<80 mgm per cent). Tangier Disease is associated with a virtual absence of high density lipoprotein from the serum and massive deposition of cholesterol in the enlarged tonsils. Bassen–Kornzweig syndrome includes a malabsorption syndrome, red cells with tentacles (acanthocytes) and a virtual absence of beta-lipoproteins from the serum.

Cerebral Lipoidoses

Several of the cerebral degenerative diseases associated with the deposition of abnormal lipids in the brain (metachromatic leucodystrophy, Krabbe's leukodystrophy) although dominated by cerebral problems include a peripheral neuropathy as part of the picture. Nerve conduction studies and nerve biopsies will often confirm the diagnosis without resort to cerebral biopsy.

All the inherited neuropathic conditions produce signs of a peripheral neuropathy; basically loss of all reflexes. The routine evaluation of all patients with neuropathy should include a careful family history, palpation of the peripheral nerves, examination of the eyes for vitreous opacities and retinitis pigmentosa and examination of the tonsils. A routine blood film, serum cholesterol and lipoprotein determination, and blood phytanic acid level should be included in the screening investigations.

In genetically determined and metabolic neuropathies a frequent finding is marked slowing of nerve conduction, which may be in the 10–20 m/sec. range (normal 38 m/sec. and higher). In other types of neuropathy slowing to the lower range of normal occurs but with the exception of Guillain–Barré syndrome this extreme slowing is rarely found.

2. Metabolically Triggered Neuropathy (Acute Intermittent Porphyria)

This rare and potentially fatal condition is due to a disorder of haemoglobin metabolism. Acute attacks may occur spontaneously but are particularly likely to be triggered by certain drugs listed in Table 5. The onset of an attack is usually marked by vomiting and severe abdominal pain, a condition easily misdiagnosed as an intra-abdominal emergency and worsened if barbiturate anaesthesia or sulphonamides are administered to the patient. The illness then affects the nervous system producing an acute psychosis or a rapidly progressive neuropathy or a combination of both. The weakness may be found mainly in the proximal muscles and the sensory loss may occur in a bathing suit distribution rather than peripherally. When these rather "non-organic" signs are coupled with the psychiatric complications the ease with which an attack can be misdiagnosed as hysteria is apparent and understandable. A careful history of drug ingestion should be taken routinely in *all* patients with *any* disorder of the central nervous system. There may be no family history until the first case is detected. Full family screening may reveal other members who have yet to have an attack and who may even have taken provocative drugs *without* developing an episode.

Table 5

DRUGS PRECIPITATING ATTACKS OF PORPHYRIA

Barbiturates
Sulphonamides
Alpha-methyl-dopa
Laevodopa
Griseofulvin
Dichloralphenazone (Welldorm)
Glutethimide (Doriden)
Phenylbutazone
Oestrogens (including the birth control pill)

The diagnosis is made by the detection of excess porphobilinogen and delta-amino laevulinic acid in the urine. Porphyrins, which are a deep red in colour, form when porphobilinogens are exposed to light and oxidation. The urine may not change colour for several hours.

Treatment is supportive and although cases occur too infrequently for controlled observations, consensus opinion suggests that chlorpromazine has a beneficial effect, possibly by an effect on liver function.

3. Infective Neuropathies

There are four neuropathies related to infective organisms. Leprosy, which is a direct infection of the nerves, diphtheria via a toxin produced in the body, Guillain—Barré syndrome possible due to an abnormal immune response to viral infections and botulinum poisoning in which the toxins produced by the organism are ingested.

Leprosy

Leprosy is probably the single most important cause of peripheral neuropathy on a world-wide scale. Fortunately it is now rare in Europe but is endemic throughout Africa and the Middle East. It is not very infective and travellers are unlikely to contract the disease, but contract workers who live in these areas for prolonged periods are at some risk. The nerves are directly infected and patches of numbness appear all over the body, but particularly on the extremities and the face. If the patient is coloured the affected patches become pale. The main nerve trunks are thickened and become pressure sensitive so that sudden pressure palsies of particularly vulnerable nerves (i.e. the ulnar and peroneal nerves) punctuate the slow development of a diffuse neuropathy. The patient therefore develops "mononeuritis multiplex" (the other causes of this condition being diabetes and polyarteritis nodosa). Pain and temperature sensation are specifically affected and severe trophic changes may occur with ulceration and necrosis of the extremities. One patient seen by the writer discovered his neuropathy when he accidentally shut his hand in the door of a Land-Rover. This was quite painless and later that day he found he could hold the injured hand in a fire without discomfort but devastating effect on his injuries! He had been completely asymptomatic until that time.

Diphtheria

In most civilised countries this disease has become a rarity due to mass immunisation. Occasional outbreaks still occur and reveal that the disease remains a very serious and often lethal infection of childhood. The neuropathy occurs in most patients to a minor degree as paralysis of accommodation and palatal weakness frequently occur in the third week of the illness. At any time up to two months after the onset an explosive neuropathy may occur with rapidly ascending paralysis, and respiratory problems. With intensive care recovery should occur, the limiting factor often being the myocarditis which complicates the illness.

Guillain—Barré Syndrome

This condition is thought to be a single response of the central nervous system to a variety of infective processes. It often follows acute upper respiratory tract or gut infections and specifically complicates glandular fever in a few cases. It may occur in association with a remote carcinoma. It can occur at any age, and the clinical findings may be very variable and hysteria is often suspected. The first symptoms are usually peripheral painful paraesthesiae but rarely accompanied by definite sensory findings. Weakness may come on quite explosively and a patient may become extremely weak over as short a period as thirty minutes, although more typically the period of advancing weakness in an acute case is some twelve to forty-eight hours. The weakness is often most marked in the proximal muscles, so that the patient may be unable to sit or stand at a time when peripheral strength is quite normal; it is this combination that may lead to a diagnosis of hysteria. In most cases the main clue, and in the writer's opinion almost diagnostic finding, is the total abolition of reflexes, even at the stage when the weakness has not become generalised. Bilateral facial weakness is quite common but easily missed unless eye closure, cheek blowing and lip pouting are routinely tested. If present this is another virtually diagnostic sign of Guillain—Barré syndrome—it is extremely rare in other forms of neuropathy.

Some twenty-five per cent of patients have significant respiratory problems and the ten per cent mortality rate is a measure of the potential danger of this disease. Patients should be moved to a unit where respiratory facilities are available. Dramatic deterioration may occur in an hour and transfer should not be delayed once the diagnosis is established.

The C.S.F. protein is typically elevated, but this may take several days to occur, and in the very acute stages of a severe attack some lymphocytes may be found in the C.S.F. raising diagnostic possibilities such as poliomyelitis.

Guillain—Barré syndrome is one of a few conditions that the writer regards as an acute neurological emergency, and yet it is often casually treated and regarded as a benign condition by those who see the occasional case that runs a mild course with recovery over a few weeks.

At the opposite extreme there is a variant of this disorder of slow onset, often over several weeks, with a tendency to persist or even slowly progress over a period of years with severe disability, and occasionally responding to steroids. In the acute type of attack ACTH may be of some benefit. In the chronic variety the author has had considerable success in two cases using cytotoxic drugs.

Botulinum Toxin Poisoning

This is an extremely lethal acute neuropathy that follows the ingestion of tinned or preserved foods contaminated by Clostridium botulinum. The illness therefore occurs in a group of people who have eaten the contaminated food within a period of three to four hours. The acute symptoms are pupillary dilatation, diplopia, slurred speech and difficulty in swallowing, followed by a rapidly descending paralysis. Polyvalent botulinum antitoxin 50,000 I.V.I. should be given immediately to block circulating toxin and full resuscitative measures instituted. The toxin blocks acetylcholine release at the neuromuscular junction and the condition is similar to myasthenia gravis in its clinical onset. The rapid deterioration should suggest the even more serious diagnosis of botulinum toxin poisoning.

4. Toxic Neuropathies

There are a wide range of drugs and chemicals, particularly heavy metals and benzene derivatives that can cause peripheral nerve damage. A full history of drug ingestion and possible chemical exposure should be part of the routine questioning in patients with peripheral neuropathy. Exposure to heavy metals, particularly lead and arsenic and organic industrial solvents may be difficult to establish unless the medical department of the patient's employers are directly approached.

5. Miscellaneous Neuropathies

This category includes several important general medical conditions including diabetes, alcoholism, renal disease and malignancy, in which the exact relationship to the underlying disease or drugs is an uncertain one. Each will be discussed as a separate entity.

Alcoholic Peripheral Neuropathy

In the world as a whole alcohol is a common cause of peripheral neuropathy but in Great Britain at least it is not a common disorder. There is dispute as to whether it is due to a direct toxic effect of alcohol or secondary vitamin B_1 deficiency. Although B_1 deficiency alone is enough to cause a neuropathy similar clinically to that of alcoholism the response to B_1 is not as dramatic in an alcoholic, even when alcohol is also withdrawn. Alcoholic neuropathy is usually very painful with spontaneous pain in the legs and hands and very marked hypersensitivity to light touch or painful stimuli. The patient cannot bear the bedclothes

to touch his feet or his feet on the ground. This part of the neuropathy usually responds within days to B_1 administration. In a severe case, symmetrical weakness and wasting with loss of reflexes may occur and recovery may take years even with adequate vitamin replacement and abstention from alcohol.

Diabetic Peripheral Neuropathy

Diabetes is probably the commonest cause of neuropathy in Great Britain. It may occur in classical adolescent onset diabetes, but occurs much more frequently in maturity onset diabetes and is often the presenting symptom of this condition. Peripheral paraesthesiae and tingling accompanied by loss of reflexes are the usual clinical findings and the neuropathy usually remains fairly mild and restricted. In a severe case marked loss of pain sensation may occur and lead to the formation of Charcot's joints particularly at the ankle.

The exact relationship to the diabetes is uncertain, but an ischaemic basis due to small vessel disease seems likely. The peripheral nerves are very sensitive to pressure and a "mononeuritis multiplex" picture due to multiple pressure palsies is common. The extraocular nerves (see Chapter 5) and the femoral nerve (see Chapter 17) are both subject to spontaneous infarction in diabetic patients.

The autonomic nerves may be involved and impotence and postural hypotension occur. The role of autonomic nerve damage in the reported intermittent and nocturnal diarrhoea of diabetes is uncertain (see also Chapter 26). Some diabetic nerve lesions are painful, particularly that associated with a femoral nerve lesion (diabetic amyotrophy) but in the majority of diabetics the neuropathy is a relatively minor problem.

Ischaemic Peripheral Neuropathy

The probable role of nerve ischaemia in diabetic neuropathy has been discussed above. Many 70–80-year-old patients complain of tingling paraesthesiae in the feet, particularly in a warm bed or on standing. This may be accompanied by definite blunting of cutaneous sensation over the feet. This is almost certainly due to poor skin nutrition affecting the cutaneous nerve filaments and nerve endings in the skin. No treatment is of any benefit.

The Neuropathy of Chronic Renal Failure

Chronic renal failure causes peripheral neuropathy. Some cases may have been due to nitrofurantoin (Furadantin) in the past but it was always argued that the nerve damage was due to the uraemia. It seems likely that this was so, as the recent advent of chronic renal dialysis in patients *not* taking antibiotics has revealed that these patients do develop peripheral neuropathy. In several centres routine periodic nerve conduction studies are used as one method of monitoring the effectiveness of dialysis.

6. Neuropathy associated with malignant disease

A mixed sensory and motor neuropathy associated with non-metastatic malignant disease occurs but is extremely rare, and is almost invariably associated with bronchial carcinoma, almost to the exclusion of other malignant disorders. Malignant lymphomas of all types may produce the same picture; in some instances due to direct infiltration of the nerves. It has become increasingly difficult to study neuropathy in malignant disease as the cytotoxic drug, Vincristine, has a marked neurotoxic effect, producing a peripheral neuropathy in approximately half the patients that receive it.

It is incumbent on the physician to examine the patient with a neuropathy for evidence of malignant disease or lymphoma. Investigations should include a chest film and a routine blood film but there is no need for full radiological screening of the bowel or kidney; the chance of finding a tumour at these sites is minimal.

Even if a primary carcinoma is found its removal appears to have no definite effect on the neuropathy; the patient usually continues to deteriorate although very rarely improvement may occur.

ELECTROMYOGRAPHY AND NERVE CONDUCTION STUDIES

The study of the electrical activity of resting and contracting skeletal muscle and conduction of the nerve impulse has become one of the most useful diagnostic tools in neurology.

At experimental level the technique has been responsible for a complete reappraisal of neuromuscular diseases, and clinically E.M.G. studies may completely alter the diagnosis and prevent a serious diagnostic error. E.M.G. and nerve conduction studies have become indispensable in the diagnosis and management of peripheral nerve and muscle disease. It is really only possible to learn these techniques by practical experience but it is worth understanding the terms used descriptively in E.M.G. reporting and these are described below. The general principles of nerve conduction studies are described and the application to specific situations shown in Figures 16.2 and 16.3.

Electromyography

Electromyography is carried out by the insertion of a twin core needle electrode into the muscle. The electrical potentials in the muscle are observed on an oscilloscope during insertion of the needle, with the muscle at rest and during full muscle contraction. The muscle to be sampled is selected depending on the clinical diagnosis. In general a mildly affected muscle is preferred to a severely affected muscle as in the latter case there may be so few surviving muscle fibres that the E.M.G. findings are confusing (see Figure 16.1).

1. *Denervation* (Figure 16.1a)

If the nerve supply to a muscle is damaged by disease of the ventral horn cell, nerve root or peripheral nerve the muscle is "denervated" and the E.M.G. findings are known as "chronic partial denervation".

Each ventral horn cell and its axon supplies a group of muscle fibres, the whole known as a "motor unit". This means that if a ventral horn cell or its neurone is damaged a discrete and limited group of muscle fibres cease to function. It has been shown that surviving neurones are capable of branching and taking over adjacent denervated muscle fibres, enlarging the size of the surviving units. These basic changes lead to the following E.M.G. findings in a denervated muscle.

a. Denervated muscle fibres are very irritable and show spontaneous electrical activity. On needle insertion the normal brief injury potentials are greatly prolonged (increased insertional activity) and occasionally continue in a burst of decreasing frequency and amplitude (a pseudo-myotonic run).

b. With the needle held still in the resting muscle transient alterations in the muscle membrane potential of 50–200 μV size and of extremely brief duration occur. These are fibrillation potentials. These may occasionally be of longer duration and monophasic and are then known as a positive sharp wave. Twitches of entire motor units produce fasciculation potentials. These are the contractions visible to the naked eye and sometimes incorrectly referred to clinically as "fibrillation". These are not necessarily pathological.

c. When the resting activity has been observed the patient is asked to contract the muscle gently while the examiner steadies the needle. Individual units are studied. The normal motor unit produces a bi- or tri-phasic potential of 2 mV size in a proximal muscle and 5 mV in the small hand or feet muscles. When a unit has been enlarged by the branching of its nerve fibre to incorporate adjacent muscle fibres two things happen. The duration and size of the unit is increased, producing a polyphasic potential that is greatly enlarged in amplitude, often reaching 5–10 mV in foot muscles and 15 mV in the small hand muscles. These are known as giant units.

Figure 16.1.

Normal Muscle

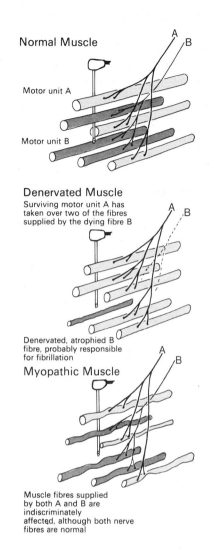

Motor unit A

Motor unit B

Denervated Muscle

Surviving motor unit A has taken over two of the fibres supplied by the dying fibre B

Denervated, atrophied B fibre, probably responsible for fibrillation

Myopathic Muscle

Muscle fibres supplied by both A and B are indiscriminately affected, although both nerve fibres are normal

Normal E.M.G.

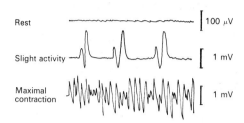

Rest — 100 μV

Slight activity — 1 mV

Maximal contraction — 1 mV

Figure 16.1A. Chronic Partial Denervation

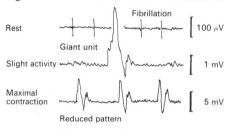

Rest — Fibrillation — 100 μV

Giant unit

Slight activity — 1 mV

Maximal contraction — 5 mV

Reduced pattern

Figure 16.1B. Myopathic E.M.G.

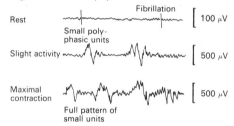

Rest — Fibrillation — 100 μV

Small polyphasic units

Slight activity — 500 μV

Maximal contraction — 500 μV

Full pattern of small units

d. The patient then contracts the muscle as hard as possible against resistance. In a normal muscle the activity is continuous as units contract and rest as others take over. The baseline sweep is completely obliterated. This is known as the interference pattern. In a denervated muscle gaps appear in the pattern marking the former position of a damaged unit in the sequence and the surviving units are often large and polyphasic. From their identical appearance it is often clear that it is the *same* giant unit repeating at regular intervals. This is known as a reduction in the interference pattern.

These findings may be patchy and in some diseases the fastest conducting fibres seem to be affected first so that the maximal findings of denervation are in the periphery of the muscle. This is a particular feature of motor neurone disease.

It must be stressed that these findings only indicate damage to the nerve fibres or ventral horn cell—the level at which the damage has occurred must be deduced from the clinical features and nerve conduction studies. Chronic partial denervation does *not* automatically indicate ventral horn cell disease.

2. *Myopathic Changes* (Figure 16.1b)

In muscle disease the situation is quite different. The disease process affects all or some muscle fibres in an entirely random way without regard to motor units. The only exception to this is in polymyositis in which the changes may be extremely patchy and full depth sampling in several areas of a muscle may be necessary before an area of typical damage is detected.

The following features are found in muscle disease:

a. Damaged muscle fibres, particularly in necrotic myopathies such as polymyositis and in Pompé's disease (see

Chapter 17), (in which glycogen storage disease affects both the muscle fibre and the ventral horn cell) may be irritable and show fibrillation which may lead to an incorrect diagnosis of denervation.

b. As the process is often patchy in individual fibres there is delayed or blocked conduction along the fibre, both dispersing the unit and reducing its size. The end result is a small (200–500 μV) polyphasic action potential. The interference pattern is usually full as part of all units survive but the small polyphasic potentials produce a very characteristic "crackling" noise on the E.M.G. amplifier.

c. In muscle disease associated with myotonia, the prolonged discharges that produce the typical stiffness of the muscles are audible as decrementing bursts of potentials that were formerly likened to "dive-bomber" noises, but in the author's view a more accurate and contemporary description would be the sound of a highly tuned Japanese motor-cycle engine. The bursts often superimpose on one another, quite unlike the brief "pseudo-myotonic" runs provoked by needle movement in irritable partially denervated muscles.

d. E.M.G. techniques have a limited place in the diagnosis of myasthenia gravis as the muscles typically affected are often inaccessible to EMG techniques.

Nerve Conduction Studies

1. The basic requirements for motor nerve conduction studies are that a suitable muscle is available and that its nerve supply can be stimulated at two points along its course. The time taken from the stimulus nearest the muscle is known as the distal latency and includes not only the time taken for the impulse to travel down the nerve but also the delay at the end plate and initiation of contraction. If the nerve is then stimulated higher up a second latency can be obtained, the difference in the time taken being an accurate measurement of the time taken for the impulse to traverse a measured length of nerve. From this the conduction velocity in metres per second is easily calculated. Very carefully documented velocity ranges for all the nerves that can be studied in this way have been reported. These are the median and ulnar nerves in the arm and the peroneal and tibial nerves in the leg. Nerves such as the radial and femoral can only be readily stimulated at one point and a latency to an appropriate muscle is all that can be measured.

In general if a muscle is denervated and it can be shown that the lesion responsible is above the proximal stimulus it is probably affecting the nerve root or ventral horn cell.

Figure 16.2. Nerve Conduction Studies in the Arm

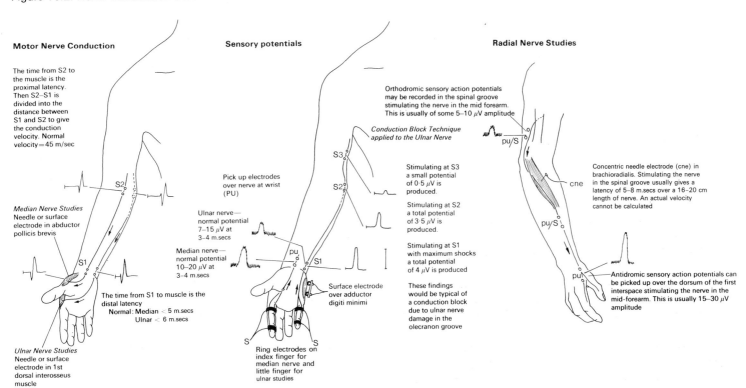

Motor Nerve Conduction

The time from S2 to the muscle is the proximal latency. Then S2–S1 is divided into the distance between S1 and S2 to give the conduction velocity. Normal velocity = 45 m/sec

S2

Median Nerve Studies
Needle or surface electrode in abductor pollicis brevis

S1

The time from S1 to muscle is the distal latency
Normal: Median < 5 m.secs
Ulnar < 6 m.secs

Ulnar Nerve Studies
Needle or surface electrode in 1st dorsal interosseus muscle

Sensory potentials

Pick up electrodes over nerve at wrist (PU)

Ulnar nerve— normal potential 7–15 μV at 3–4 m.secs

Median nerve— normal potential 10–20 μV at 3–4 m.secs

pu

S1

Surface electrode over adductor digiti minimi

Ring electrodes on index finger for median nerve and little finger for ulnar studies

Conduction Block Technique applied to the Ulnar Nerve

S3

S2

Stimulating at S3 a small potential of 0·5 μV is produced.

Stimulating at S2 a total potential of 3·5 μV is produced.

Stimulating at S1 with maximum shocks a total potential of 4 μV is produced

These findings would be typical of a conduction block due to ulnar nerve damage in the olecranon groove

Radial Nerve Studies

Orthodromic sensory action potentials may be recorded in the spinal groove stimulating the nerve in the mid forearm. This is usually of some 5–10 μV amplitude

pu/S

cne

Concentric needle electrode (cne) in brachioradialis. Stimulating the nerve in the spinal groove usually gives a latency of 5–8 m.secs over a 16–20 cm length of nerve. An actual velocity cannot be calculated

pu/S

pu

Antidromic sensory action potentials can be picked up over the dorsum of the first interspace stimulating the nerve in the mid-forearm. This is usually 15–30 μV amplitude

Figure 16.3. Nerve Conduction Studies in the Leg

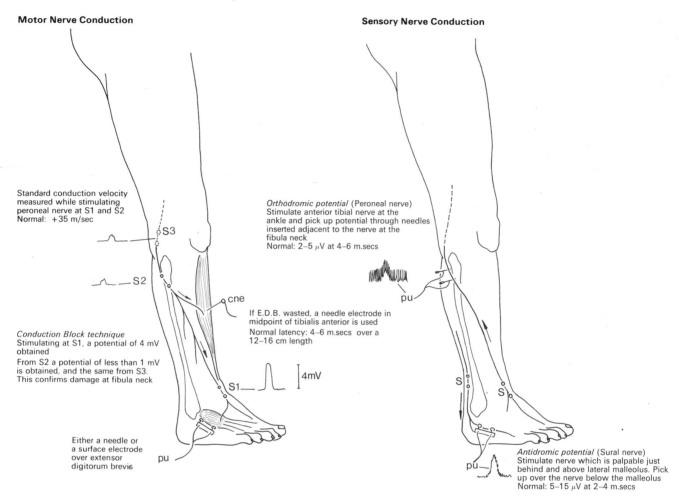

Motor Nerve Conduction

Standard conduction velocity measured while stimulating peroneal nerve at S1 and S2
Normal: +35 m/sec

S3

S2

cne

Conduction Block technique
Stimulating at S1, a potential of 4 mV obtained
From S2 a potential of less than 1 mV is obtained, and the same from S3. This confirms damage at fibula neck

If E.D.B. wasted, a needle electrode in midpoint of tibialis anterior is used
Normal latency: 4–6 m.secs over a 12–16 cm length

S1

4mV

Either a needle or a surface electrode over extensor digitorum brevis

pu

Sensory Nerve Conduction

Orthodromic potential (Peroneal nerve)
Stimulate anterior tibial nerve at the ankle and pick up potential through needles inserted adjacent to the nerve at the fibula neck
Normal: 2–5 μV at 4–6 m.secs

pu

S

S

Antidromic potential (Sural nerve)
Stimulate nerve which is palpable just behind and above lateral malleolus. Pick up over the nerve below the malleolus
Normal: 5–15 μV at 2–4 m.secs

pu

The position of electrodes and velocities for the arm and legs are shown in Figures 16.2 and 16.3.

2. Nerve action potentials can be measured in two ways orthodromically or antidromically. Here the main requirement is a nerve near enough to the surface to be picked up by a surface electrode or anatomically constant in position allowing needle electrodes to be inserted next to the nerve. Both the median and ulnar nerve action potentials can be detected at the wrist by stimulating the interdigital nerves of the appropriate fingers. Nerve action potentials in the leg present a great problem. The techniques are shown in Figures 16.2 and 16.3.

3. In the case of ulnar nerve lesions at the elbow or the peroneal nerve lesions at the fibula neck due to compression some patients do *not* demonstrate slowed conduction through the damaged area. A very useful ancillary test is the study of quantitative muscle action potentials. Using max-imal shocks the full muscle potential produced from stimulation at the wrist or ankle is measured. The nerve is then stimulated just below the elbow or fibula neck. A slight reduction of potential of some ten per cent is normal. Then the nerve is stimulated *above* the elbow or in the popliteal fossa respectively. A dramatic drop in the potential is often seen indicating that some fifty to seventy-five per cent of fibres are *not* functioning in the damaged segments even though the velocity in the surviving fibres is normal (see Figures 16.2 and 16.3). Using this technique the actual point of damage may be detected at a position where the nerve is almost inexcitable.

There is no standard examination for any patient referred for E.M.G. and nerve conduction studies. The clinical problem is considered and a combination of muscle sampling and nerve studies are performed appropriate to the situation.

Chapter 17

DISEASES OF MUSCLE AND THE MUSCLE END PLATE

Muscles are subject to a wide range of inherited, degenerative, metabolic and toxic disorders. There is a marked similarity to peripheral nerve disease in that a wide range of disorders produce a limited group of symptoms and signs. Differential diagnosis depends on a careful family history, careful documentation of the extent and distribution of the muscle abnormalities and an awareness of all the diagnostic possibilities.

1. MUSCULAR DYSTROPHY

Muscular dystrophy is characterised by an inherited degeneration of various muscle groups that begins after a period of apparently normal muscle development and function. In some varieties the onset is delayed until adulthood. Although still regarded as a primary muscle disorder clinical and electro-physiological evidence has suggested a neurogenic component. A full discussion of these controversial views is beyond the scope of the present text.

Although clinical features often allow a confident diagnosis to be made it is essential that full confirmatory studies including electrophysiological tests and muscle biopsy are performed. The diagnosis must be certain for prognostic purposes and to allow genetic counselling to be firmly based. Occasionally, patients are seen who have been given a lethal prognosis, and who are later shown to have a restricted form of myopathy or a neuropathic disease such as Kugelberg–Welander syndrome.

The muscular dystrophies include:

a. Duchenne muscular dystrophy—
   1. Sex-linked disease of males with dominant inheritance.
   2. Non-sex-linked autosomal recessive in males and females.

b. Beckers muscular dystrophy—
   1. A mild sex-linked form of muscular dystrophy in males.

c. Limb-girdle dystrophy—
   1. Pelvi-femoral type (Leyden–Mobius variety).
   2. Scapulo-humeral dystrophy.

d. Facio-scapulo-humeral dystrophy (Landouzy–Dejerine).

e. Dystrophia myotonica (Steinert's disease).

f. Myotonia congenita (Thomsen's disease).

g. Ocular dystrophies.

General Clinical Features of Muscular Dystrophy

1. There is usually a positive family history. It is always worth remembering that family histories can be unreliable or impossible to obtain. Only a *positive* family history has any significance.

2. The distribution and sequence of muscle damage will vary widely depending on the type of dystrophy. Indeed, these features form the basis of the classification of muscular dystrophy (see Figures 17.1–17.5).

3. In muscular dystrophy the muscles become weak *before* significant wasting is apparent. This is because the degenerating fibres are often replaced by fat, and the muscles may even appear hypertrophied. Such muscles have a stodgy, doughy feel. This is quite the reverse of neural disease in which the atrophy proceeds faster than weakness.

4. Reflexes are often depressed or absent very early in the course of muscular dystrophy and long before the muscle is significantly wasted. This is one of the features that has led to the suggestion that there is a neurogenic component.

5. In the terminal stages of muscular dystrophy it may be impossible to make a clinical diagnosis as the widespread muscle wasting, weakness and loss of reflexes could equally well indicate a diffuse neurogenic disorder.

The sequence and distribution of weakness in the various types of muscular dystrophy are indicated in Figures 17.1–17.5, and the other features are summarised in the legend of each diagram.

2. CONGENITAL MYOPATHIES

For many years the term "floppy infant" was used to describe a group of muscular disorders, present from birth in which the child was hypotonic and showed delayed motor activity and development. The disabilities may be sufficiently severe to threaten the child's survival. A wide range of disorders may be responsible. In some cases the condition is merely evidence of severe cerebral damage, as spasticity and choreo-athetoid movements *cannot* develop until 1–2 years

Figure 17.1. Clinical Features of Duchenne Dystrophy

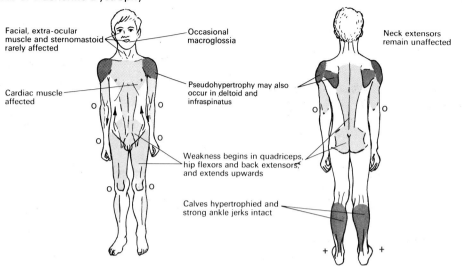

Facial, extra-ocular
muscle and sternomastoid
rarely affected

Occasional
macroglossia

Cardiac muscle
affected

Pseudohypertrophy may also
occur in deltoid and
infraspinatus

Weakness begins in quadriceps,
hip flexors and back extensors,
and extends upwards

Neck extensors
remain unaffected

Calves hypertrophied and
strong ankle jerks intact

DUCHENNE (Pseudohypertrophic) MUSCULAR DYSTROPHY

1. Males, inherited as sex-linked recessive (very rare female cases reported).
2. Onset between 3 and 10 years of age.
3. No abortive cases, most die within ten years of onset.
4. Onset in proximal muscles of leg, especially quadriceps and lower trunk muscles; later shoulder girdle and then extends peripherally. Contractures occur early and are severe.
5. Important early signs include loss of reflexes except the ankle jerk which usually remains intact and excludes a neuropathy.
6. The diaphragm, neck muscles, extraocular and facial muscles very rarely involved.
7. Other features include macroglossia in some cases and pseudohypertrophy usually of the calves but occasionally of the deltoid and infraspinatus.
8. Bone thinning, scoliosis, pathological fractures, fatty infiltration of the heart and respiratory infections are important complications that may lead to death.
9. Thirty per cent of affected patients have an I.Q. of less than 75.
10. The carrier state may be detected by serum enzyme studies and E.M.G. In the patient early on enzymes are very high with a later fall into normal range when atrophy is severe.

of age. Werdnig–Hoffman disease may be so severe at birth that floppy paralysis is already present. Dystrophia myotonica may be another cause of the "floppy infant" syndrome; although the usual onset is in the second or third decade.

This leaves several other disorders that appear to be due to a myopathic process, ranging from a benign variety with delayed but normal motor development, to a progressive myopathy. The routine use of muscle biopsy including electron microscopy and histochemistry has revealed several different pathologies.

Currently four varieties of congenital myopathy have been identified.

1. Central core disease: (abnormal structure and absence of muscle enzymes in the central areas of muscle fibres).

2. Nemaline-rod myopathy: (thread-like structures are found in the muscle fibres).
3. Myotubular myopathy: (the muscle fibres have a tubular structure similar to foetal muscle).
4. Congenital fibre-type disproportion: (abnormal ratio of type 1 and type 2 muscle fibres).

All these conditions cause a slowly progressive proximal weakness usually more severe in the legs. The nemaline-rod-myopathy is associated with kyphoscoliosis, pes cavus and a long thin face. The myotubular type may affect the extra-ocular muscles and in some cases may be associated with a long thin face. Congenital fibre-type disproportion causes very severe floppy weakness easily misdiagnosed as Werdnig–Hoffman disease. Even in this latter disorder some degree of improvement begins after two to three years, and most patients with these disorders survive into adulthood.

Figure 17.2. Clinical Features of Limb-Girdle Dystrophy

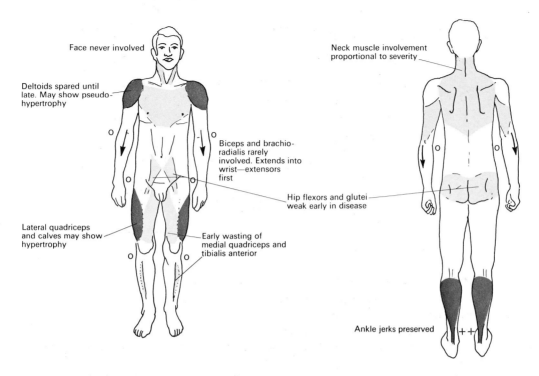

Face never involved

Deltoids spared until late. May show pseudo-hypertrophy

Biceps and brachio-radialis rarely involved. Extends into wrist—extensors first

Lateral quadriceps and calves may show hypertrophy

Early wasting of medial quadriceps and tibialis anterior

Neck muscle involvement proportional to severity

Hip flexors and glutei weak early in disease

Ankle jerks preserved + +

LIMB-GIRDLE DYSTROPHY

1. Males/females equally affected, autosomal recessive but occasionally dominant or sporadic.
2. Onset between 10 and 30 years of age.
3. Abortive cases with incomplete picture occur with mainly pelvic or shoulder girdle involvement. Usually causes disability over ten to twenty years after onset.
4. Onset may be in either pelvic or shoulder girdle and may remain confined to these areas or apparently static for years. In late cases considerable peripheral wasting and weakness may occur. Contractures are unusual.
5. Proximal reflexes are often impaired and as in Duchenne dystrophy the ankle jerks are usually preserved until late in the disease.
6. Cardiac involvement is extremely rare; and facial muscles are only slightly affected if at all.
7. Pseudohypertrophy may occur in the calves and deltoids and strikingly in the lateral quadriceps often associated with early and gross wasting of the medial thigh.
8. There are no special complications and life span is unaffected.
9. Intelligence is normal.
10. The serum enzymes are slightly elevated or normal.

Figure 17.3. Clinical features of Facio-Scapulo-Humeral Dystrophy

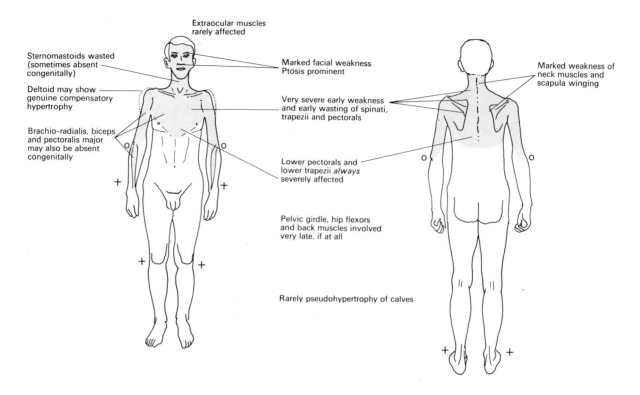

Extraocular muscles rarely affected

Sternomastoids wasted (sometimes absent congenitally)

Deltoid may show genuine compensatory hypertrophy

Brachio-radialis, biceps and pectoralis major may also be absent congenitally

Marked facial weakness Ptosis prominent

Very severe early weakness and early wasting of spinati, trapezii and pectorals

Lower pectorals and lower trapezii *always* severely affected

Pelvic girdle, hip flexors and back muscles involved very late, if at all

Rarely pseudohypertrophy of calves

Marked weakness of neck muscles and scapula winging

FACIO-SCAPULO-HUMERAL DYSTROPHY (Landouzy–Dejerine)

1. Males/females equally affected, autosomal dominant, occasionally recessive.
2. Onset at any age between 10 and 40 years of age.
3. Mild abortive cases common. Siblings or parents of a case often have only facial weakness.
4. Weakness begins in the face, then involves the shoulder girdle, particularly the lower trapezii and pectoralis, triceps and biceps. Pelvic girdle is rarely significantly involved and very late if at all. Contractures very rare.
5. Reflexes only impaired at biceps and triceps. Progression extremely slow. Disability is relatively minor.
6. Pseudohypertrophy is rare; the deltoids are often enlarged by true hypertrophy to compensate for other weak muscles.
7. Special features include congenital absence of pectoralis, biceps or brachioradialis. Occasionally tibialis anterior may be the only muscle involved outside the shoulder girdle.
8. Normal life span.
9. Normal intelligence.
10. Serum enzyme studies usually normal.

Figure 17.4. Myotonia Congenita (Thomsen's Disease)

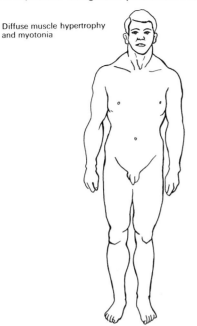

Diffuse muscle hypertrophy
and myotonia

MYOTONIA CONGENITA (Thomsen's Disease)

1. Both sexes affected. Inherited as an autosomal dominant.

2. Myotonia is present from birth and first noticed as a peculiar cry, difficulty in feeding or inability to re-open the eyes while having the face washed.

3. Muscle hypertrophy becomes apparent in the second decade but athletic ability is poor due to slowness and stiffness of movement. Once mobile the stiffness eases and some patients can compete in long-distance events. The myotonia is much worse in the cold and this makes winter games such as football virtually impossible.

4. The muscle hypertrophy is the result of almost continual involuntary isometric exercise.

5. The myotonia becomes less severe with age and often responds well to procaineamide or quinidine. Patients are well advised to pursue an indoor occupation. One patient of the writer's was a glazier. He was unable to work in winter as whenever he offered up a piece of glass into a window frame he was unable to let go, much to the consternation of his helper!

6. There are no associated abnormalities and the condition has no effect on life expectancy.

Figure 17.5. Clinical features of Dystrophia Myotonica

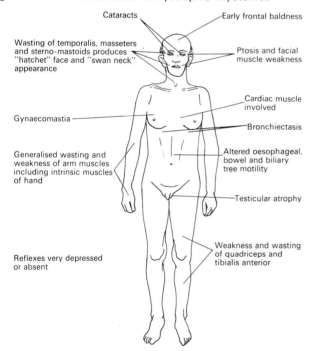

Cataracts

Early frontal baldness

Wasting of temporalis, masseters and sterno-mastoids produces "hatchet" face and "swan neck" appearance

Ptosis and facial muscle weakness

Cardiac muscle involved

Gynaecomastia

Bronchiectasis

Generalised wasting and weakness of arm muscles including intrinsic muscles of hand

Altered oesophageal, bowel and biliary tree motility

Testicular atrophy

Weakness and wasting of quadriceps and tibialis anterior

Reflexes very depressed or absent

4. The onset may be either dominated by weakness or myotonia or a combination of both. Difficulty in releasing the grip may present problems if delicate skills are required or pure weakness if manual work is involved. In some patients with leg weakness difficulty in kicking a ball or pseudo-drop attacks due to quadriceps weakness may be presenting symptoms. In most cases the flexor muscles of the arms are myotonic and the extensors weak.

5. Important additional clues to the diagnosis are numerous. These include frontal baldness (in females this may be disguised by a wig), loss of facial expression and ptosis, marked wasting of masseters and temporalis giving a haggard, wasted appearance to the face, cataracts and dysarthria due to myotonia of the tongue. Wasting of the sterno-mastoids to the point of disappearance is a prominent early feature and patients may have difficulty in lifting the head from a pillow. The neck is thinned producing a "swan neck". If the tongue is percussed on a tongue depressor or the thenar eminence percussed a slow myotonic contraction of the muscle is seen.

6. Numerous other abnormalities occur including gynaecomastia, gonadal atrophy, cardiac abnormalities, and motility disorders of the entire bowel and biliary tree. Respiratory infections are common due to muscular difficulties and occasionally abnormalities in immune globulins. Many patients have a low I.Q. and dementia may occur in the course of the disease.

7. The diagnosis is usually unmistakable on clinical grounds alone and the E.M.G. changes of myotonia are easily detectable in almost any muscle.

DYSTROPHIA MYOTONICA (Myotonic muscular dystrophy)

1. Males/females both affected. Inherited as an autosomal dominant in most cases.

2. Onset at any age is possible including congenital, but most patients develop disease between 20 and 30 years of age.

3. There is a general impression that the disease shows incomplete penetrance and it has been claimed that cataracts in a previous generation are minimal evidence of the disease. It is also possible that the disease appears earlier in successive generations *but* this may merely reflect earlier recognition. These points are all subject to considerable controversy.

LATE DISTAL DYSTROPHY

1. Males more frequently affected than females. Inherited as an autosomal dominant in Sweden. Very rare in other countries and usually sporadic in these cases.

2. Onset at forty to fifty years of age.

3. Progresses to moderate disability in fifteen years.

4. Starts in small hand muscles and leg—and extends proximally but girdle involvement is very rare. The legs are very similar to those in Charcot—Marie—Tooth disease which is distinguished by absent sensation.

5. There are no associated features.

Figure 17.6. Glucose-Glycogen Metabolism in Muscle

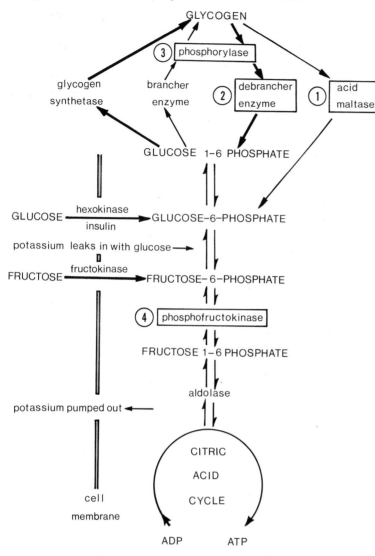

The following glycogen storage disorders produce muscle disease. The enzyme block is indicated on the figure
1. Pompé's disease (Type II glycogenosis)
2. Cori's disease (Type III glycogenosis)
3. McCardle's Syndrome (Type V glycogenosis)
4. Tarui's disease (Type VII glycogenosis)
Note also the leak of potassium into the cell during glucose uptake and the active pump mechanism which keeps the intracellular potassium down (see the periodic paralyses)

3. METABOLIC MYOPATHY

A complete discussion of muscle metabolism is beyond the immediate scope of the present text. For brevity discussion will be confined to generalisations which give an idea of the biochemical function of muscles on which discussion of the different types of myopathy can be based.

There are three main metabolic considerations:

1. Protein metabolism must be normal to maintain the contractile proteins. In some endocrine myopathies contractile protein abnormalities may contribute to muscle weakness.
2. The metabolism of energy production in the muscle must be intact. This basically means that glucose availability and the glycogen breakdown pathways must be normal. Several muscle disorders are based on either glucose assimilation disorders or enzyme deficiencies in the glycogen pathway.
3. The importance of normal sodium, potassium and calcium metabolism in maintaining resting membrane potentials and in the contractile mechanism is critical in the induction and cessation of contraction.

The metabolic pathways and inter-relationships of these metabolic activities are summarised in Figure 17.6.

The metabolic myopathies tend to cause chronic progressive muscle weakness, but in the initial stages episodes of sudden severe weakness during or following exertion are the most typical feature. The distinction can often be made on a typical history of the acute episodes.

Muscle Disease due to Abnormal Glycogen Metabolism

Although there are seven glycogen storage disorders only four are associated with muscle disease.

1. *Pompe's Disease (Type II glycogenosis)*

This is a disease of infancy and invariably fatal. In recent years however a few cases of a mild form of this disorder have been recognised in adults. In the infantile form the heart, liver, kidneys and the C.N.S. itself are also affected. Either cardiac failure or muscle weakness may be the first evidence of the disease. The neurological condition is very hard to distinguish from Werdnig—Hoffman disease including the fact that the E.M.G. shows profuse fibrillation—an indication of ventral horn cell disease or denervation. This is said to be due to co-existent ventral horn cell infiltration. The clinical clues lie in cardiac damage and often a very large tongue. These do not occur in Werdnig—Hoffman disease but the latter feature may suggest cretinism.

2. *Debranching Enzyme Disease (Limit dextrinosis) (Type III glycogenosis)*

In this variety the main infiltration and damage is to the liver causing hypoglycaemia. A mild proximal myopathy with hypotonia is present in infancy and a few adult cases have been reported—with a clinical appearance easily mistaken for motor neurone disease.

3. Myophosphorylase Deficiency (McArdle's Syndrome) (Type V glycogenosis)

The abnormality in this condition is confined to the skeletal muscles. The abnormality is apparent only on exertion as the defect blocks the glycogen-glucose conversion. Because the enzyme has no role in glycogen synthesis there is only a minimal excess of glycogen in the muscle. The disorder causes easy fatiguability and severe muscle cramping with breakdown of muscle proteins leading to myoglobinuria. As in all metabolic muscle disorders (see later) there is a tendency for the patients to develop permanent girdle muscle weakness later in life. The disease is inherited as an autosomal recessive. The classical investigation is to exercise the forearm muscles with a cuff on the arm so that the muscle is ischaemic. This increases the need for anaerobic glycolysis and the muscle promptly goes into severe cramp. If a venous sample of blood is taken from the exercised arm there is no rise in the blood lactate level and E.M.G. sampling of the muscles in cramp will reveal electrical silence—quite the reverse of normal muscle cramp.

The disorder is extremely rare. Few neurologists have seen more than two or three examples of the condition.

4. Phosphofructokinase Deficiency (Tarui's Disease) (Type VII glycogenosis)

The clinical details of this disease are virtually identical to McArdles syndrome but in this case the block in the glycogen-glucose pathway is several stages lower down (see Figure 17.6).

4. MUSCLE DISEASE DUE TO ABNORMAL POTASSIUM HANDLING

These conditions are known as the periodic paralyses and are associated with alteration in serum potassium levels. The defect however probably lies in muscle membrane permeability, the serum potassium levels reflecting massive uptake or loss of potassium from the muscles. There are three types.

1. Familial Hypokalaemic Periodic Paralysis

This is inherited as an autosomal dominant affecting males more than females. The condition becomes evident between 10 and 20 years of age and tends to remit after 35 years of age. Attacks typically occur after rest, usually on waking in the morning. They specifically occur if a heavy carbohydrate meal or excessive exercise were taken on the previous evening. It is thought that an excess of potassium enters the muscle during the high rate of glucose uptake following a meal or after exercise. The serum potassium falls, weakness becoming apparent at a level of 3·5 mEq/L and maximal at 2·5 mEq/L, suggesting that it is the high intracellular potassium that causes the weakness rather than the serum level. It is extremely unusual for a patient to die in an attack as the diaphragm, respiratory muscles and eye muscles are normally unaffected. This is because the continual activity of these muscles even during sleep keeps pumping potassium out of the cells; further evidence that it is the intracellular potassium that is critical in causing weakness. Attacks usually last eight to twenty-four hours.

An attack may be relieved by 10 gms. of potassium chloride in water taken orally.

2. Adynamia Episodica Hereditaria (Gamstorp's Disease)

This disease is characterised by the sudden onset of weakness some thirty minutes after exercise. If the patient senses the stiffness and weakness coming on further exercise may delay the onset but the attack when it comes is then more severe. Proximal muscles are particularly affected and often become stiff and myotonic. Attacks start between 5 and 15 years of age and tend to remit after 20 years of age. Each attack lasts thirty minutes to two hours. A chronic proximal myopathy often develops after the disease itself has remitted.

The weakness is probably due to release of potassium from the muscles as it occurs when the serum level is only 5 mEq/L. In patients with potassium retention weakness does *not* occur until a serum level of 8 mEq/L.

Attacks may be prevented by the use of acetazolamide 50—100 mgs. daily and acute attacks terminated by 1—2 gms. of calcium chloride I.V.I.

3. Normokalaemic Periodic Paralysis

This very rare condition occurs in infancy between 2 and 10 years of age. The attacks consist of sudden episodes of flaccid quadriplegia, that may last from one to three weeks. They may respond to sodium chloride and can be prevented by the use of salt-retaining steroids such as fludrocortisone. The relationship of this disorder to potassium metabolism is obscure.

5. SECONDARY METABOLIC AND ENDOCRINE MYOPATHIES

Some features of endocrine myopathy are due to co-existent electrolyte disturbances so that some degree of overlap is necessary in discussing these problems.

Electrolyte Disturbance

Several disorders of sodium metabolism cause cerebral

symptoms that dominate the clinical features. Milder disorders contribute to muscle weakness in adrenal disease as discussed later.

Hypokalaemia

Hypokalaemia of less than 2·5 mEq/L causes severe flaccid tetraparesis. The most frequent causes are:

Conn's syndrome (aldosterone secreting adrenal tumour).
Renal disease (Fanconi syndrome, renal tubular acidosis).
Potassium losing enteritis and severe diarrhoea.
Excessive diuretic therapy (thiazide diuretics).
Carbenoxolone therapy (liquorice extract used in peptic ulcer disease).

An immediate serum potassium determination is indicated *in any* patient with acute or subacute flaccid paraparesis. One patient with Conn's syndrome was only diagnosed when a *third* attack of acute paralytic poliomyelitis was thought to be an unlikely diagnosis!

Hyperkalaemia

Hyperkalaemia greater than 7 mEq/L causes a severe ascending quadriplegia that may mimic Guillain–Barré syndrome. It is extremely rare for the extraocular muscles to be affected. The most frequent causes are:

Renal failure.
Excessive administration of potassium salts in I.V. infusions.
Aldosterone antagonists (spironolactone).

In these patients there is a much greater risk that the cardiotoxic effect of hyperkalaemia will kill the patient before the onset of paralysis.

Hypocalcaemia

Chronic hypocalcaemia causes attacks of tetany and muscle weakness. In infancy convulsions, papilloedema and calcification of the basal ganglia may occur. Hypocalcaemia should be carefully excluded in any young patient who is developing cataracts. Causes include primary or secondary hypoparathyroidism, renal disease or bladder diversion procedures, deficient diet or lack of Vitamin D.

Hypercalcaemia

Hypercalcaemia tends to cause striking cerebral dysfunction or psychosis of acute onset. A slower onset causes quite severe but variable proximal muscle weakness. This is usually combined with brisk reflexes which may raise the diagnostic possibility of motor neurone disease. The most frequent cause is primary hyperparathyroidism due to a parathyroid adenoma. It may also occur in patients with metastatic malignancy who have osteolytic metastases or occasionally as a primary disorder without bone metastases. Multiple myeloma in particular may cause diffuse bone destruction and hypercalcaemia. Sarcoidosis, excessive intake of Vitamin D, milk alkali syndrome and idiopathic hypercalcaemia of infancy are other possible causes.

Endocrine Disease

Thyroid Disease

There are several ways in which the thyroid gland may be associated with muscular disorders.

Myasthenia gravis is often associated with thyrotoxicosis (in ten per cent of cases) and routine thyroid investigations are indicated in any patient with myasthenia gravis.

Hypokalaemic periodic paralysis occurs in association with thyrotoxicosis particularly in the Japanese but also in other ethnic groups.

The most frequent complication is thyrotoxic myopathy which particularly affects the shoulder girdle (spinati, deltoid and triceps) or pelvic girdle (hip flexors and quadriceps). It often occurs as the only *overt* manifestation of the disease and more often in males (even though thyrotoxicosis occurs three times as commonly in females). The clue to this diagnosis is the retention of reflexes, which are often very brisk. The picture is similar to hypercalcaemic myopathy in this respect.

Extra-ocular muscle disease in thyrotoxicosis has been described in Chapter 5.

Myxoedema causes proximal muscle weakness as part of the general slowing down, but the more dramatic neurological complication of this disorder is cerebellar degeneration (see Chapter 11). Proximal muscle weakness also occurs in cretins.

Adrenal Disease

In Cushings syndrome very striking wasting and weakness of the pelvic girdle and thigh muscles occurs. A similar picture is produced by the use of fluorinated steroids, especially triamcinolone.

In Addison's disease general lethargy, muscle cramps and weakness are an integral part of the disease. This is usually due to the hyponatraemia.

Conn's syndrome with hypokalaemic muscle weakness has been discussed above.

Parathyroid Disease

The effects of parathyroid disease on muscle have already been described in the section on disordered calcium metabolism.

6. MUSCLE DISEASE DUE TO DRUGS

Four drugs in general use may cause muscle disorders. Carbenoxolone (liquorice extract) used in the treatment of peptic ulceration and thiazide diuretics both cause loss of potassium and can cause very acute severe muscle weakness.

All steroid drugs, particularly fluorinated steroids and chloroquine may cause a progressive proximal myopathy. Even steroids used under occlusive dressings may cause systemic toxicity or wasting and weakness of the muscles under the dressing.

Within the last two years penicillamine has found increasing use in the treatment of rheumatoid and psoriatic arthropathy. Within recent months examples of both myasthenic syndromes and polymyositis apparently caused by the drug have been reported. The writer has had one patient with both anticholinsterase-sensitive weakness and polymyositis who had been on penicillamine for over a year, thought to be another example of this problem.

7. INFLAMMATORY MUSCLE DISEASE

Muscles are remarkably resistant to infection and with the exception of gas gangrene caused by Clostridium Welchii bacterial infection is rare. Sarcoidosis may also cause mild to severe muscle disease but the exact role of infection in this peculiar disease and its rarity do not justify more detailed consideration. Muscle inflammation in viral disease is exemplified by Bornholm disease (epidemic pleurodynia) and the general myalgia and listlessness of influenza may mimic acute poliomyelitis. Parasitic involvement is very rare in Great Britain with Trichinella spiralis (trichinosis—particularly affecting the extra-ocular muscles) and Taenia solium (cysticercosis—usually asymptomatic cysts in trunk muscles in a patient who has become an accidental intermediate host in the life cycle of the pork tape worm) are the only disorders worth mentioning. The latter condition usually causes epilepsy due to cerebral cysts, but plain x-rays of the trunk muscles to show the calcified cysts are important in establishing the diagnosis.

Muscle tenderness, severe aching and very severe deep burning, tearing pains in the muscles often described by the patient "as if the flesh were being torn from the bone" are the main symptoms of a peculiar disease known as "polymyalgia rheumatica". The E.S.R. is markedly elevated and an almost immediate response to indomethacin or steroids gives strong support for this diagnosis. The relationship of the disease to rheumatoid arthritis is uncertain but a special feature is that some forty per cent of patients go on to develop temporal arteritis. Prolonged observation is therefore necessary.

The most important inflammatory muscle disease is polymyositis.

Polymyositis

The importance of this disorder lies not only in the muscle problem, which may be considerable, but also in the possibility of serious underlying disease. There are several complicated classifications based on a combination of age and type of underlying disorder which includes malignant disease, collagen-vascular disease and Sjörgen's syndrome.

As with all neurological disorders the beginner's problem is less one of classification but more of recognising the condition in the first place. Polymyositis shares with porphyria and Guillain—Barré syndrome the distinction of being easily misdiagnosed as a functional disorder or hysteria.

Some of the difficulty stems from the name and usual descriptions which suggest that the muscles are very tender and weak and make the diagnosis obvious. This is unfortunately quite inaccurate as less than half the patients have demonstrable muscle tenderness and the weakness may be no greater than enough to make the patient feel rather listless with a tendency to fatigue easily; symptoms easily dismissed as due to depression or anxiety.

General Clinical Features

1. Muscle weakness is the usual presenting symptom and usually affects the pelvic girdle first. This causes difficulty climbing stairs or getting up from a chair.

2. This is followed by shoulder girdle weakness with difficulty reaching objects on shelves, washing the face or brushing the hair. Weakness of the neck muscles and dysphagia are very common at this stage but facial weakness and extraocular muscle weakness is extremely rare (an important distinguishing feature from myasthenia gravis).

3. Pain and tenderness of the affected muscles occurs in less than half the patients and is almost invariably found in the shoulder girdle muscles.

4. Systemic symptoms such as weight loss, anorexia, fever and lassitude occur more frequently in childhood polymyositis.

5. Atrophy of the affected muscles is late and mild and it is always difficult to detect atrophy in the plump pelvic area.

6. Evidence of collagen vascular disease such as Raynauds phenomenon, arthralgia, pneumonitis and renal damage are found in twenty-five to thirty per cent of cases.

7. Tendon reflexes are preserved until very late in the course of the disease.

Figure 17.7. Clinical Features of Progressive Ocular Myopathy

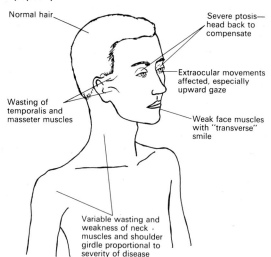

Normal hair

Severe ptosis—head back to compensate

Extraocular movements affected, especially upward gaze

Wasting of temporalis and masseter muscles

Weak face muscles with "transverse" smile

Variable wasting and weakness of neck muscles and shoulder girdle proportional to severity of disease

PROGRESSIVE OCULAR MYOPATHY (including oculo-pharyngeal muscular dystrophy)

1. Both sexes affected. Dominant or sporadic inheritance.
2. Clinical features range from ptosis alone to ptosis with eye movement disorder and facial weakness, and in some twenty-five per cent of cases shoulder girdle involvement.
3. Fifty per cent have dysphagia and the term oculo-pharyngeal muscular dystrophy has been proposed for this group.
4. Some families include retinitis pigmentosa, visual difficulties, endocrine abnormalities, cardiac involvement and cerebellar abnormalities. Electrical and histological studies confirm neuropathic rather than myopathic changes in some patients.
5. The disorder may lie somewhere between the muscular dystrophies and metabolic neuropathies such as Refsum's disease, and clinically must be distinguished from dystrophia myotonica.

8. The association with skin changes and its significance depends on the patient's age. The combination is known as dermatomyositis. The skin rash consists of a lilac-coloured rash over the cheeks and eyelids and thickened, reddened skin over the interphalangeal joints.

9. Dermatomyositis is the usual pattern of the disease in childhood but is *never* associated with underlying malignant disease in this age group. Systemic symptoms however, are very common in childhood, and the disorder may be associated with bowel perforation, intestinal obstruction and the deposition of calcium in the skin and subcutaneous tissues.

10. In adulthood only fifty per cent of patients show skin changes but the considerable risk of underlying malignant disease is almost confined to this group. There is also a marked sex difference. Over the age of 50, seventy per cent of males with dermatomyositis are eventually found to have underlying malignant disease. In females the risk is only twenty-five per cent. Underlying malignant disease occurs in the following sites; carcinoma of the stomach, breast, bronchus and ovary. Bowel tumours underlie some thirty per cent of cases and in contrast to the situation with peripheral neuropathy full bowel investigation *is* indicated in patients over fifty years of age with dermatomyositis, if no tumour in the breast or lung can be demonstrated.

CASE REPORT

A 58-year-old man returned from abroad to live with his family. He related that he had been slowing down physically for two years. This had been ascribed to depression following his wife's death and he had been on anti-depressants. On his arrival he showed marked physical inertia and had a persistent cough with profuse watery sputum. On examination he clearly had parkinsonism but the most dramatic finding was gross weakness and wasting of the proximal muscles. A chest x-ray revealed a cavitating carcinoma of the right upper lobe and E.M.G. studies showed findings consistent with polymyositis. He responded well to levodopa and prednisone but died a few weeks later while having radiotherapy.

This is almost certainly an example of malignancy-associated polymyositis although the good response to steroids was unusual.

All groups may be treated with steroids with the expectation of a good response in childhood and in the idiopathic cases in middle age but little or no response in patients with underlying malignant disease. In children a myasthenic syndrome may be superadded to the dermatomyositis and a tensilon test is indicated if the child's clinical status worsens or fluctuates.

8. MYASTHENIA GRAVIS AND MYASTHENIC SYNDROMES

Like many diseases *classical* myasthenia gravis is easy to diagnose; but in common with other disorders the *first* symptoms can be very difficult to recognise. In the case of myasthenia this is usually because the typical features of variability and fatiguability may *not* be obvious and the patient may present with a fixed mild ptosis or eye movement disorder that may be misdiagnosed as an incomplete extra-ocular nerve palsy. If the bulbar muscles are affected by a non-variable weakness motor neurone disease or a brain-stem vascular accident may be suspected. At the opposite extreme attacks of diplopia or dysarthria may be so brief that a breaking-down squint or a transient brainstem ischaemic attack may be considered. Finally there is the problem of the tensilon test. A basic requirement of the test is a measurable degree of weakness in a specific muscle that can be easily observed; this may not always be possible and in the early stages of the disorder myasthenic muscles may not respond to tensilon, or to longer acting anticholinesterases given as a clinical trial. One patient of the author's failed to respond to tensilon or prostigmine over a period of ten weeks. Quite suddenly the affected bulbar muscles became tensilon sensitive and good therapeutic control became possible.

As already indicated variable ptosis of one or other eyelid or variable diplopia are the most frequent presenting symptoms closely followed by weakness of chewing, dysarthria or difficulty in swallowing. In a severe case respiratory difficulty may occur, but the usual indication for tracheostomy in the management of myasthenia is to protect the airway from inhalation of food when swallowing is severely impaired. Limb symptoms are a late and relatively minor symptom in the majority of myasthenics. It is unusual for the reflexes to be altered, in fact they are often brisker than normal. The drug management of myasthenia is discussed in detail in Chapter 24.

Myasthenia may occur transiently in ten per cent of children born to myasthenic mothers. If the mother has needed large doses of anticholinesterases during labour the child may be born with cholinergic blockade. The latter is unusual as in general myasthenia tends to improve during pregnancy.

In childhood myasthenia is quite rare, but is invariably associated with severe generalised weakness quite unlike the adult form. Otherwise the clinical features are similar to the adult. In childhood myasthenia there is a good possibility that a spontaneous remission will occur. As noted above the condition may complicate dermatomyositis in this age group.

In adults with long-standing well-controlled disease a proximal "myasthenic myopathy" may supervene, and in most cases progressive atrophy of the maximally affected muscles with diminishing responsiveness to anticholinergic drugs occurs.

In all cases thyrotoxicosis should be excluded. This occurs in ten per cent of males and twenty per cent of females with myasthenia gravis. Routine and special x-ray investigations to exclude a thymic tumour are indicated, particularly in young patients with severe myasthenia in whom the possibility of thymectomy as a method of treatment is being considered.

Myasthenic Syndrome

This condition is also known as the Lambert–Eaton syndrome and usually occurs in association with an oat-cell carcinoma of the lung. The weakness is mainly found in the proximal muscles of the pelvic and shoulder girdles. Neck and trunk muscles are affected but involvement of the bulbar or extra-ocular muscles is unusual. Unlike myasthenia gravis repeated activity of the muscle leads to increasing strength rather than weakness. The condition sometimes responds to guanidine hydrochloride which is thought to act by releasing acetylcholine at the motor end plate. Although only half the patients have a detectable malignancy at diagnosis close follow-up is necessary as the syndrome may precede the identification of the underlying malignant disease by several years.

Chapter 18

DIAGNOSIS OF ROOT AND NERVE LESIONS AFFECTING THE ARM

Most clinical students and many doctors are reluctant to attempt to make an accurate diagnosis of nerve root or peripheral nerve lesions in the arm due to deficient anatomical knowledge. There is also a widely held misconception that plexus lesions are a frequent cause of disease affecting the nerve supply of the arms. The anatomy of the brachial plexus is intimidating enough to daunt anyone who encounters a patient with a suspected plexus lesion! In fact, plexus lesions are quite rare in most civilised countries with a frequency proportional to the deliberate or accidental misuse of fire arms and knives. There are few disease processes that primarily affect the brachial plexus.

In this chapter the anatomical and clinical difference between nerve root and peripheral nerve lesions will be compared and contrasted. A final section on plexus lesions is included containing a specially constructed diagram of the brachial plexus based on a functional approach.

The clinical problem can usually be reduced to a simple consideration; is the pain or weakness in the territory supplied by a single nerve root or a single peripheral nerve or one of its branches. Definitive diagnosis usually depends on a very careful evaluation of the motor system as in the arm motor findings are much more reliable than sensory findings for reasons to be discussed later. For this reason the comparative tables (see Tables 6 and 7) are based on a simple evaluation of the motor supply of the arm, tested by ten movements, which in all but the most exceptional cases should provide all the information required for accurate localising diagnosis.

THE VULNERABLE AREAS OF THE NERVE SUPPLY TO THE ARM

Figure 18.1 shows the entire course of each of the roots and peripheral nerves supplying the arm. Emphasis has been given to those areas where the relationship of the neural structures to bone or muscle may predispose to traumatic damage. Note that the radial nerve is vulnerable at three positions along its course, the ulnar nerve at two positions and the median nerve only at the wrist. In spite of this, damage to the median nerve at the wrist and the ulnar nerve at the elbow are the peripheral lesions most often encountered. When one considers the cervical roots; C5 and C6 are those most often affected by cervical spondylosis, and C7 by acute disc lesions. Involvement of roots above and below these levels is relatively unusual and involvement of the C2, 3 or C8 and D1 roots requires careful consideration of other diagnostic possibilities. D1 root damage is quite a common consequence of altered anatomy in the area of the apical pleura, due to a cervical rib or invasion by neoplastic disease in the upper part of the lung.

CLINICAL EVALUATION OF SENSORY SYMPTOMS AND SIGNS

We have already noted the unreliability of sensory phenomena in the arms and this probably stems from the complex central representation of the limb and considerable overlapping of nerve territories at the periphery. Root pains may range from tingling paraesthesiae in a well-localised distribution to very severe pain which the patient cannot localise accurately (see Figure 18.2). Individual root irritation causes pain in the following distributions:

C5 root pain occurs across the shoulder and in the lateral arm and does not radiate below the elbow. A confirmatory clue is often an aching pain down the medial scapula border. (This scapula pain may also occur with C6 and C7 root irritation, but much less frequently.)

C6 root pain causes deep aching pain in the biceps muscle which spreads down the lateral fore-arm, involving the thumb and index fingers, on both the palmar and dorsal aspects.

C7 root pain is inherently diffuse as the C7 root supplies the periosteum of the bones of the arm with a long cutaneous distribution down the centre of both the front and back of the arm. There is usually deep aching in the triceps muscle with pain down the front and back of the central forearm, radiating particularly into the middle finger but often spreading into both the index and ring fingers. When C7 root pain is very severe patients often complain that the *entire* arm is hurting.

C8 root pain is relatively unusual. It radiates from just below the olecranon down into the little ring fingers.

D1 root irritation causes a deep aching sensation felt in the shoulder joint and axilla and occasionally down the medial side of the arm to the olecranon.

Table 6   COMPARATIVE DATA ON ROOT AND NERVE LESIONS IN THE ARM

ROOTS	C5	C6	C7	C8	D1
Sensory supply	Lateral border upper arm	Lateral forearm including thumb	Over triceps, mid-forearm and middle finger	Medial forearm to include little finger	Axilla down to the olecranon
Sensory loss	As above	As above	Middle fingers	As above	As above
Area of pain	As above and medial scapula border	As above esp. thumb and index finger	As above and medial scapula border	As above	Deep aching in shoulder and axilla to olecranon
Reflex arc	Biceps jerk	Supinator jerk	Triceps jerk	Finger jerk	None
Motor deficit	Deltoid Supraspinatus Infraspinatus Rhomboids	Biceps Brachioradialis Brachialis (Pronators and supinators of forearm)	Latissimus dorsi Pectoralis major Triceps Wrist extensors Wrist flexors	Finger flexors Finger extensors Flexor carpi ulnaris (thenar muscles in some patients)	*All* small hand muscles (in some thenar muscles via C8)
Causative lesions	Brachial neuritis Cervical spondylosis Upper plexus avulsion	Cervical spondylosis Acute disc lesions	Acute disc lesions Cervical spondylosis	Rare in disc lesions or spondylosis	Cervical rib Outlet syndromes Pancoast tumour Metastatic carcinoma in deep cervical nodes

Table 7

NERVES	AXILLARY	MUSCULO-CUTANEOUS	RADIAL	MEDIAN	ULNAR
Sensory supply	Over deltoid	Lateral forearm to wrist	Lateral dorsal forearm and back of thumb and index finger	Lateral palm and lateral fingers	Medial palm and 5th and medial half ring finger
Sensory loss	Small area over deltoid	Lateral forearm	Dorsum of thumb and index (if any)	As above	As above but often none at all
Area of pain	Across shoulder tip	Lateral forearm	Dorsum of thumb and index	Thumb, index and middle finger. Often spreads up forearm	Ulnar supplied fingers and palm distal to wrist. Pain occasionally along course of nerve
Reflex arc	Nil	Biceps jerk	Triceps jerk and supinator jerk	Finger jerks (flexor digitorum sublimis)	Nil
Motor deficit	Deltoid (Teres minor cannot be evaluated)	Biceps Brachialis (coracobrachialis weakness not detectable)	Triceps Wrist extensors Finger extensors Brachioradialis Supinator of forearm	Wrist flexors Long finger flexors (thumb, index and middle finger) Pronators of forearm. Abductor pollicis brevis	All small hand muscles excluding abductor pollicis brevis. Flexor carpi ulnaris. Long flexors of ring and little finger
Causative lesions	Fractured neck of humerus. Dislocated shoulder. Deep I.M. injections	Very rarely damaged	Crutch palsy. Saturday night palsy. Fractured humerus. In supinator muscle	Carpal tunnel syndrome Direct trauma to wrist	Elbow: trauma, bed rest, fractured olecranon. Wrist: local trauma, ganglion of wrist joint

Figure 18.1. Clinically Relevant Anatomy of the Nerve Supply to the Arm

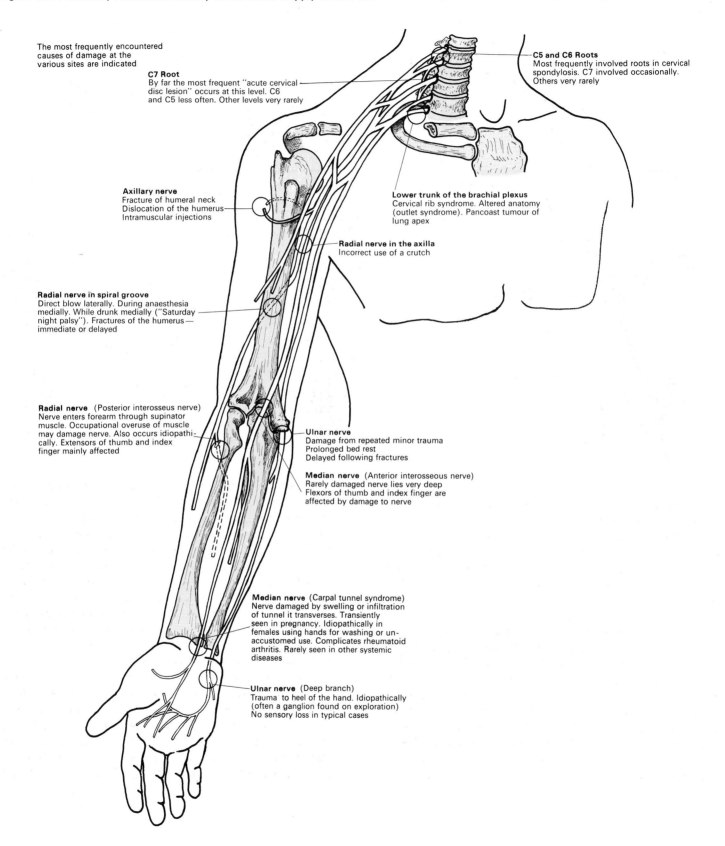

The most frequently encountered causes of damage at the various sites are indicated

C5 and C6 Roots
Most frequently involved roots in cervical spondylosis. C7 involved occasionally. Others very rarely

C7 Root
By far the most frequent "acute cervical disc lesion" occurs at this level. C6 and C5 less often. Other levels very rarely

Axillary nerve
Fracture of humeral neck
Dislocation of the humerus
Intramuscular injections

Lower trunk of the brachial plexus
Cervical rib syndrome. Altered anatomy (outlet syndrome). Pancoast tumour of lung apex

Radial nerve in the axilla
Incorrect use of a crutch

Radial nerve in spiral groove
Direct blow laterally. During anaesthesia medially. While drunk medially ("Saturday night palsy"). Fractures of the humerus — immediate or delayed

Radial nerve (Posterior interosseus nerve)
Nerve enters forearm through supinator muscle. Occupational overuse of muscle may damage nerve. Also occurs idiopathically. Extensors of thumb and index finger mainly affected

Ulnar nerve
Damage from repeated minor trauma
Prolonged bed rest
Delayed following fractures

Median nerve (Anterior interosseous nerve)
Rarely damaged nerve lies very deep
Flexors of thumb and index finger are affected by damage to nerve

Median nerve (Carpal tunnel syndrome)
Nerve damaged by swelling or infiltration of tunnel it transverses. Transiently seen in pregnancy. Idiopathically in females using hands for washing or unaccustomed use. Complicates rheumatoid arthritis. Rarely seen in other systemic diseases

Ulnar nerve (Deep branch)
Trauma to heel of the hand. Idiopathically (often a ganglion found on exploration) No sensory loss in typical cases

Figure 18.2. Distribution of Root Pain and Paraesthesiae

Figure 18.3. Distribution of Pain and Paraesthesiae in Peripheral Nerve Lesions

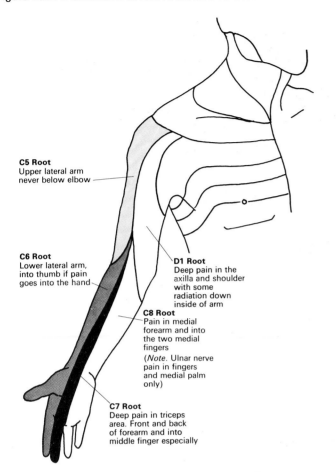

C5 Root
Upper lateral arm never below elbow

C6 Root
Lower lateral arm, into thumb if pain goes into the hand

D1 Root
Deep pain in the axilla and shoulder with some radiation down inside of arm

C8 Root
Pain in medial forearm and into the two medial fingers
(*Note*. Ulnar nerve pain in fingers and medial palm only)

C7 Root
Deep pain in triceps area. Front and back of forearm and into middle finger especially

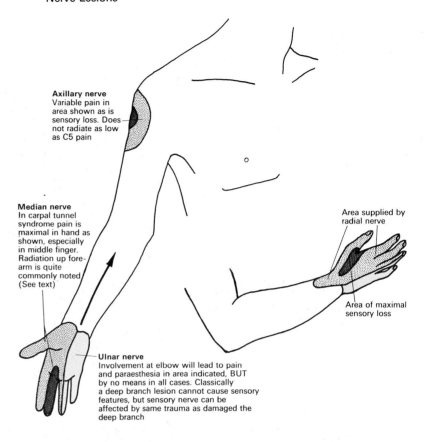

Axillary nerve
Variable pain in area shown as is sensory loss. Does not radiate as low as C5 pain

Median nerve
In carpal tunnel syndrome pain is maximal in hand as shown, especially in middle finger. Radiation up fore-arm is quite commonly noted (See text)

Ulnar nerve
Involvement at elbow will lead to pain and paraesthesia in area indicated, BUT by no means in all cases. Classically a deep branch lesion cannot cause sensory features, but sensory nerve can be affected by same trauma as damaged the deep branch

Area supplied by radial nerve

Area of maximal sensory loss

When one comes to consider the sensory symptoms due to involvement of peripheral nerves there are two special considerations (see Figure 18.3).

1. The area supplied by the radial nerve is so readily overlapped by other nerve supplies that detectable sensory loss is quite unusual and sensory symptoms may be confined to slight tingling over the dorsum of the thumb and index finger.

2. On purely anatomical grounds compression of the median nerve at the wrist should produce pain only in the lateral palm and three and a half fingers. In fact, many patients with carpel tunnel syndrome complain that the pain radiates up the central forearm to the elbow and occasionally to the shoulder. Many patients insist that at the height of the pain the fifth finger is also involved. The reasons for this are not clearly understood, but certainly the pain in all the fingers of the hand may well be related to the large number of sympathetic nerve fibres to the blood vessels of the hand, which are almost exclusively carried in the median nerve.

This probably accounts for the fact that most patients with pain in *all* fingers claim that at the height of an attack of pain, the fingers blanch and appear to be swollen, rather like Raynaud's phenomenon. In most patients with peripheral involvement of the median or ulnar nerves, appropriate sensory impairment may be found. Two-point discrimination sensation in the fingers is a particularly useful test to detect minimal sensory loss, but it must be realised that in many instances quite severe compression of either the median or the ulnar nerve may occur in the absence of any sensory symptoms or any sensory findings. It is this feature that can make diagnosis so difficult on occasions.

In the case of root involvement, although the pain may be exceptionally severe, it is very unusual to be able to document any definite sensory loss and extremely unusual for the sensory loss if found, to occupy the entire anatomical area supplied by a root. For example in the case of C6 some numbness over the dorsum of perhaps the index finger and thumb may be detected, even though the area in the forearm

Figure 18.4. Shoulder and Arm Movements

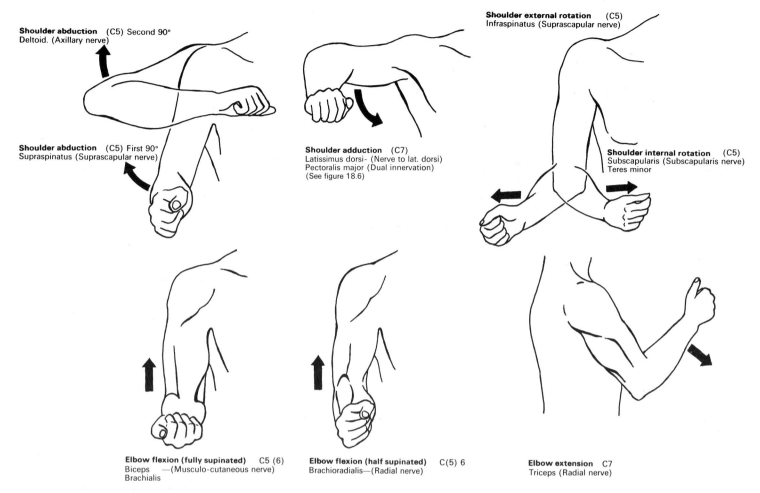

Shoulder abduction (C5) Second 90°
Deltoid. (Axillary nerve)

Shoulder abduction (C5) First 90°
Supraspinatus (Suprascapular nerve)

Shoulder adduction (C7)
Latissimus dorsi- (Nerve to lat. dorsi)
Pectoralis major (Dual innervation)
(See figure 18.6)

Shoulder external rotation (C5)
Infraspinatus (Suprascapular nerve)

Shoulder internal rotation (C5)
Subscapularis (Subscapularis nerve)
Teres minor

Elbow flexion (fully supinated) C5 (6)
Biceps —(Musculo-cutaneous nerve)
Brachialis

Elbow flexion (half supinated) C(5) 6
Brachioradialis—(Radial nerve)

Elbow extension C7
Triceps (Radial nerve)

supplied by the root may appear to have normal sensation. In general, it should be stated that the failure to demonstrate sensory loss in any situation where there is pain in the arm should *not* be taken as evidence that the patient's symptoms are on a functional basis. It is for this reason that the motor findings are so important.

CLINICAL EVALUATION OF MOTOR FUNCTION IN THE ARM

For diagnostic purposes it is important to forget the multiplicity of roots contributing to the formation of individual peripheral nerves, particularly the radial and median nerves. One must think instead of the fact that each movement of the arm is controlled almost exclusively by a single root. It is not even necessary to remember all the muscles contributing to that movement. The only other consideration then becomes "which nerve carries the root to this or that muscle group?"

Thus for each of the basic movements of the arm there is a root value and a peripheral nerve value. These are indicated in Figures 18.4 and 18.5. It follows that each reflex in the arm also has a root value and a peripheral nerve value. If the reader will refer to the figures it will be noticed that the traditional methods used for testing arm function, the grip and opposition of the thumb and fifth finger are not included. A little thought will show that these movements involve several muscle groups, multiple nerves and multiple roots in their performance. Their diagnostic value is almost nil in terms of differentiating root and nerve lesions.

Special points that need to be emphasised in regard to testing of motor function in the arm are as follows.

1. A C5 root lesion will weaken all 180° of shoulder abduction. An axillary nerve lesion, affecting only the deltoid muscle, will weaken only the second 90° of movement. This should not be confused with the frozen shoulder syndrome in which severe pain prevents the second 90° of movement.

Figure 18.5. Forearm and Hand Movements

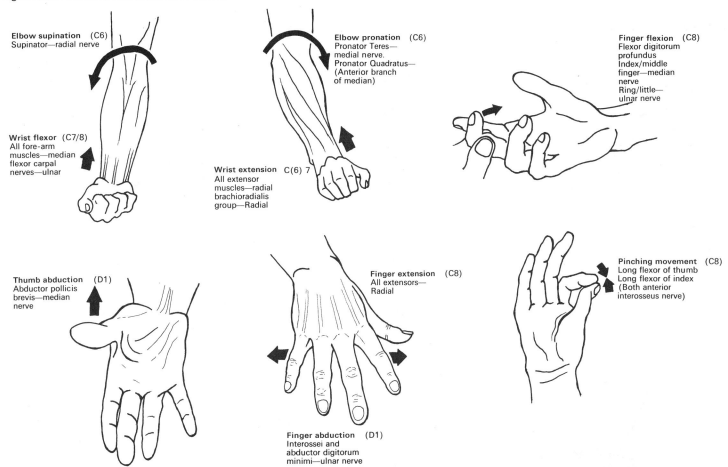

Elbow supination (C6)
Supinator—radial nerve

Wrist flexor (C7/8)
All fore-arm
muscles—median
flexor carpal
nerves—ulnar

Elbow pronation (C6)
Pronator Teres—
medial nerve.
Pronator Quadratus—
(Anterior branch
of median)

Wrist extension C(6) 7
All extensor
muscles—radial
brachioradialis
group—Radial

Finger flexion (C8)
Flexor digitorum
profundus
Index/middle
finger—median
nerve
Ring/little—
ulnar nerve

Thumb abduction (D1)
Abductor pollicis
brevis—median
nerve

Finger extension (C8)
All extensors—
Radial

Finger abduction (D1)
Interossei and
abductor digitorum
minimi—ulnar nerve

Pinching movement (C8)
Long flexor of thumb
Long flexor of index
(Both anterior
interosseus nerve)

2. A C6 root lesion will produce weakness of elbow flexion in both the supine position (produced by biceps and brachialis) and in the half supinnated position (produced by brachioradialis muscle). A musculo-cutaneous nerve lesion (an extremely rare event) would only weaken the biceps and brachialis muscles. A radial nerve lesion will only weaken the brachioradialis muscle (as far as the elbow flexion is concerned).

3. A C7 root lesion causes weakness of shoulder adduction, elbow extension, wrist extension and wrist flexion because it contributes to both the radial and the median nerves. By contrast a radial nerve lesion cannot affect shoulder adduction or wrist flexion and in addition will also affect the brachioradialis muscle. This clinical distinction between a C7 root lesion and a radial nerve lesion is extremely important.

4. A C8 root lesion (relatively rare) will cause weakness of the long extensors and flexors of the fingers and many would add the small hand muscles. This latter feature is extremely controversial and it would appear that in some patients there is some contribution from C8 root to small hand muscles, but in the majority the small hand muscles are almost exclusively innervated by the D1 root.

5. A D1 root lesion will cause wasting and weakness of *all* the small hand muscles. An ulnar nerve lesion also causes wasting of the small hand muscles but spares the abductor pollicis brevis muscle as this is supplied by the D1 root but via the median nerve. Unfortunately, in some two to three per cent of otherwise normal persons *all* the small hand muscles are innervated by the ulnar nerve. This is a considerable diagnostic trap as in these instances *all* the small hand muscles will be wasted and a D1 root lesion or even more seriously, motor neurone disease may be diagnosed in error, when the patient has a simple ulnar nerve lesion.

It must be remembered that this is only a diagnostic guide; several movements have not even been considered. This is solely because their inclusion complicates the presentation without significantly improving the diagnostic value. In practice the information given will enable a confident conclusion to be arrived at in the majority of cases. To enhance the value of this approach we will now consider the different clinical conditions that should be considered after an initial history and examination has given some idea as to the diagnosis.

CLINICAL FEATURES OF CONDITIONS CAUSING ROOT AND NERVE LESIONS IN THE ARMS

Root Avulsion Syndromes

These conditions rarely cause differential diagnostic problems as the causative trauma is usually only too obvious. There are two basic syndromes:

1. Erb—Duchenne type of paralysis, which is due to avulsion of the C5 and C6 roots. This is usually the result of pressure applied to the shoulder, and may occur following motor-cycle accidents or in infancy during a forceps delivery, if the shoulders are stuck and the head is pulled too hard. This leads to loss of abduction of the shoulder and flexion at the elbow. This means that the arm hangs limply at the side and cannot be flexed, and therefore the hand cannot be placed into a useful, functional position, although hand function itself is perfectly normal.

2. The second type, known as Klumpke paralysis, occurs when the D1 and C8 roots have been avulsed. This tends to occur during falls when the patient makes an attempt to grasp something and the arm is pulled up while the body continues moving. A similar situation is sometimes encountered when the arm is trapped in a moving machine. In this instance there is gross loss of use of all the instrinsic muscles of the hand, and the long finger flexors and extensors so that although the arm can be moved normally into any position, there is no useful function in the hand itself. In both types severe causalgic pain in the affected areas often complicates root avulsion due to recent trauma.

Root lesions due to Cervical Spondylosis

Root lesions due to spondylosis have been discussed in detail in Chapter 15. We will mention them briefly in the present section. We have already noted that C5 and C6 are the two roots most likely to be affected. This leads to an almost diagnostic combination of reflex changes. The biceps and supinator jerks being carried by the C5 and C6 roots are usually depressed or absent and the triceps jerk is usually strikingly increased in a typical case. This is due to the local damage to the spinal roots at C5 and C6, blocking the reflex

arcs, and the narrowing of the canal at this level causing some degree of cord compression enhancing the triceps jerk which is passing through the C7 reflex arc just below the level of the compression. In some instances all three reflexes are absent in both arms. As already mentioned, root lesions apart from C5, C6 and C7 are relatively rare and if other roots are involved other diagnostic possibilities should be kept in mind. Cervical spondylosis is a physiological result of ageing and it is extremely dangerous to accept that root lesions or progressive problems in the cervical cord are due to spondylosis because of plain film changes, and careful investigation is indicated in the majority of cases.

Acute Cervical Disc Lesions

Acute cervical disc lesions are relatively uncommon compared to the very frequent occurrence of lumbar disc lesions. They fall into two main groups.

1. Those injuries occurring in an otherwise normal spine, usually the result of a sports injury in a young person. This is almost invariably strictly unilateral. The patient develops very severe neck pain with radicular pain in a typical root distribution, which may or may not be associated with weakness of the muscles innervated by the affected nerve root. The C7 root is most often affected by a traumatic disc lesion.

2. The second type of injury occurs in a person who already has an abnormal neck due to cervical spondylosis. In these patients sudden flexion or extension of the neck, following a simple trip or in a rear end collision in a car may produce acute root symptoms or even serious cord damage. In these instances root symptoms are often bilateral and may affect multiple roots and the cord damage may be so severe as to cause an acute tetraparesis. The potential seriousness of even minor trauma affecting the cervical spine in this way in patients with severe pre-existing spondylosis cannot be over-emphasised.

CASE REPORT

A 72-year-old man was given barbiturate sleeping pills. Under their influence he fell downstairs and became tetraparetic. He had the typical signs of acute C5/6 root lesions and a mild spastic paraparesis without sensory loss. His plain films showed very gross spondylotic damages and a very narrow canal at C4/5 level. In spite of skilled care he died of bronchopneumonia six days following the incident.

Brachial Neuritis (Serum Neuritis, Neuralgic Amyotrophy)

This is a classical neurological condition that was originally recognised as a sequel to immunisation procedures involving the injection of sera into the deltoid muscle. The condition is not due to any direct trauma to the peripheral nerves. It is believed to be an inflammatory process occurring in the roots. In a typical case very severe pain over the C5 dermatome is followed in two to three days by rapid wasting and weakness of all the C5 and C6 innervated muscles. In a particularly severe case there may also be involvement of the sterno-mastoid and upper trapezius and C7 innervated groups. Occasionally the condition may occur bilaterally simultaneously. In general the prognosis is extremely good. Cases showing definite evidence of recovery within five to six weeks usually make a full recovery over a period of three to six months. Those taking several months before any sign of recovery is apparent may take eighteen months to two years before maximal recovery is made and this is often incomplete. This seems to be a particular problem in patients who have severe co-existent cervical spondylosis.

The Cervical Rib Syndrome

Twenty years ago textbooks contained whole chapters devoted to what were known as the "outlet syndromes". At that time cervical spondylosis and carpal tunnel syndrome were not even recognised entities. With the recognition of the latter conditions the outlet syndromes have almost vanished from the diagnostic repertoire. The only unequivocal survivor is the cervical rib syndrome, and to this we may add the situation where a normal first rib is displaced upwards by distortion of the thorax. This may occur in patients with thoracic scoliosis or following artificial pneumothorax or thoracoplasty. The symptoms produced may be due to either neural or vascular damage.

The Neural Picture: The neural picture is extremely interesting. The sensory symptoms comprise a deep aching pain in the axilla and down the ulnar border of the arm, often into the hand, in other words, in the territory of both C8 and D1. The motor signs, however, are dominated by damage to the D1 root and in particular to those fibres destined to supply the abductor pollicis brevis muscle to the exclusion of the other small hand muscles. This leads to a situation where the main pain is in the ulnar innervated fingers, but the main wasting and weakness is in the median innervated abductor pollicis brevis muscle. Many patients have had their median nerve decompressed at the wrist for this syndrome, when in fact a careful evaluation of sensory symptoms should have made the diagnosis of carpal tunnel syndrome untenable. On electromyography the situation can be easily confirmed and the findings comprise an electromyographic "syndrome". This consists of evidence of denervation of the abductor pollicis brevis muscle with a normal median nerve action potential, coupled with normal ulnar innervated muscles in the hand, but an absent ulnar action potential at the wrist. On

these electromyographic findings alone, even if no cervical rib can be demonstrated on plain x-ray it is worth exploring the lower roots of the brachial plexus in the neck, as damage due to abnormal fibrous bands may be found in this situation.

The Vascular Syndrome: The vascular syndrome is a result of the fact that the abnormally high rib also displaces the axillary artery upwards. This causes an area of stenosis with the risk of the development of post-stenotic dilatation. Clot may form on the wall of the dilated vessel. Small fragments of clot then become detached and pass down the brachial artery into the hand. This causes acute embolic episodes resembling Raynaud's phenomena which may subsequently cause ischaemic changes in the fingers. In this situation there may be no abnormal neurological findings, but an incorrect diagnosis of carpal tunnel syndrome may be made when the patient relates the history of repeated attacks of severe pain in the hand, associated with blanching, and swelling of the fingers.

It is worth restating that the outlet syndromes described in the older books appear to be of doubtful validity. In fifteen years the writer has not seen a single example of a surgically proven lesion of the roots in the neck caused by simple muscle displacement. A cervical rib or an abnormal fibrous band associated with an unusually elongated transverse process of the C7 vertebra appear to be the only valid causes of the so-called outlet syndrome.

Lesions of the Radial Nerve

The radial nerve in the axilla is often damaged by the incorrect use of a crutch, in which the patient takes his weight on the axilla. It should be pointed out, however, that the correct use of the crutch, in which the patient takes his weight on the heel of the hand can damage the deep branch of the ulnar nerve in the palm!

Damage to the radial nerve in the axilla usually causes weakness of all the radial innervated muscles; the triceps, wrist extensors, finger extensors and brachioradialis.

Damage lower down may be produced in two ways. First by direct trauma to the radial nerve in the spiral groove on the lateral aspect of the upper arm. This may occur accidentally or be deliberately inflicted as in the schoolboy trick in which the outer aspect of the arm is punched hard, which causes an acute wrist drop. The nerve may be similarly damaged on the medial aspect of the arm in a "Saturday night palsy". This occurs in people who are inebriated or heavily sedated and go to sleep with their arm hanging over the back of a chair or over the edge of the bed. Fractures of the midshaft of the humerus may involve the nerve either acutely during the actual fracture or later if there is over-exuberant callus formation. In this situation, although the nerve palsy may appear to be progressive, it is unusual for permanent damage to result and rarely is surgical exploration of the nerve necessary. Lesions at mid-humerus level usually spare the triceps muscle, the weakness being confined to the wrist extensors, brachioradialis and the finger extensors. Damage to the nerve in the axilla or upper arm, although associated with aching, tingling or numbness in the radial nerve cutaneous distribution, very rarely causes detectable sensory loss as the territory is so readily overlapped by the adjacent ulnar and median nerves. If any sensory loss can be detected it is usually over the dorsum of the thumb and index finger. The terminal motor branch of the radial nerve is the posterior interosseus nerve and this enters the forearm by penetrating the supinator muscle. Damage to the posterior interosseus nerve causes weakness of the wrist extensors and in particular, the extensors of the index finger and thumb. This lesion may occur idiopathically or follow the unaccustomed use of a screw-driver. Cases involving damage to the nerve at this point have also been described following Indian bar wrestling in which the opponents rest their elbows on the table and try to force one another's hand over backwards, and in orchestral conductors, as a rather unique occupational hazard. Presumably, in these cases direct entrapment of the nerve by the contracting supinator muscle is the cause.

In older textbooks it is stated that lead poisoning specifically damages the posterior interosseus nerve. It may well be that the nerve was predisposed to damage by lead poisoning, but it seems probable that occupational over-use of the supinator muscle by house painters led to the localisation of the damage to this nerve.

Lesions of the Ulnar Nerve

The ease with which the ulnar nerve may be damaged at the elbow is well known from the common experience of hitting the "funny-bone". The fact that ulnar nerve palsies may result from repeated and apparently trivial trauma of this sort is less appreciated. Simple alteration in personal habits, such as the substitution of a modern wooden armed chair for a soft armchair may lead to the insidious onset of an ulnar nerve palsy. Driving with the arm resting on the door sill is another frequently encountered cause of an ulnar nerve palsy of this type. Patients confined to bed often use their elbows to shuffle about in bed and the insidious development of bilateral ulnar nerve palsies is a common sequel. Damage occurs idiopathically in women who have a larger carrying angle at the elbow than men and in whom repeated flexion and extension of the arm is more likely to stretch the nerve around the olecranon. A variant of this anatomical deformity

leads to the condition known as a "tardy ulnar palsy". In this situation the patient invariably suffered a supra-condylar fracture of the humerus in childhood, resulting in a slight developmental deformity of the elbow. As the years pass an insidious ulnar nerve palsy develops and it may be twenty to thirty years before its presence is recognised. In any situation in which insidious damage to the nerve has occurred there may be a remarkable absence of sensory phenomena. Although one would anticipate tingling and numbness in the ulnar fingers, quite severe and even complete loss of motor function in ulnar innervated muscles may occur in the total absence of any sensory symptoms. If one remembers that in two to three per cent of people *all* the small hand muscles are innervated by the ulnar nerve there is a real possibility of motor neurone disease being diagnosed when the patient is merely suffering from a simple painless ulnar nerve palsy. Lesions at the elbow ought theoretically to produce weakness of flexor carpal ulnaris and the medial part of the flexor digitorum profundus. For reasons that are far from clear it is quite unusual for these muscles to be affected and even more complicated is the fact that damage to the nerve at the elbow seems specifically to affect fibres destined to innervate the first dorsal interosseus muscle. Therefore, the patient may present with striking weakness and wasting of the first dorsal interosseus muscle with almost complete sparing of the abductor digiti minimi muscle on the medial side of the hand. In this situation the possibility of an ulnar nerve lesion at the wrist is suspected but this is rarely the case.

At the wrist the nerve divides into a superficial sensory part and a deep motor branch. Repeated trauma to the heel of the hand (using the heel of the hand to shut a sticking car door, or the use of a chuck key by a lathe worker etc.) will crush the nerve against the carpal bones. This usually produces wasting and weakness of all the ulnar innervated small hand muscles in the absence of sensory involvement. Again if the patient has an all ulnar innervated hand total wasting and weakness of *all* the intrinsic muscles of the hand may be found and an incorrect diagnosis of motor neurone disease made. Occasionally, the nerve may also be affected at the wrist by a ganglion arising from the joint and if there is no history of trauma to the heel of the hand it is worth exploring the nerve to exclude this possibility. In general whenever the intrinsic muscles of the hand are involved early exploration and attempts to decompress the nerve should be made as if wasting is allowed to persist delayed surgery produces very unsatisfactory results.

Lesions of the Median Nerve

The median nerve is well protected from trauma in the arm itself. Rarely the anterior interosseus nerve, given off from the median nerve just below the elbow, may be damaged in forearm fractures or dislocations of the elbow. An anterior interosseus nerve lesion (Kiloh–Nevin syndrome) causes weakness of the long flexors of the thumb and index finger. At the carpal tunnel, however, the nerve is extremely vulnerable and probably the commonest peripheral nerve lesion encountered is the carpal tunnel syndrome. It is difficult to realise that this condition was first recognised in the mid 1940s and only put on a firm electro-physiological basis in the mid 1950s. It is instructive to remember that some physicians denied the existence of this condition for a whole decade after its original description and insisted that all pain in the hand was due to "outlet syndromes". The striking clinical feature of carpal tunnel syndrome is that the pain is particularly severe during the night. The patient typically wakes with severe pain in the median innervated part of the hand and the symptoms are fairly readily relieved by swinging the arm or flexing and extending the wrist. Both these features are important diagnostic clues and however atypical the description of the pain may be, night pain in the arm should be assumed to be due to carpal tunnel syndrome until proved otherwise. Conversely, pain that is primarily present on waking in the morning is usually due to a cervical root irritation from spondylosis. The peculiarities of the distribution of sensory symptoms in carpal tunnel syndrome have already been pointed out in the introductory part of this chapter.

Sensory findings may be quite marked with total loss of sensation in the median innervated area of the hand or may be normal in spite of quite severe pain. Motor involvement is usually confined to the abductor pollicis brevis muscle as the other muscles supplied by the median nerve either have dual innervation from the ulnar nerve or can be readily substituted by long forearm muscles and it is usually only the wasting and weakness of abductor pollicis brevis that can be easily and convincingly demonstrated.

From a clinical point of view it is sufficient to test abductor pollicis brevis correctly as shown in Figure 18.5 and then to be certain that the ulnar innervated muscles are functioning normally.

Lesions of the Long Thoracic Nerve of Bell

A unique problem in the arm is the long thin nerve that supplies a solitary but important muscle; the serratus anterior. This muscle normally holds the scapula flat against the back, and stabilises the shoulder joint during abduction of the arm.

Patients notice they cannot hold the arm on the affected side up straight and have difficulty combing their hair and putting on clothes. Relatives notice the striking protrusion of the shoulder blade.

There are no specific causes; recent cases seen by the author, occurred after log cutting, exposure to cold and as a consequence of an episode of neuralgic amyotrophy. Recovery seems to be slow and incomplete.

The diagnostic problems presented by root and nerve lesions affecting the arm have been outlined. The wide disparity between what actually happens and what ought to happen on purely anatomical grounds has been emphasised. A simplified method of evaluating the arm directly applicable to these circumstances has been outlined. In most instances electro-diagnostic studies can be of considerable value and details of the techniques used and the results to be anticipated are described in Chapter 16.

Brachial Plexus Lesions

As noted in the introduction to this chapter pathological processes affecting the brachial plexus are rare. Traumatic lesions are certainly the most frequent cause and the only non-traumatic condition presenting a diagnostic problem is damage to the plexus caused by radiation of the axillary area for carcinoma of breast, the decision required usually being whether the problem is due to metastatic disease requiring more radiotherapy or due to radiotherapy itself. In the writer's experience there are four main sites of plexus damage producing fairly typical clinical pictures (see Figure 18.6).

a. Lesions of the Upper Trunk

Damage to this area which is the most superficial part of the plexus, often occurs with stab or bullet wounds in the neck. C5 and C6 are destroyed leaving the patient with numbness of the lateral arm, forearm and hand with loss of abduction, internal and external rotation of the shoulder, elbow flexion and radial wrist extension due to weakness in the extensor carpi radialis longus and brevis. The biceps and supinator jerks are absent. Note that the lesion is distal to the roots and spares the rhomboid muscles which are supplied by a branch from the C5 root and serratus anterior which is supplied by branches from C5, C6 and C7 roots.

b. Lesions of the Lower Trunk

Damage to this area has already been described to some extent in connection with cervical rib syndrome. This is also the area of the plexus that is damaged by carcinoma of the lung apex extending through the apical pleura (Pancoast's syndrome) and metastatic disease in the axillary glands, from malignant disease from the breast or elsewhere. The clinical

Figure 18.6. Scheme of the Anatomy of the Brachial Plexus showing the eventual destination of all Root Components

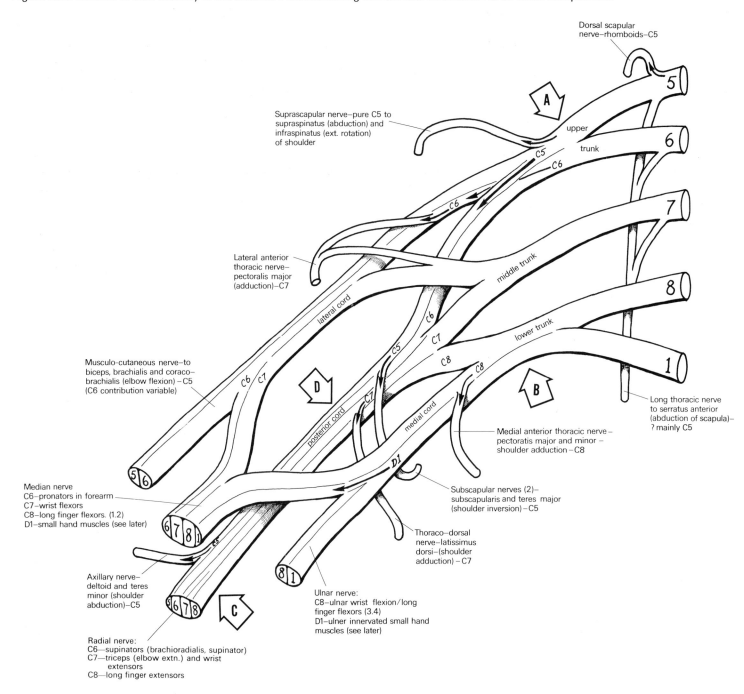

Dorsal scapular nerve–rhomboids–C5

Suprascapular nerve–pure C5 to supraspinatus (abduction) and infraspinatus (ext. rotation) of shoulder

Lateral anterior thoracic nerve– pectoralis major (adduction)–C7

Musculo-cutaneous nerve–to biceps, brachialis and coraco– brachialis (elbow flexion) – C5 (C6 contribution variable)

Median nerve
C6–pronators in forearm
C7–wrist flexors
C8–long finger flexors. (1.2)
D1–small hand muscles (see later)

Axillary nerve– deltoid and teres minor (shoulder abduction)–C5

Radial nerve:
C6—supinators (brachioradialis, supinator)
C7—triceps (elbow extn.) and wrist extensors
C8—long finger extensors

upper trunk

middle trunk

lower trunk

lateral cord

posterior cord

medial cord

Long thoracic nerve to serratus anterior (abduction of scapula)– ? mainly C5

Medial anterior thoracic nerve– pectoralis major and minor – shoulder adduction–C8

Subscapular nerves (2)– subscapularis and teres major (shoulder inversion)–C5

Thoraco–dorsal nerve–latissimus dorsi–(shoulder adduction) – C7

Ulnar nerve:
C8–ulnar wrist flexion/long finger flexors (3.4)
D1–ulner innervated small hand muscles (see later)

picture consists of pain and numbness down the medial arm and forearm into the little and ring fingers of the hand. Weakness of finger flexors and extensors and the small hand muscles follows and as noted above, is particularly likely to affect the abductor pollicis brevis first. There may also be some wasting and weakness of pectoralis major but this muscle has dual innervation and this finding is variable.

c. *A Radial Nerve Lesion in the Axilla*

This has already been discussed under crutch injuries to the nerve in the lower axilla and radial nerve damage may also occur following stab wounds and neoplastic disease in the axillary glands. A complete radial nerve palsy including weakness of the triceps muscle is found.

d. *Lesions of the Posterior Cord*

Lesions of the posterior cord in the author's experience seem to follow small calibre, low velocity bullet wounds to the plexus. The bullet traverses the region of the plexus and impacts against the inner surface of the scapula and the posterior cord seems to be particularly likely to be damaged. The picture is often a transient one with later recovery. A posterior cord lesion is easy to diagnose as it is essentially a radial nerve palsy combined with an axillary nerve lesion. Therefore, there is inability to extend the elbow, extend the wrist and fingers and weakness of the second 90° of shoulder abduction due to paralysis of the deltoid muscle.

Radiation Damage to the Plexus

Patients who have received irradiation to the lymphatic nodes adjacent to the plexus as prophylaxis against metastasis from a carcinoma of the breast, sustain damage to the C7 root with lesser involvement of C6 and C8. The numbness and weakness is of sudden onset and is progressive over a few weeks only. There is no pain and this is quite an important point against the diagnosis of malignant infiltration of the plexus. Three weeks' observation to establish that the lesion is static confirms that the damage is probably due to the irradiation and not due to malignant infiltration; although prolonged careful observation is necessary.

Chapter 19

DIAGNOSIS OF ROOT AND NERVE LESIONS AFFECTING THE LEG

In the previous chapter dealing with root and nerve lesions affecting the arm three points were emphasised:

1. Anatomical features that place nerves in vulnerable positions in fibrous tunnels against bone or traversing muscles.
2. Bizarre sensory disturbances that defy anatomical explanation and make sensory symptoms somewhat unreliable.
3. The reliability of motor signs, both the reflexes and muscle weakness in assessing nerve and root injuries.

When we come to consider the situation in the leg there are some striking differences:

1. The peripheral nerves are much less vulnerable to everyday trauma, and with the exception of the peroneal nerve at the fibula neck, are infrequently damaged compared with the nerves in the arm.
2. In root disease sensory symptoms are extremely reliable in indicating which root is affected. Furthermore, the two common peripheral nerve lesions, both the lateral cutaneous nerve of the thigh and the peroneal nerve produce pain and discomfort in an anatomically accurate area, making for easy diagnosis.
3. In general, motor signs in lumbar and sacral root disease are extremely unreliable due to the fact that most muscles have a nerve supply derived from two roots, making wasting and weakness extremely difficult to detect.

There are also several anatomical features that require re-emphasis at this stage. All the nerve roots supplying the leg arise from the spinal cord above L1 vertebral level and each root then traverses several inches in the spinal canal before reaching its exit foramen. It is therefore obvious that even if there is evidence of a single nerve root being affected, one cannot be certain at which level in the canal the damage has occurred, and the L5 root, for example, could be damaged anywhere over a six-inch intra-dural course. In practice the root is most commonly damaged in the region of its exit foramen by disc lesions but it is the failure to recognise the possibility that the damage could be higher if no local lesion can be demonstrated that occasionally leads to diagnostic errors.

The problems of the diagnosis of intra-dural lesions of the lumbar and sacral roots are fully discussed under cauda equina lesions in Chapter 15.

The clinical term "sciatica" also requires definition. It must be realised that "sciatica" is a symptom and not a disease. It is *not* inevitably due to disc disease and may be the presenting symptom of *serious* intra-pelvic disease. The cutaneous distribution of the sciatic nerve does not extend up the posterior thigh or on to the buttock. "Sciatica" means pain in the leg and is no more specific than that.

ANATOMICAL FEATURES OF THE NERVE SUPPLY OF THE LEG

The highest components of the nerve supply to the leg arise from roots L2, L3 and L4, and emerge from the vertebral canal just below the diaphragm to enter the fibres of origin of the psoas muscle (see Figure 19.1). These three roots form the lumbar plexus and the branches of the plexus have to reach the front of the leg. The first branch, the lateral cutaneous nerve of the thigh, does so by skirting around the pelvic brim and exits under the lateral part of the inguinal ligament. The femoral nerve remains on the lateral side of psoas muscle and passes with the muscle under the inguinal ligament into the anterior part of the thigh. The obturator nerve lies on the medial side of the psoas muscle and comes into close relationship with the uterus in the pelvis before emerging through the obturator foramen. Here it is subject to damage during obstetric procedures. The lumbar plexus therefore supplies the hip flexors, thigh adductors, knee extensors and skin over the anterior medial and lateral thigh and via the saphenous branch of the femoral nerve a long promontory of skin down the medial side of the leg including the medial surface of the ankle.

The rest of the leg is supplied by the sacral plexus which is derived from L4, L5, S1 and S2 roots. This plexus is formed over the sacro-iliac joint and almost immediately leaves the pelvis via the greater sciatic foramen. Its main branches, the gluteal nerves, the sciatic nerve and the posterior cutaneous nerve of thigh, then lie directly behind the hip joint. It is obvious that fractures of the upper femur, particularly those involving the acetabulum, represent a considerable threat to

Figure 19.1. Anterior View of the Pelvic Cavity Showing the Course of the Nerve Supply to the Leg

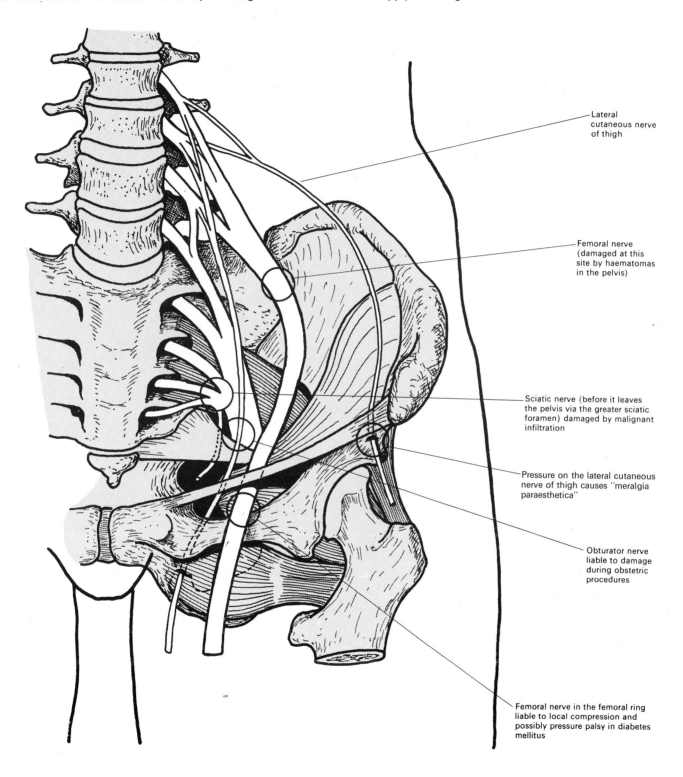

Lateral cutaneous nerve of thigh

Femoral nerve (damaged at this site by haematomas in the pelvis)

Sciatic nerve (before it leaves the pelvis via the greater sciatic foramen) damaged by malignant infiltration

Pressure on the lateral cutaneous nerve of thigh causes "meralgia paraesthetica"

Obturator nerve liable to damage during obstetric procedures

Femoral nerve in the femoral ring liable to local compression and possibly pressure palsy in diabetes mellitus

Figure 19.2. Posterior View of the Pelvis Showing the Nerves to the Posterior Part of the Leg

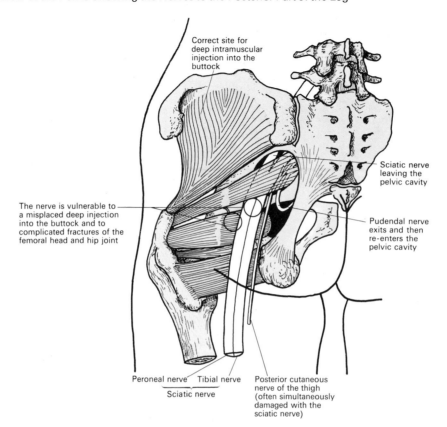

Correct site for deep intramuscular injection into the buttock

Sciatic nerve leaving the pelvic cavity

The nerve is vulnerable to a misplaced deep injection into the buttock and to complicated fractures of the femoral head and hip joint

Pudendal nerve exits and then re-enters the pelvic cavity

Peroneal nerve   Tibial nerve
Sciatic nerve

Posterior cutaneous nerve of the thigh (often simultaneously damaged with the sciatic nerve)

these nerves. They are also liable to damage from a misplaced intra-muscular injection in the buttock. The correct position for such an injection is shown in Figure 19.2.

The sciatic nerve is formed of two discrete components—the peroneal (lateral popliteal) and the tibial (medial popliteal) nerves. Even when the whole nerve is traumatised the peroneal component is much more likely to be damaged than the tibial component. The reason for this is not entirely clear, but this feature has considerable clinical significance. Following the separation into individual nerves in the lower thigh the tibial nerve remains deep and is very rarely damaged (Figure 19.3). The peroneal nerve, however, has to gain access to the anterior and lateral compartments of the leg, and in doing so becomes extremely vulnerable as it crosses the fibula neck. The subsequent division of the peroneal nerve into the anterior tibial and musculocutaneous nerves has little practical significance as damage to the nerves below the fibula neck is extremely rare. The terminal digital branches of the tibial nerve are subject to trauma as they lie under the metatarsal heads, leading to the condition known as Morton's metatarsalgia.

CLINICALLY IMPORTANT FEATURES OF THE SENSORY SUPPLY TO THE LEG

The Peripheral Nerve Supply

The area supplied by the lateral cutaneous nerve of the thigh is indicated in Figure 19.5; note that the area does not cross the midline of the thigh and compare this with the area supplied with the L2 root, shown in Figure 19.4. Secondly, note the long promontory of skin supplied by the saphenous branch of the femoral nerve. This is important as sensory loss following sciatic nerve injuries cannot produce complete stocking sensory loss below the knee, and one should always look for an area of preserved sensation on the medial side of the leg. The sciatic nerve itself supplies a relatively small area of the skin of the leg. Unless the posterior cutaneous nerve of the thigh is simultaneously injured the patient will not have numbness over the back of the thigh. A peroneal nerve pressure palsy at the fibula neck has many similarities to a radial nerve palsy in the arm, as it causes a foot drop, and the similarity extends to the fact that sensory loss is also relatively unusual with peroneal nerve lesions.

208

Figure 19.3. Diagram to Show the course and Bony Relations of the Nerve Supply of the Leg

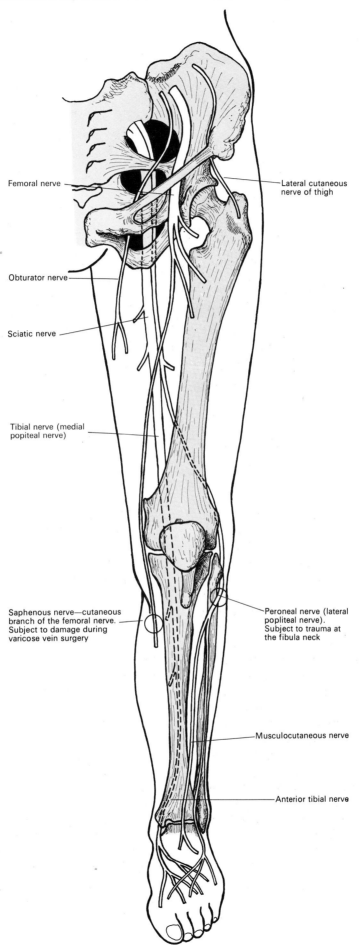

Femoral nerve

Lateral cutaneous
nerve of thigh

Obturator nerve

Sciatic nerve

Tibial nerve (medial
popliteal nerve)

Saphenous nerve—cutaneous
branch of the femoral nerve.
Subject to damage during
varicose vein surgery

Peroneal nerve (lateral
popliteal nerve).
Subject to trauma at
the fibula neck

Musculocutaneous nerve

Anterior tibial nerve

The area normally involved if such loss is present is shown on the figure.

The Root Supply

Refer to Figure 19.4. Note that the distribution of lumbar roots L2, L3 and L4 is in a spiral across the front of the thigh and down on to the medial side of the leg. This should be contrasted with the distribution of the cutaneous nerves of this area, which are essentially straight up and down the thigh. When one considers the rarity of disc disease above L4 level it is immediately apparent that pain in the anterior thigh should *not* be ascribed to disc disease. This point has been amplified further in the section on cauda equina lesions in Chapter 15. The L4 root is the highest root that may be affected by disc disease and even this is relatively rare. The pain produced radiates across the front of the knee on to the medial side of the leg down to the medial malleolus. L5 is the root most commonly affected by disc disease and the typical radiation of the pain is across the buttock, down the back of the thigh on to the lateral side of the leg and on to the dorsal and ventral aspects of the foot. Pain in the big toe seems to be particularly typical of an L5 root lesion. S1 root irritation produces pain down the back of the leg on to the side of the leg as L5, but the pain in the foot is confined to the lateral side. In either case, it is exceptional to find definite sensory loss although slightly altered perception of sensation over the dorsum of the foot in the case of the L5 root lesion or behind the lateral malleolus with an S1 root lesion may be found. The lower sacral roots S2 to S5 supply the skin of the inner posterior thigh, the inner buttocks and the genitalia. Sensation over these areas should be carefully checked in all patients complaining of pain in the posterior thigh or genitalia, and in patients with sphincter disturbances.

Figure 19.4. Cutaneous Distribution of Nerve Roots in the Leg

Figure 19.5. Cutaneous Nerves in the Leg

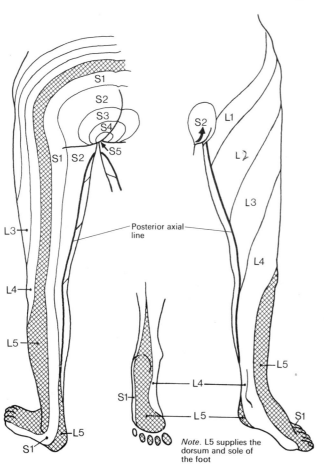

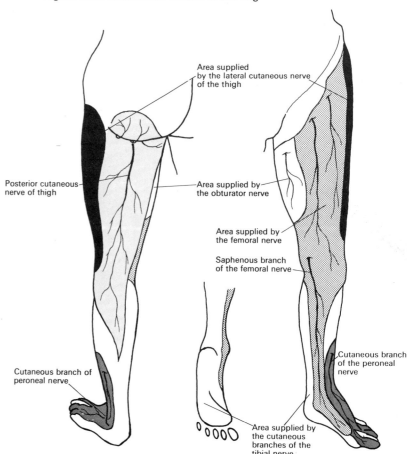

Table 8   COMPARATIVE DATA ON ROOT AND NERVE LESIONS IN THE LEG

ROOTS	L2	L3	L4	L5	S1
Sensory supply	Across upper thigh	Across lower thigh	Across knee to medial malleolus	Side of leg to dorsum and sole of foot	Behind lateral malleolus to lateral foot
Sensory loss	Often none	Often none	Medial leg	Dorsum of foot	Behind lateral malleolus
Area of pain	Across thigh	Across thigh	Down to medial malleolus	Back of thigh, lateral calf— dorsum of foot	Back of thigh, back of calf— lateral foot
Reflex arc	None	Adductor reflex	Knee jerk	None	Ankle jerk
Motor deficit	Hip flexion	Knee extension Adduction of thigh	Inversion of the foot	Dorsiflexion of toes and foot (latter L4 also)	Plantar flexion and eversion of foot
Causative lesions (in order of frequency)		Neurofibroma Meningioma Neoplastic disease Disc lesions very rare (except L4 <5 per cent *all*)		Disc lesions Metastatic Malignancy Neurofibromas Meningioma	

Table 9

NERVES	OBTURATOR	FEMORAL	SCIATIC NERVE	
			PERONEAL DIVISION	TIBIAL DIVISION
Sensory supply	Medial surface of thigh	Antero medial surface of thigh and leg to medial malleolus	Anterior leg, dorsum of ankle and foot	Posterior leg, sole and lateral border of foot
Sensory loss	Often none	Usually anatomical	Often just dorsum of foot	Sole of foot
Area of pain	Medial thigh	Anterior thigh and medial leg	Often painless	Often painless
Reflex arc	Adductor reflex	Knee jerk	None	Ankle jerk
Motor deficit	Adduction of thigh	Extension of knee	Dorsiflexion, inversion and eversion of the foot (+lateral hamstrings)	Plantar flexion and inversion of foot (+medial hamstrings)
Causative lesions	Pelvic neoplasm Pregnancy	Diabetes Femoral hernia Femoral artery aneurysm Posterior abdominal neoplasm Psoas abscess	Pressure palsy at fibula neck Hip fracture/dislocation Penetrating trauma to buttock Misplaced injection	Very rarely injured even in buttock Peroneal division more sensitive to damage

CLINICALLY IMPORTANT FEATURES OF THE MOTOR SUPPLY TO THE LEGS

The correct methods of testing leg movements and their root and nerve values are show in Figures 19.6 and 19.7.

The Peripheral Nerve Supply

The femoral nerve is partially responsible for hip flexion as it innervates the iliacus muscle and wholly responsible for knee extension as it innervates the entire quadriceps muscle. A lesion affecting the femoral nerve in the pelvis will weaken hip flexion as well as knee extension. Unfortunately, lesions in the abdomen will often interfere with psoas muscle contraction directly and may make hip flexion too painful for the patient to attempt. However, if psoas is weak, or attempts to use it cause severe pain, either is a strong indication that the lesion causing the femoral nerve palsy is intra-abdominal

so that from a strictly practical point of view no distinction as to the cause of the hip flexor weakness need be made.

The obturator nerve supplies the obturator externus muscle (lateral rotation of the thigh) and the adductor muscles of the thigh. Its function can be simply tested by the patient's ability to hold the legs together against resistance.

The peroneal nerve supplies part of the biceps femoris (the lateral ham-string muscle), the muscles in the anterior and lateral compartment of the leg and extensor digitorum brevis of the dorsum of the foot. This is the small muscle that can be detected just below and anterior to the lateral malleolus when the toes are dorsiflexed.

The tibial nerve supplies the bulk of the ham-string muscles, the muscles of the posterior compartment of the leg and all the small foot muscles with the exception of extensor digitorum brevis.

Figure 19.6. Movements of the Leg

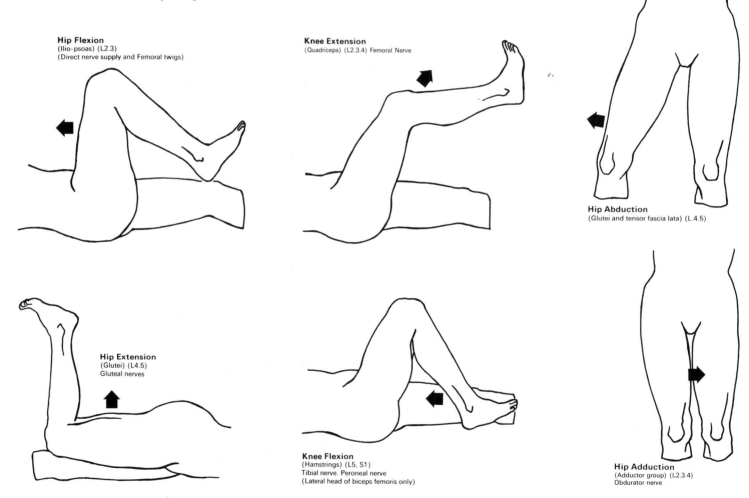

Hip Flexion
(Ilio-psoas) (L2.3)
(Direct nerve supply and Femoral twigs)

Knee Extension
(Quadriceps) (L2.3.4) Femoral Nerve

Hip Abduction
(Glutei and tensor fascia lata) (L.4.5)

Hip Extension
(Glutei) (L4.5)
Gluteal nerves

Knee Flexion
(Hamstrings) (L5, S1)
Tibial nerve. Peroneal nerve
(Lateral head of biceps femoris only)

Hip Adduction
(Adductor group) (L2.3.4)
Obdurator nerve

The Root Supply

The L2 root is predominantly responsible for hip flexion. Knee extension is usually unaffected even though it is generally stated that the quadriceps receive a contribution from L2, L3 and L4.

L3 root lesions cause weakness of both knee extension and thigh adduction, and it would appear clinically that the main motor innervation of the adductor muscles and the quadriceps is derived from L3.

L4 root lesions, although causing depression or absence of the knee jerk, rarely seem to lead to definite weakness of the quadriceps muscle. Clinically it would appear that its main importance in respect of the quadriceps is conveying the reflex arc. The important point about the L4 root is that it is the exclusive root supply to the inverters of the foot (tibialis anterior, in the anterior compartment of the leg and tibialis posterior, in the posterior compartment of the leg).

The L4 contribution to these muscles reaches them via the peroneal and tibial nerves respectively. Therefore, although in an L4 lesion a little weakness of dorsiflexion and plantar flexion of the foot may be apparent, there is striking weakness of inversion of the foot. A patient with a bilateral L4 root lesion walks in a most peculiar way, with the feet flapping on the ground, as if extremely flat footed.

In an L5 root lesion *if* any weakness is detectable, it is usually maximal in the toe extensors, particularly the extensor of the big toe. Because both L4 and S1 contribute to the innervation of the muscles responsible for plantar and dorsiflexion of the foot, it is unusual to be able to detect any weakness of these movements. Both L4 and L5 roots contribute to the nerve supply of the gluteal muscles, but wasting and weakness in these very powerful and bulky muscles may be extremely difficult to detect. In the case of an S1 root lesion the ankle jerk is usually abolished. Again,

Figure 19.7. Movements of the Foot

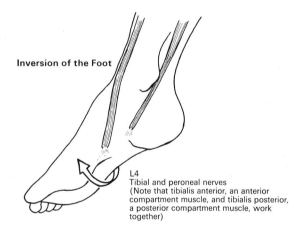

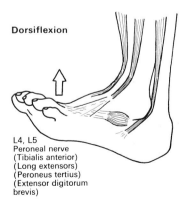

Plantar Flexion

S1, S2
Tibial nerve
(Gastrocnemii)
(Tibialis posterior)

Inversion of the Foot

L4
Tibial and peroneal nerves
(Note that tibialis anterior, an anterior compartment muscle, and tibialis posterior, a posterior compartment muscle, work together)

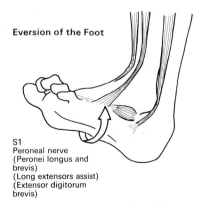

Dorsiflexion

L4, L5
Peroneal nerve
(Tibialis anterior)
(Long extensors)
(Peroneus tertius)
(Extensor digitorum brevis)

Eversion of the Foot

S1
Peroneal nerve
(Peronei longus and brevis)
(Long extensors assist)
(Extensor digitorum brevis)

weakness may be extremely difficult to detect and eversion of the foot is the best movement to test. In a severe S1 lesion there may be weakness of plantar flexion and of the ham-string muscles. The ham-strings present much the same problems as the glutei—they are such large powerful muscles that weakness and wasting may be extremely difficult to detect in the early stages of an S1 root lesion.

When examining power in the legs in any patient who has either back or abdominal pain it is necessary to make considerable allowances for inhibition caused by the pain. In general, if the patient is encouraged to make one maximal effort, however severe the pain, it is usually possible to establish whether or not strength is normal, and most patients will make this effort if they are told how important it is from a diagnostic point of view. In patients with leg pain it is not permissible to dismiss the motor examination as "impossible due to pain", as important localising evidence may be missed if the examination is incomplete.

SPECIFIC CLINICAL CONDITIONS AFFECTING THE NERVES AND NERVE ROOTS OF THE LEG

Meralgia Paraesthetica (lateral cutaneous nerve of the thigh)

This common condition produces a peculiar numb, tingling sensation in the upper lateral thigh. In the male it may be noticed when the hand is placed in the pocket because of the peculiar sensation that is provoked. The condition is most often encountered in obese patients who have lost a lot of weight (it is theorised that the sagging anterior abdominal wall pulls on the nerve) or may occur spontaneously without clear reasons. The writer has seen two examples of the condition in young males as a consequence of a young lady sitting on their laps! The condition quite often remits spontaneously and surgery should be deferred for three months in most instances to give it time to do so.

Femoral Nerve Lesions

The femoral nerve may be damaged in the upper abdomen by primary or secondary neoplasms or a psoas abscess. In the lower abdomen it may be damaged by an intra-pelvic haematoma. Direct trauma to the nerve during arterial catheterisation or by a femoral aneurysm can occur. Diabetics appear to be particularly prone to develop a femoral neuropathy. This condition is sometimes known as diabetic amyotrophy of Garland. It is characterised by the onset of very severe pain in the front of the thigh, which may radiate down the medial side of the leg to the medial malleolus. Within a few days or weeks of the onset of pain, which may require narcotics for its control, the patient suddenly develops complete weakness and wasting of the quadriceps muscle, making walking impossible. Usually as the weakness appears the pain tends to remit. The condition almost invariably eventually improves although four to six months may elapse before any recovery is apparent. Occasionally it is not the femoral nerve itself but the L2, L3 and L4 roots which seem to be affected, producing a picture of more widespread weakness and wasting including the hip flexors. With the exception of these diabetic patients femoral nerve lesions are extremely rare.

Sciatic Nerve Lesions

The sciatic nerve may be damaged in the pelvis by the direct spread of neoplasms of the rectum and genito-urinary tract. The nerve may also be compressed in the later stages of pregnancy. In the buttock, complicated hip fractures, penetrating trauma, especially by gunshot or knife wounds, and misplaced deep intra-muscular injections are the most frequent causes of sciatic nerve damage. An unusual feature of damage at this site, already mentioned earlier, is that the peroneal division is six times as likely to be damaged as the tibial division in spite of non-selective trauma to the whole nerve trunk. The practical importance of this may be seen in the following example.

A patient with severe traumatic damage to the hip may be impossible to examine initially and open joint surgery is performed. Subsequently it is discovered that the patient has a foot drop. The question will then arise as to whether this occurred as a result of pressure on the peroneal nerve during surgery, or as a result of any plaster casting that has been carried out or whether it was primarily injured in either the trauma or the subsequent surgery.

The marked difference in prognosis both in time and potential degree of recovery is extremely important. Clinically, the writer has found that the most useful sign is the detection of wasting and weakness in the biceps femoris. This is the part of the ham-string muscle supplied by the peroneal nerve and is unaffected by a peroneal nerve lesion at the fibula neck. Furthermore, one can elicit both medial and lateral ham-string reflexes by tapping the appropriate tendons and the lateral reflex invariably disappears in this situation.

Misplaced injections into the sciatic nerve are especially disastrous, as not only is there weakness of dorsiflexion and plantar flexion of the foot, but often very severe causalgic pain results, making it impossible for the patient to tolerate the leg splints necessary to compensate for the weakness.

Peroneal Nerve Lesions

This is probably the commonest nerve lesion in the leg and is due to compression of the nerve at the fibula neck. This may occur in quite normal persons following a sharp blow to the nerve, or while sitting with the legs crossed for a prolonged period. However, in all cases care should be taken to exclude any possible cause of impaired nutrition of the nerve. In Great Britain diabetes is probably the commonest cause, but polyarteritis nodosa should also be excluded and other collagen vascular diseases such as rheumatoid arthritis. In all these situations other peripheral nerves may be damaged by compression, particularly the ulnar nerve, and when multiple palsies occur in this way the condition is known as mono-neuritis multiplex. Leprosy is the commonest cause of this situation in appropriate areas of the world. Pressure on the peroneal nerve may occur while resting in bed, particularly if there has been marked weight loss or from a leg plaster. The patient complains of inability to dorsiflex or evert the foot. There is little or no sensory loss in most cases. It is important to distinguish the condition from a painless L5 root lesion and this may be extremely difficult unless one can detect weakness or wasting in the calf muscles. Electromyography is extremely useful in this situation.

Nerve lesions in the legs are relatively rare compared with the arm. Root lesions occur with a much greater frequency and are often related to serious intra-pelvic or abdominal disease, and it is quite wrong and extremely dangerous to assume that all leg pain is due to a simple disc lesion. It is essential to have a clear grasp of the anatomy of the lumbar and sacral nerve roots to be aware of the clinical clues that suggest the more ominous pathological possibilities. In the writer's view, the single most ominous symptom in a patient with back pain radiating into the leg is that the pain is worst at *rest*, particularly in bed at night. This is in marked contrast to simple disc disease in which rest is the main relieving factor.

Chapter 20

HEADACHE

Many student texts contain long classifications of the causes of headaches that seem to indicate that the differential diagnosis of headache is a mere formality.

With the exception of all but the most classical cases of migraine, this implication is certainly unjustified. The degree of overlap between both the aetiological factors and some of the features of the headache may make differential diagnosis extremely difficult. For example, many patients with headache who are referred as "diagnostic problems" are suffering from migraine headaches, the diagnostic difficulty usually having arisen because the headache was not frontal, strictly unilateral or throbbing in nature. All these features do occur in classical migraine, but none of them need to be present for the diagnosis of migraine headache to be made. When we consider aetiological factors, the main problem is the role played by tension in an individual case. Just because the patient is tense, it does not automatically follow that he had tension headache. Migraine is often precipitated by tension, and any patient who has had a series of bad migraine headaches soon becomes tense. Failure to appreciate the nature of the headache will lead to prolonged ineffectual therapy with tranquilisers, and deny the patient the possible symptomatic relief he could obtain with ergot preparations.

There are considerable similarities in the diagnostic approach and aetiological factors in patients with headache and face pain and the reader is strongly recommended to read this and the subsequent chapter in sequence.

General Considerations Concerning Headaches

There is a widely held misconception, not confined to the general public, that the most common causes of headache are eye strain and sinus disease. Very few patients are referred who have not already had their eyes tested and many have also had their sinuses x-rayed.

Refractive errors cause pain in and around the eye when the eyes are used for unusually long periods or in poor light. Refractive errors cannot cause intermittent severe headaches *not* linked to the use of the eyes for close work or reading. Occasionally serious delays are caused by referral to opticians, as it takes several weeks for the patient to obtain new glasses and discover that they do not relieve the headache.

Many patients complain of life-long "sinus headache" often abbreviated to the more colloquial "sinus". Close questioning usually reveals a typical history of migraine. Sinus disease causes pain in the affected sinus. The pain may be referred to other areas of the face and head, but the underlying pain in the sinus is identifiable. The suggestion that chronic *sub-clinical* sinus infection can cause recurrent severe headaches over decades is no longer acceptable.

The term "ordinary headaches" is also often used by patients. This term seems to mean headaches that have been sufficiently infrequent or so short-lived that the patient has never bothered to seek advice. It is essential to try to establish the nature of such headaches, and not accept the patient's own diagnosis.

The possibility that a headache is due to something serious does *not* increase in proportion to the severity of the headache. In fact, the most severe headaches are usually due to migraine, and many of the patients who are harbouring cerebral tumours complain of a "dull" or "muzzy" head, only on direct questioning. It is not often that the headache itself prompts the patient to seek medical advice.

X-rays of the skull, although greatly respected by patients, rarely give help in the investigation of headache. The views taken can be restricted to an AP and a lateral skull and often even these can be dispensed with if a confident clinical diagnosis has been made. Normal skull x-rays do not exclude anything. The most important investigation in the evaluation of headache is the history.

MIGRAINE HEADACHE

In the introductory paragraphs the emphasis placed on the recognition of migraine headache will be apparent. This is because migraine or migraine variants are responsible for the headache in a majority of patients referred to hospital.

The difficulty in making the diagnosis may be due to atypical features of the headache, and this cannot always be avoided. However, it is frequently due to the uncritical acceptance of the patient's history that he has only had "sinus" or "ordinary" headache previously. Headache apparently starting at the age of 55 years may create a diagnostic problem, but when seen in the setting of life-long migraine (hitherto called "sinus") the diagnosis is easy. Ascribing a causal role to tension, when the tension is secondary to the headache itself, is another error. Although

Figure 20.1. Classical Migraine
(Hemicrania)

Figure 20.2. Occipital-Orbital Migraine

Figure 20.3. Orbital Migraine

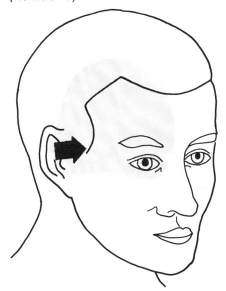

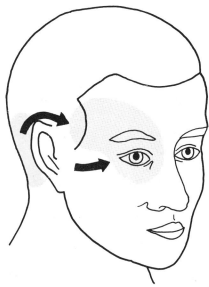

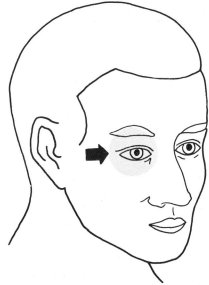

The headache starts in the temple on one side and spreads to involve the whole side of the head. It is a pulsatile headache, and any or all of the common migraine concomitants may occur. It usually remains strictly unilateral but may occur on either side on subsequent occasions. Usually self limited lasting from 30 minutes to several hours

This is the type of headache most often requiring hospital referral. The onset is less dramatic, often a dull ache in the occipital area which extends forward around the temple, or deep into the area behind the eye. A dull bursting ache behind the eye is an important diagnostic clue. The pain may also be bilateral in this type, although the pain on one side is usually worse than the other
Other migraine concomitants may not be present and the headache may last several days

This is a minor variant of migrainous neuralgia. The pain is predominantly a deep nagging ache behind the eye with occasional stabs of pain "like a needle in the back of the eye"
Photophobia is common and light or sudden movement provokes the pain. This variety is seen (in the author's opinion) as a common variant of the vascular headache produced by the birth control Pill (see text)

the tension component may well require appropriate therapy with valium, it is unlikely that this will succeed, if the underlying headache is due to migraine, as the concomitantly prescribed simple analgesics *will not* relieve the headache that is causing the tension. This is because in the majority of migraine sufferers simple proprietary analgesics and even narcotics do *not* significantly alleviate the pain.

Several features of migraine that are rarely stressed are the tendency for attacks to be present on waking in the morning, especially at weekends. This often seems to be related to relaxation and "lying-in" and may be aborted by following a normal working day routine at weekends. The ultimate expression of these relaxation migraine attacks is found in patients who only get headaches during their holidays!

Site of the Headache (Figures 20.1, 20.2 and 20.3)

Classical migraine is frontal-temporal in site and usually unilateral. There should be little difficulty in diagnosis with this type of headache. The headache site shown on Figure 20.2 causes most difficulty. Such stress is laid on the tension in neck muscles that is held to be responsible for tension

headache that it is assumed that occipital headache is invariably due to tension. In fact many cases of otherwise typical migraine start in the occipital area and radiate forward to the "classical" frontal site. The variant shown in the figure is less typical, and creates a diagnostic problem. The pain starts sub-occipitally and radiates forward to the temple or deep in behind the eye. It is usually bilateral, although one side is more severely affected than the other. The most severe pain may be indicated by the patient clutching both temples and describing a "bursting" feeling. Throbbing may not occur, or may only be felt deep in the eye, and may be provoked by exertion or bright lights.

The third variety (Figure 20.3) is often ascribed to sinus disease. The pain is essentially confined to a position deep in behind the eye. It may be bilateral, and is aggravated by bright light. It is more or less continual over weeks with periodic exacerbations. It is usually referred to as migrainous neuralgia. It often supervenes in a patient with a previous history of migraine, and is more frequently seen in females (unlike cluster headache which is almost confined to males). This type of headache seems particularly to be produced by the birth control Pill. These patients may complain of a feeling as if a pin or a red-hot needle were being jabbed into the back of the eye. In any young female with this variant the possibility that it is due to the Pill must be considered.

Type of Pain

It is worth noting briefly that although throbbing is, of course, a typical feature of migraine, the headache does not have to be of this variety for the diagnosis to be made. Even in a classical case throbbing may only occur as the headache develops, the eventual pain being more or less constant. In the second and third varieties it is unusual for throbbing to be a prominent feature, but the deep bursting pain in the eye must be emphasised as it is not only the diagnostic feature in these cases but often provides a diagnostic clue in the case of the facial migraine syndromes to be discussed in the next chapter.

In the author's opinion these peculiar prickling sensations, likened by one patient to a bunch of stinging nettles in the eye, are virtually diagnostic of migraine. They occur in all the variants and may require specific questioning to remind the patient of their occurrence. This is best discovered by asking if the patient has noticed any special sensations or feelings in the eye, while avoiding more specific suggestions. The description is so characteristic that however atypical the rest of the history the diagnosis of migraine is certain.

Associated Symptoms

In descriptions of classical migraine great emphasis is placed on dramatic prodromata such as fortification spectra. These are zig-zag lines or circles that have the appearance of a plan of the castle and its fortifications. These are by no means a universal accompaniment of the headache, and although they ought to occur at the onset of the attacks when the blood vessels are in spasm, quite often they occur at the height of the actual headache. Perhaps the most common visual symptoms are photophobia and slight blurring of vision. Some patients specifically complain that their headaches are caused by bright light, and working under strip lighting, or driving a car in bright sunshine are commonly cited as specific provoking factors.

The majority of patients feel extremely nauseated during an attack, but severe vomiting is an unusual and often isolated event. Indeed, it is a useful general rule that if vomiting is a new feature of attacks, the possibility of more serious disease should be considered. If there is *no* previous history of migraine the recent onset of headache associated with vomiting should be regarded as due to a posterior fossa tumour until proved otherwise.

Intense irritability, noise intolerance and anxiety are present to a greater or lesser degree in all attacks and the sufferer seeks a quiet dark room.

Other Important Variants

Childhood Migraine

Attacks of pallor, nausea and vomiting with occasional complaints of blurred vision, so-called "abdominal migraine" usually occur in childhood. It is unusual for the child actually to complain of headache until about ten years of age.

Occasionally exceptional five-year-olds are able to give remarkably accurate descriptions of their attacks if allowed to do so by their parents. One little boy called his attacks "headaches with colours", others call them "giddy heads" or "a pain above the eye". The parents' description of a pale, listless and sleepy child leaves little doubt as to the diagnosis. As in the adult, attacks may be precipitated by exertion and some athletically inclined children fond of games and physical education have these classes ruined by the onset of their attacks. Unlike adults, however, the attacks may be extremely brief, often as short as fifteen to twenty minutes with sudden and complete recovery.

In the early teens the variant that has been called "basilar migraine" occurs. In this type, attacks of brain stem ischaemia dominate the picture. One 13-year-old boy seen by the author was referred because of five episodes of teichopsia (flashing lights) followed by hemianopia and tetraplegia, each lasting nearly thirty minutes, occurring over the previous two years. All had been followed by a typical migraine headache and between attacks typical migraine without the ischaemic symptoms had occurred.

Cluster Headaches (Figure 20.4)

This syndrome is in many ways even more typical than classical migraine, and yet is frequently misdiagnosed. It occurs almost exclusively in middle-aged males who have usually *not* previously suffered from migraine headaches. The headache is frontal and strictly unilateral. The pain in the eye is particularly severe and may reduce strong men to tears. The affected eye becomes bloodshot and waters throughout the attack. The nose is also congested and nasal discharge occurs.

Perhaps the most characteristic feature is that the attacks are often strictly nocturnal, wake the patient from sleep and may last from thirty minutes to two hours. More than one attack may occur in one night. During the day attacks are very infrequent, but many patients notice specific pro-

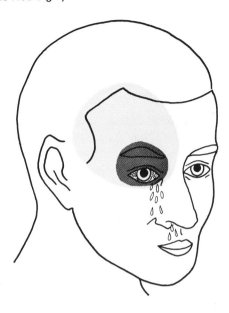

Figure 20.4. Cluster Headache
(Migrainous Neuralgia)

Almost exclusively a disease of middle-aged males. Often occurs without a prior history of migraine. Attacks last 30 minutes to two hours and are mainly nocturnal
Pain is excruciating in and around the eye. Eye may become bloodshot and nose "stuffed up". Lacrimation and nasal watering occur. Especially likely to be provoked by alcohol between attacks. Bout lasts 6–12 weeks and may recur at the same time each year. Excellent response to ergot

vocation by alcohol. A series of attacks may last from six to twelve weeks (in clusters, hence the name of the syndrome) and may occur at the same time each year for several years. Occasionally, attacks are prolonged. Cases persisting twenty-six and fourteen months respectively with no relief until the appropriate treatment was initiated have been seen by the writer. These patients are often suspected of harbouring an intracranial aneurysm, but the periodicity of the symptoms and relative brevity of each individual episode of severe pain are the important diagnostic clues.

"Status Migrainosus"

This condition is best described as chronic mild migraine. The distribution of the headache is similar to that shown in Figure 20.3. The episode is usually initiated by a stressful situation, but by the time the patient is seen the initial stress is often no longer operative, but the headache itself has become the stress! This variety of headache is sometimes called "tension migraine". The importance of treating the headache as well as the tension with anti-migraine drugs is worth reiterating.

In this group of patients reassurance that the patient does not have a cerebral tumour is a vital part of management. Patients are often frightened to voice their fear, but this is such a constant worry in this group that it is worth specifically telling the patient that the possibility has been considered and excluded.

Exertional Migraine

This is a rarely discussed, but quite frequent, variant of migraine of some importance. It is invariably diagnosed as subarachnoid haemorrhage. It may occur during any exertion, but is most often noticed during sexual intercourse. It is usually a fairly typical migraine headache of explosive suddenness noticed at climax or just after. It may occur in either partner and the writer has encountered two examples of simultaneous headache in both partners. If the patient attends hospital he is likely to be subjected to an immediate L.P. to exclude subarachnoid haemorrhage. A problem arises if the patient is seen several weeks after an episode. The condition occurs often enough for fairly confident reassurance that this was *not* a "small bleed" to be given if the headache had cleared completely by the next day. A similar headache following the heading of a football by professional footballers has recently been reported.

Migraine with Vertigo

Occasionally the vertigenous component of migraine with vomiting may be so severe that the headache is overlooked. The importance of the past history cannot be over-estimated. A 53-year-old woman was referred for investigation of severe attacks of vertigo, that usually occurred while she was in bed. At the end of each attack there was a generalised throbbing headache. Her past history revealed that she had had migraine since she was 14 years old, *always* associated with vertigo, and the only difference in the present episodes was that the vertigo was more severe than the headache. Her symptoms were completely relieved by anti-migraine prophylactic drugs (see also Chapter 6).

Management of Migraine Headaches

Simple analgesics give little or no relief in migraine. Patients will often claim that they are helpful, but usually this is not substantiated by further questioning. Effective analgesics give appreciable relief within thirty minutes. Patients with migraine may take six to eight aspirins over several hours, and when the headache eventually clears mistakenly ascribe the recovery to the tablets they have taken. Opiates should never be used. Notwithstanding the obvious addictive potential they do not give any relief of the headache, and usually compound the patient's misery by provoking vomiting. Once the headache is well established, parenteral ergotamine is rarely effective and carries some risk. If the patient can get to sleep, even for only thirty minutes or so, this will often terminate the attack. The writer's preferred treatment in the acute established attack is 50 mgs. promethazine (Phenergan) intramuscularly, which not only sedates the patient but is an effective anti-emetic.

If the patient has isolated attacks with a recognisable prodrome, any one of the standard oral preparations of ergotamine are suitable, provided it is taken as soon as possible after the onset. The headache is unlikely to respond to any drug once it is established. If vomiting is a feature, a preparation containing an anti-emetic is useful, or the ergot may be given as a suppository. If there is any nausea at all it is unlikely that preparations that have to be chewed or dissolved in the mouth will be tolerated, due to the vile taste of ergotamine.

If attacks are occurring several times a week, an attempt at prevention should be made. In ascending order of effectiveness clonidine 0·05 mgs. t.d.s., Bellergal® 1 t.d.s. or methysergide maleate 1 mg, t.d.s. may be tried. (The long-term risks of the latter drug should be remembered and very carefully considered before initiating treatment.)

In the variety called "status migrainosus" any of the prophylactics mentioned above coupled with a tranquilliser such as valium should be used. As the headache in this situation is virtually continual there is little point in using the standard ergotamine preparations.

Cluster headache responds dramatically to ergotamine and an ergotamine suppository before retiring may be the only therapy needed.

If this fails, or attacks are also occurring during the day, methysergide maleate is the drug of choice. As the length of cluster headache attacks is self-limited there need be little concern over the risks of long-term usage of this drug. Therapy should be continued two weeks *beyond* the last episode of pain to avoid an early relapse.

Further details of the use of anti-migraine drugs and their toxic effects are to be found in Chapter 24.

In the case of headache due to the Pill the patient should be advised to stop taking the Pill. Almost invariably, if the Pill is solely responsible, the headache ceases entirely within two weeks of stopping the Pill. In view of the possible relationship of Pill-induced headache to vascular accidents occurring in patients on the Pill it would seem advisable to avoid the use of ergot in any form in these cases.

There are so many different agents available for the treatment of migraine that the different therapeutic regimes that can be used are legion. The methods outlined above are

those preferred by the author. The fact that even the use of appropriate drugs cannot guarantee a cure should certainly be made known to the patient. At best about half the patients' attacks can be alleviated. The failure of ergotamine to relieve any given headache cannot be taken as proof that the headache is not due to migraine.

TENSION HEADACHE (Figure 20.5)

The typical tension headache is a headache that starts as a tight feeling in the suboccipital muscles and then spreads over the top of the head as a "tight" feeling. However, many of the cases that are referred to hospital have failed to respond to tranquillisers. These cases often have additional symptoms including giddiness, lack of concentration and pain deep behind the eyes. In the writer's opinion such cases are on the border-line between tension headache and tension-migraine, and it is usually worth a trial of anti-migraine prophylactics in addition to the tranquillisers, even if the vascular component is minimal. Deep aching pain in the eye seems to be an important feature that singles out those cases that may respond to such a combined regime.

Figure 20.5. Tension (Muscle Contraction) Headache

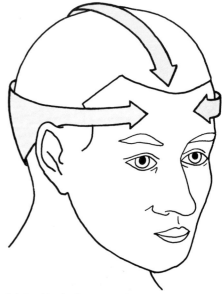

Pain is said to be due to spasm in the scalp and sub-occipital muscles. The muscles are said to be tender and knotted, but this is extremely difficult to evaluate. In general the description of tightness like a "band" or "scalp too tight" is a frequent clue. (This is in contrast to the "bursting feeling" complained of by migraine sufferers.) These patients are usually overtly anxious and respond to minor tranquillisers

Reassurance that the patient does not have a cerebral tumour is usually required in these patients. Often the anxiety has been compounded by a "friend" informing the patient that they knew someone with just that sort of headache who died!

PSYCHOTIC HEADACHES (Figure 20.6)

This is an unfortunate term as the patients are not "psychotic" in the usual sense of the word. Their symptoms are remarkably constant. There is a pain in the head, often localised to a discrete area, often able to be covered by a penny piece and usually indicated with one finger. The sensation described is the feature that has delusional overtones. Expressions such as "I can feel the lump just inside the skull", "there are worms crawling about inside the head" or "the bone is going rotten" are frequently voiced. Reassurance is always greeted by "Well, I know *you* cannot

Figure 20.6. Psychotic Headache

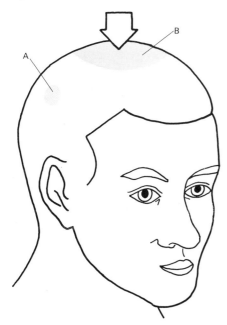

(A) A specific spot on the head is singled out and bizarre complaints such as "bone is going bad" "worms crawling under the skin", are quickly followed by an invitation to feel the increasingly large lump. Usually nothing other than normal bulge in the skull is palpable. No amount of reassurance or investigation helps. Antidepressants may have limited success in reducing the complaints but it is rare for the pain to go away. This condition should always be suspected if the patient offers to locate the headache with one finger

(B) A relentless pressure feeling over the vertex is typical of simple depressive headache

find anything but *I* know there is something there!" Such patients regularly invite the examiner to feel the lump overlying the painful area, and the patient, and often the spouse, will confirm that some evenings a lump as big as a hen's egg appears transiently. These patients willingly undergo repeated contrast studies, if someone willing to do them can be found, and are never reassured by negative tests. Occasionally patients are seen who have had the symptom for thirty years or more, and it would appear that none are ever cured.

PRESSURE HEADACHE

A "typical" pressure headache is one that occurs on waking, is aggravated by bending or coughing, produces a "bursting" sensation in the head and does not respond well to analgesics. Unfortunately all these features may occur in migraine, so that the diagnosis is not a straightforward one. Many patients with such headaches are extensively investigated and no abnormality is found. Headaches that occur only on coughing fulfil some of the criteria, and again the decision to embark on full investigation of this symptom requires careful clinical judgement. Seeing many patients with headache one soon becomes impressed with the fact that very few patients with headache have serious disease. Conversely patients who actually have cerebral tumours often require a direct question to elicit the fact that they have had "muzzy heads" in the mornings for several weeks. It is usually a more dramatic neurological symptom that prompted their seeking medical advice.

One can only draw consolation from the fact that of all patients referred with headache as the sole symptom a very small number indeed have a cerebral tumour. In the last fourteen months only two of over 400 patients in this category, seen by the writer, had cerebral tumours. In an even larger reported series only one of 1,600 consecutive patients had a cerebral tumour. This is not to suggest that vigilance is not required but it is a great relief to patients to know that tumours are *not* the commonest cause of headache!

TEMPORAL ARTERITIS (Figure 20.7)

In some ways the name of this syndrome is an unfortunate one as it gives the impression that the temporal artery is the only vessel involved in this disease. The typical situation is that an elderly patient (invariably over sixty years of age) develops pain and tenderness over an obviously swollen temporal artery on one or both sides. The other superficial

Figure 20.7. Temporal Arteritis

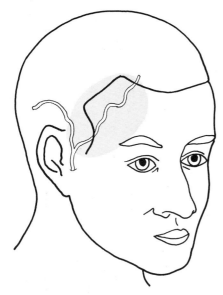

Although swelling, redness and tenderness of the temporal artery, and a headache in the distribution of the artery are the hallmarks of the disease—this is only in a classical case. A diffuse headache can occur. The occipital artery may be involved and an identical picture of tenderness and swelling is produced. The age of the patients, invariably over 60 years old, should help exclude migrainous neuralgia or facial migraine syndromes. General malaise and high ESR are diagnostic

arteries of the head may also be involved, and occipital pain with local tenderness may easily be misdiagnosed as "tension headache". Although the condition is a rare one it is best to assume that all headache starting after the age of sixty years is temporal arteritis until proved otherwise. For practical purposes this can be readily excluded by performing an immediate E.S.R. If this is elevated, immediate admission for biopsy confirmation is necessary in view of the high risk of blindness developing if steroids are not given. In addition to the local headache a generalised dull headache or a deep "burning" headache is often described, and it is only by maintaining a high index of suspicion in elderly patients with headache that the condition may be recognised in some cases. The tendency for the headache to be particularly severe in bed at night and to be associated with anorexia and general malaise are important additional diagnostic clues. Some patients (as many as thirty per cent in some series) also give a history of very severe tearing or burning pains in the limbs, often affecting muscles rather than joints. This condition is called "polymyalgia rheumatica" and may need treatment with steroids.

POST-TRAUMATIC HEADACHES

This condition has been left until last as its features underline many of the problems already discussed. There are three distinct varieties. Patients who have had serious trauma with a fracture or surgical intervention not surprisingly have severe headaches. These are intermittent and severe when they occur, and are relieved to some extent by simple analgesics. There is often local tenderness at the site of injury which may be relieved by local anaesthetic injection.

Patients with less serious trauma, and occasionally quite trivial head injury, may experience chronic headaches. One of these is fairly typically of the tension variety, and may be related to the stresses of the actual events leading to the head injury, or to the possibility of compensation. The other is fairly easily identified as a migraine, and occurs post-traumatically in patients with no prior history of headaches of this variety. These respond to ergot.

Case History

As an example of the complexities of post-traumatic headache, and to reiterate the importance of assessing *the type of headache* before any judgement as to the aetiology is made, the following case is of interest.

CASE REPORT

A 32-year-old American truck driver suffered a serious injury as the result of a well-known hazard of changing the wheels on a 40-ton truck. The wrong bolts were removed and the outer wheel rim flew into the patient's face and chest. This pushed his face back to the extent that the maxillae were under the skull base. His chest was "stove in" as the American surgeons' report so aptly described. Extensive maxillofacial surgery restored his face to some extent and he was seen nine months later with a continual excruciating headache. Not surprisingly the headache was bifrontal, continual and not responding to four-hourly demerol (a synthetic narcotic). The striking part of the history was the dull aching in the backs of the eyes and photophobia. In spite of the obvious severity of the known facial trauma a diagnosis of post traumatic headache of the migrainous variety was made. He had been previously suspected of malingering or tension due to the fact that as the error was his he would not get compensation and he owed several thousand dollars in medical bills. In spite of all these additional factors he was pain-free within twenty-four hours of starting therapy with ergot, and remained so for three months until he was lost to follow-up.

Post traumatic headache and post traumatic syndromes are considered in greater detail in Chapter 23.

In conclusion the history is the most important if not the *only* thing that matters in a patient with a headache. Snap judgements should not be made. A systematic approach which should be identical for every patient should be used if important details are not to be overlooked.

Table 10

QUESTIONNAIRE APPROACH TO HEADACHE DIAGNOSIS

HEADACHE	MIGRAINE		CLUSTER	TENSION	PSYCHOTIC	PRESSURE	TEMPORAL ARTERITIS
	CLASSICAL	ATYPICAL					
Age and sex pattern	Any age both sexes	Females> males, middle age	Almost exclusively males 30–50 years	Any sex Any age	Both sexes Middle age	No specific features	Both sexes Over 60 years
Site	Frontal Unilateral	Fronto-temporal or occipital, often bilateral	Strictly frontal and in eye	Around whole head	Often local painful spot or pressure on vertex	Dull bursting ache of whole head	Superficial, usually unilateral
Nature	Throbbing	Dull ache, stabbing pain in the eye	Severe stabbing pain in eye	Tight band	Heavy weight on top of head	Very low grade ache	Burning quality
Special features	Classically pulsatile	Although bilateral maximal pain behind one eye	Bloodshot eye with lacrimation and rhinorrhoea	Worse under stress	Present continually preventing activity	None	Associated with tenderness over scalp
Diurnal pattern	Often on waking and weekends	Waking or later in day	Almost exclusively nocturnal and like clockwork	Worse towards end of day	Present all the time	Mainly on waking, clear by midday	Usually much worse in the night
Aggravating factors	Often none Alcohol in some	Bright light Noise Tension	Alcohol	Stress Anxiety Fear of tumour	None	Bending Coughing Sneezing	Touching affected area brushing hair
Relieving factors	Rest Dark Room Ergotamine Sleeping	Rest Dark Room Prophylactic drugs	None— attacks last 20 minutes– 2 hours	Tranquillisers, holidays	Anti-depressants	Better if standing	Specific response to steroids
Associated features	Visual phenomena Nausea Vomiting	Dull relentless pain	None	Other features of anxiety	Weight loss Crying Inability to sleep	Vomiting Visual blurring	Weight loss General lassitude General muscle aching

223

Chapter 21

FACE PAIN

In the previous chapter the problem of headache was discussed and special emphasis was given to the importance of the history in the differential diagnosis. This is also the situation when we consider the symptom of pain in the face but unlike headaches, several of the conditions causing facial pain are nearly always "typical" in their historical features. This is particularly true of trigeminal neuralgia. Unfortunately, there are several popular misconceptions about facial pain. Prominent among these is the feeling that any pain that is not identifiable as trigeminal neuralgia is automatically due to the condition called "atypical facial pain". In fact in many ways "atypical facial pain" is just as "typical", historically, as trigeminal neuralgia. This underlines the importance of the history. In the case of headache no anatomically discrete areas of involvement are demanded, and the "headache" is allowed to spread on to the neck or well on to the face without much concern as to the anatomical substrate. In considering face pain an accurate knowledge of the anatomy of the fifth cranial nerve is essential, and this information is provided in Figure 21.1.

A brief discussion of the role of disease of the teeth and the sinuses in the context of face and head pain is necessary. A diseased tooth in the upper jaw can cause headache on the same side, that is not in direct continuity with the pain in the tooth. A diseased tooth in the lower jaw may cause considerable pain in the mandibular division of the nerve including pain felt deep in the ear. In both cases it must be stressed that the pain in the involved tooth dominates the picture—there is no difficulty in recognising that the pain is coming from a tooth. A similar situation exists in respect of sinus disease. Experimental work has shown that the lining of the sinuses is relatively pain insensitive, and that the bulk of the severe pain in sinus disease is due to the congestion of the nasal mucosa and the turbinates. As such involvement produces symptoms of nasal congestion and discharge the diagnosis should be obvious. This means that in the absence of such symptoms the time-honoured search for evidence of chronic sub-clinical sinus infection as the explanation for attacks of pain in the face is unnecessary.

On the premise that there was such a thing as chronic sub-clinical sinus infection causing face pain, various aetiological hypotheses were suggested. The most popular of these held that various autonomic nerves and ganglia were "irri-tated" by such infection and caused pain. Entities such as vidian neuralgia, ciliary neuralgia, spheno-palatine neuralgia, and petrosal neuralgia were described, and a variety of surgical procedures were designed to ablate the offending nerves. All these conditions are now known to be variants of facial migraine and we can add cluster headache and Sluder's lower-half headache to the list. As these conditions are subject to runs of attacks with long remissions the apparent success of surgical treatment is explained. Critical evaluation of these treatment methods has failed to substantiate the claims made for them.

In spite of the recognition of facial migraine and the psychological aetiology of atypical facial pain many patients with chronic facial pain are still subjected to extensive dental work and sinus drainage procedures, showing that these discredited theories of facial pain die hard, and that belief in their existence is not confined to the laity.

The Anatomy of the Fifth Cranial Nerve (Figure 21.1)

The central representation of the fifth cranial nerve is extremely complex and has been described in Chapter 15. The

Figure 21.1. Trigeminal Nerve Supply to Face

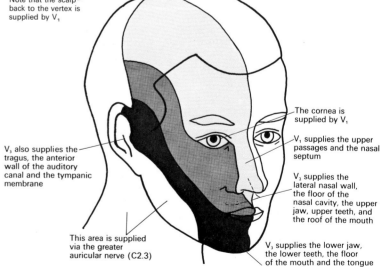

Note that the scalp back to the vertex is supplied by V₁

The cornea is supplied by V₁

V₁ supplies the upper passages and the nasal septum

V₃ also supplies the tragus, the anterior wall of the auditory canal and the tympanic membrane

V₂ supplies the lateral nasal wall, the floor of the nasal cavity, the upper jaw, upper teeth, and the roof of the mouth

This area is supplied via the greater auricular nerve (C2.3)

V₃ supplies the lower jaw, the lower teeth, the floor of the mouth and the tongue (not taste)

exact distribution of the peripheral fifth nerve is of some importance. The important points are as follows:

1. The upper limit of the territory supplied by the nerve is the vertex, and a line drawn from here to the top of the ear on each side indicates the posterior boundary.

2. The lower border of the territory supplied by the fifth nerve is not indicated by the line of the edge of the jaw, but by a line as shown. Notice the large area supplied by the cervical roots, covering the angle of the jaw and the lateral cheek.

3. The boundaries between the three divisions are not horizontal but sweep up towards the temple as shown. The large area of the temple that is supplied by the mandibular division accounts for the spread of toothache from the lower jaw into this area as mentioned in the introduction.

4. The distribution to the mucous membranes of the nasal cavity and the oral cavity is indicated on the diagram. Attention is drawn to the fact that pain inside the nose and in the tongue can and does occur in trigeminal neuralgia. Taste sensation is conveyed from the tongue in the lingual branch of the mandibular division, but the fibres, from the chorda tympani, join the nerve so far peripherally that they are rarely affected in fifth nerve lesions.

5. The second (Maxillary) and third (Mandibular) divisions of the nerve lie in the soft tissues of the nasopharynx as they emerge from the skull base and are particularly likely to be involved by neoplasms arising in this area (see also Chapter 6).

TRIGEMINAL NEURALGIA (TIC DOULOUREUX)

Although great stress is quite rightly placed on the fact that the pain in this condition *never* extends outside the territory of the fifth nerve, it is not sufficiently appreciated that it is unusual for the pain to involve a whole division at any one time, let alone the entire territory of the nerve. It is also worth pointing out at this stage that the first (Ophthalmic) division is involved in *only* five per cent of cases. The practical point that emerges from this is that one of the least likely causes of pain in the eye or forehead is tic douloureux.

The main pain occurs in two zones. These are the mouth-ear zone (affected in about sixty per cent of cases) and the nose-orbit zone (affected in thirty per cent of cases). In the case of pain in the mouth-ear zone (Figure 21.2) the pain spreads from the region of the lower canine tooth back to a position felt deep in the ear (less frequently the pain may go from the ear to the jaw). Quite often the pain also spreads around the hinge, as shown, into the upper jaw, and therefore is along the line of the boundary between the second and third divisions and is not confined to the third division. The second, nose-orbit zone (Figure 21.3), is

Figure 21.2. Mouth-ear zone Trigeminal Neuralgia
This is the distribution of the pain in almost 60 per cent of cases

Figure 21.3. Nose-orbit Trigeminal Neuralgia
This is the distribution in 30 per cent of the cases

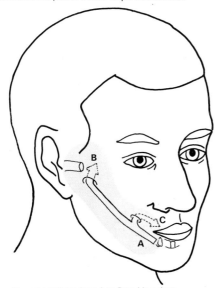

The pain radiates from A to B and is a deep sensation. It may also involve C at the heights of the pain. Less frequently it may shoot from B to A or C
Chewing, smiling, or hot and cold fluids in the mouth are the main triggering factors
The ophthalmic division (V₁) is involved in less than five per cent of cases

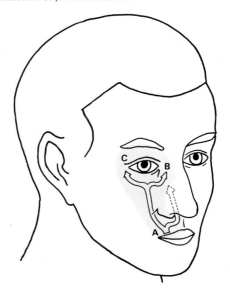

The pain shoots from A (the upper canine) to around the eye to B and or C. The areas B and C may also be 'trigger points'
The main trigger areas for this distribution are touching the alar of the nose, the outer 1/3 of the upper lip, and hot and cold fluids in the mouth

characterised by pain that shoots up from the nostril to the inner and/or outer orbit. The eye itself is not involved in the pain, but may be surrounded by it. Patients often describe this pain as similar to the feeling of a "red hot poker pushed up the nose". It is only from such descriptions that one gets some idea of the agony of this condition. It will be noticed that the pain starts in the second division but spreads into the first division as high as the eyebrow. It very rarely extends above the eyebrow. At the height of the pain the patient may find it difficult to locate the pain accurately, but the initial jabs of pain occur in the zones described above and can usually be accurately localised.

The pain of tic douloureux is also characteristic. It starts as a feeling, like "electricity", "red-hot needles" or "a machine-gun firing red hot bullets" into the affected zone. This builds up into an excruciating pain that is felt *deep* in the face, and is basically confined to the zones described. It only lasts for a few seconds, but is then replaced by a very unpleasant ache or a burning sensation. The pain is not continual although at the height of a bad attack episodes may merge so that the patient is never entirely pain-free. Attacks may vary from one every few minutes to one or two a day. The frequency usually bears some relationship to how easily attacks are "triggered". This is the third feature of the condition.

Attacks affecting the mouth-ear zone are usually triggered by the use of the jaw. Chewing, smiling, yawning, or hot or cold fluids touching the lower canine tooth are frequent provoking factors. They are rarely triggered by cutaneous stimuli. Pain in the nose-orbit zone is typically provoked by the well-known cutaneous trigger points. These are found at the alar of the nostril, the outer third of the upper lip, and at the medial end of the eyebrow. Hot and cold fluids in the mouth are also affective stimuli, as are blowing the nose and attempting to clean the teeth.

At the height of a very severe attack of tic douloureux, the sensitivity may be so great that a draught on the face, eye movement, a stumble or a sudden noise may be sufficient to provoke a burst of pain. Patients in this state are impossible to examine, and the involuntary start as any attempt is made to approach the affected side of the face is almost diagnostic of the condition, as is the distraught, unkempt haggard appearance due to the inability to wash, shave or clean the teeth.

The natural history of the condition is for attacks to occur with increasing frequency, although initially there may be periods of months to years between episodes. This fact governs the therapeutic approach to the condition. A full discussion of therapy is beyond the scope of this text, but one or two points are worth making concerning the use of carbamezepine (Tegretol). Although for long-term use in young patients there are drawbacks, the short-term use of the drug, to relieve the patient of his symptoms as quickly as possible, is indicated in all cases. There is also the added advantage that it will permit a proper examination to be made of the fifth cranial nerve which is impossible at the height of an attack. Once the patient's symptoms are under control one can enter into full discussion as to the best method of management. The writer would recommend a starting dose of 100 mg. only. Many patients, especially the very elderly, are very sensitive to the tendency of the drug to produce vertigo and vomiting. This adds considerably to the patient's misery, especially if the dosage has also been inadequate to relieve the pain. The dose can be increased over a few days to as much as 200 mg. q.d.s. A higher dose than this will invariably cause side-effects, but if it relieves the pain such side-effects as occur may be tolerable. The drug is effective in about eighty per cent of cases. It is worth remembering that before this agent became available Epanutin (Dilantin U.S.P.) was of some value, and the writer has come across several patients in whom Epanutin (Dilantin U.S.P.) was more effective than Tegretol. Symptomatic tic douloureux and its recognition are described in Chapter 6.

ATYPICAL FACIAL PAIN (Figure 21.4)

Referring back to the two psychologically determined types of headache, there are two analogous types of facial pain. These are the conditions known as atypical facial pain and psychotic facial pain.

Atypical facial pain is usually misdiagnosed as dental or sinus disease in the first instance, and many patients are edentulous by the time they are referred for a neurological opinion. The mistake is made because the first symptom is almost invariably pain in one or other maxillary region. The pain is described as deep, burning and continual. There is no jabbing onset of pain as occurs in tic douloureux. In spite of patients' insistence as to the unbearable severity of the pain, their affect is often inappropriate, and the facial appearance is quite unlike that of the patient with tic. The pain usually extends in three directions as shown in the figure. It radiates back behind the ear, down on to the neck or across the opposite maxillary area. All these sites of extension of the pain immediately exclude tic douloureux, and ought to relieve any concern that the pain is on an organic basis as it transgresses the anatomical boundaries of the fifth cranial nerve. Eventually the pain may involve the whole head and neck bilaterally, and one patient even complained that the pain sometimes spread down into the limbs. In general the longer the history the more bizarre the distribution of the pain. As some patients take several years to reach a neuro-

Figure 21.4. Atypical Facial Pain

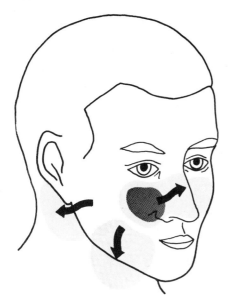

Mainly middle-aged females. Underlying
depressive illness is usually present
The pain usually starts in the upper jaw
Early spread is to the other side and back to
below and behind the ear
Finally spread onto the neck and the entire
half head may occur

Figure 21.5. Facial Migraine Syndromes

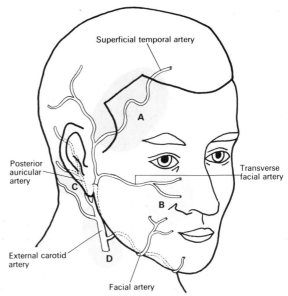

A A situation mimicking temporal arteritis. The
vessel may be visibly oedematous and very
tender
B Sluder's lower-half headache: pain at root
of the nose, usually with nasal obstruction
and deep eye pain
C Mastoid pain: a variation of Sluder's
headache and may co-exist with pain in B
D Carotidynia: tender, throbbing pain in
region of main vessel (see discussions in
text)

logist some very florid symptoms may be present by the time
the patient is seen. At this stage delusional overtones often
appear in the description of the pain, with complaints such
as "the bone is going rotten", or, large transient swellings of
the face are reported. The patients often *clutch* their face,
unlike the patients with tic who shield their face, but are very
careful not actually to touch it.

Psychotic face pain may be an extension of this condition
(just as psychotic headache may supervene in a patient with
tension headache) or it may occur acutely in pure form. In
these cases the pain is confined to a single area (the tongue
is a favourite site) and delusional complaints appear early. In
addition to the usual pain and non-existent swellings or
discolorations of the tongue, an underlying cancerphobia is
often present.

In atypical facial pain, if the case is correctly diagnosed
early, a good response to combinations of tranquillisers and
anti-depressants may be obtained. Once the delusional
overtones appear the chances of significant alleviation of the
symptoms is virtually nil. The same is true of psychotic facial
pain, although in this case no blame for this failure can be
ascribed to a delay in the referral of the patient.

The temptation to advise surgical denervation of the face

in patients suffering from psychotic face pain must be
avoided. Either the pain is unrelieved, or is replaced by the
extremely unpleasant and organic symptom of anaesthesia
dolorosa—a painful numbness of the denervated area.

FACIAL MIGRAINE SYNDROMES (Figure 21.5)

Reference has already been made to the many eponymous
and autonomic neuralgias that are all variants of migraine
affecting the facial vasculature. They include the condition
known as cluster headache discussed in the previous chapter. It will be remembered that nasal congestion and pain deep
in the eye were features of that condition. This is also true of
the facial migraine variants, and patients should be questioned as to the presence of the symptoms of eye pain and
nasal blockage during episodes of facial pain. Sluder's lower
half headache although quite rare is the most typical of these
conditions. The pain is described as a dull bursting pain with
an occasional throbbing component. This occurs either at
the base of the nose or in the region of the mastoid, and
occasionally in both sites simultaneously. Pain deep in
behind the eye is usually present, although nasal congestion
is variable, as indeed it is in cluster headache. The same

condition affecting the temporal artery may be accompanied by visible swelling, and tenderness of the artery. This may be misdiagnosed as temporal arteritis, unless the age of the patient is taken into account. Carotidynia, an episodic throbbing pain in the neck, is probably due to swelling and tenderness of the carotid artery. Slight pressure on the vessel causes pain but firm pressure may completely relieve the symptoms. In all the facial migraine syndromes the important clues are retro-orbital pain of stabbing type or a dull bursting feeling in the mastoid bone. These syndromes occur in both sexes, mainly between the ages of 25 and 45 years. Ergotamine may give some relief, and methysergide maleate is extremely effective in bringing a series of attacks to an end.

POST-HERPETIC NEURALGIA (Figure 21.6)

This rarely presents a diagnostic problem as the causative herpetic lesion is usually obvious. However, at the onset of Herpes Zoster, in the three to five days between the onset of the initial pain and the eruption of the vesicles, there is a considerable diagnostic problem. Ophthalmic herpes occurs

in the elderly and the initial pain in the forehead may mimic temporal arteritis. The E.S.R. is not too helpful as in several cases seen by the author the E.S.R. was elevated, even though the subsequent diagnosis proved to be Herpes Zoster. A daily examination for vesicles seems the correct approach to this problem in the absence of an obviously swollen, tender temporal artery. As the vesicles appear the pain may diminish. If it does not do so it is essential to use the strongest analgesics necessary to control the pain. There is a strong suspicion that inadequate pain relief at this stage predisposes in some way to the subsequent development of the post-herpetic neuralgia syndrome. As the patients are often old and lonely the administration of anti-depressants with the analgesics to prevent a depressive reaction probably has some merit. When the condition develops, as it does in about ten per cent of patients with ophthalmic herpes, the pain alters to a continual dull burning sensation with exacerbations provoked by touching the eyebrow or brushing the hair. It is not the scars that are sensitive, it is the normal skin between them. The scars are anaesthetic. The pain may remit after twelve to eighteen months, but this is by no means certain, and those patients with persistent pain present a

Figure 21.6. Post Herpetic Neuralgia

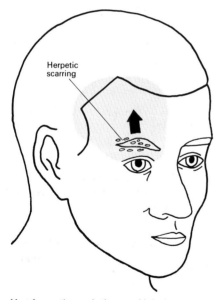

Most frequently seen in the very elderly. It occurs mainly with first division herpes; although the whole zone hurts, the pain in the eyebrow and around the eye is especially severe
The thin papery white scars are anaesthetic. The tender areas are the patches of intact skin between the scars. Pain is continual and burning, with severe pain added by touching the eyebrow or brushing the hair
The condition shows a tendency to spontaneous remission

Figure 21.7. Costen's Syndrome (temporo-mandibular arthritis)

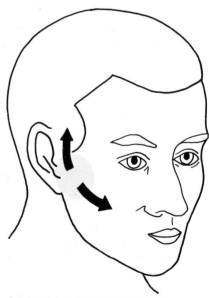

Pain is mainly in the temporo-mandibular joint, spreading forwards onto the face and up into the temporalis muscle
The joint is tender to touch and pain is provoked by chewing or just opening the mouth
The pain ceases almost entirely if the mouth is held shut and still

distressing and formidable therapeutic problem. The suicide risk is high, and in the absence of effective therapy the use of narcotic analgesics may be necessary. Occasionally an excellent response even after years of pain may be obtained by using a combination of Imiprimine 25 mgs. t.d.s. and Phenytoin 100 mgs. t.d.s., even when narcotics have failed.

COSTEN'S SYNDROME (Temporo-mandibular Osteoarthritis) (Figure 21.7)

This condition causes pain in the temporo-mandibular joint which is maximally and often only present when the patient is chewing. The joint itself is usually tender to palpation, although it is possible to mistake this for tenderness of the temporal artery. The pain may radiate forward into the face or upward into the temporalis muscle. The condition can be relieved by prosthetic devices that prevent overclosure of the bite. The problem arises, as with tooth and sinus disease, when it is assumed that disease of the joint can cause pain in the face without the joint itself being painful. Patients with atypical facial pain and the migrainous facial pain syndromes are often suspected of having this condition on this invalid premise.

OTHER CAUSES OF FACIAL PAIN

Although temporal arteritis has already been mentioned several times we must add the situation where the arteries to the muscles of mastication, including the tongue, are involved in the process. In these cases the patient may present with "intermittent claudication" of the masseter muscles, or in the tongue. The age of the patient is always a clue to this condition, and the diagnosis must always be considered in any patient over the age of 60 years who has headache or face pain.

Anginal pain is known to radiate up into the neck and lower jaw, in addition to the more typical radiation down the arms.

Table 11   QUESTIONNAIRE APPROACH TO FACIAL PAIN

TYPE OF PAIN	TRIGEMINAL NEURALGIA	ATYPICAL FACIAL PAIN	MIGRAINE FACE PAIN	POST HERPETIC NEURALGIA	COSTEN'S SYNDROME
Age/sex	Female male 3:1 R>L 5:1; over 50 years old	Females>males aged 30–50 years	Any age males> females	Very elderly females >males over 70 years old	Elderly females
Site	Lower jaw→ears Upper lip→nose Eye. Strictly unilateral	Maxillary area whole face, often other side also	May be anywhere but clue is deep eye pain or a feeling as if the mastoid swollen	Over V1 distribution usually most severe in eyebrow	In or just anterior to temporo-mandibular joint
Nature	Pain like hot needles —for seconds followed by severe pain	Described as continual, unbearable, intolerable	Throbbing pulsatile quality, lacrimation and conjunctival injection may occur	Very severe pain of non-stop type	Severe aching pain in joint radiating forwards
Special features	Unilateral nature of pain Occurs in isolated attacks	Extensive/bilateral Continual nature Interferes with sleep	Very sporadic attacks with clear gaps between	Tender area between the white scars of herpes	Over T.M. joint Only present on eating
Aggravating factors	Hot/cold fluids in mouth. Blowing nose. Chewing, smiling, talking	None, *but* may complain of triggering after many consultations	Alcohol	Touching affected area Cold draughts	Chewing Yawning
Relieving factors	Tegretol (Carbamezepine) Epanutin (Dilantin U.S.P.) (diphenyl-hydantoin) Surgical treatment	Antidepressants	Ergot derivatives Methysergide Maleate (Deseril G.B.) (Sansert U.S.P.)	Epanutin (Dilantin U.S.P.) (diphenyl-dantoin) Antidepressants Narcotics if necessary	Bite correction Surgery

CASE REPORT

A 73-year-old lady was seen with quite severe bilateral pain in both upper and lower jaws, which came on while walking, especially on cold days. Shortly after the onset of this pain a gripping feeling in the chest was noticed. The pain in the jaws was the presenting symptom and the seat of the worst pain. Cardiological advice was sought, and the diagnosis of cardiac pain referred to the jaws was confirmed.

Malignant disease in the skull base, often due to direct extension from a carcinoma of the nasopharynx, tends to involve the fifth nerve. Pain in the second and third division, or a patch of numbness on the face should be regarded as due to nasopharyngeal carcinoma until proved otherwise.

Tumours in the cerebello-pontine angle will invariably damage the root of the fifth nerve. This may produce a picture like tic douloureux but this is decidedly unusual. Careful examination in such a case will usually reveal other signs, such as a depressed corneal response, which are incompatible with the diagnosis of tic. However, tic douloureux does complicate two structural conditions in this area: Paget's disease, and basilar impression (due to senile osteoporosis). Both conditions alter the anatomy of the tip of the petrous bone which may irritate the trigeminal nerve root.

Aneurysmal dilatation of the carotid artery in the cavernous sinus will damage the first division of the fifth nerve causing severe pain in the forehead and eye. This is accompanied by multiple extraocular nerve palsies and a bloodshot eye and the diagnosis is quite obvious. It occurs mainly in hypertensive elderly females (see Chapter 5).

In this chapter, as in the case of headache, with the exception of the E.S.R., the whole diagnosis is based on the history—there are no special investigations that indicate the diagnosis. There is *no* alternative to sitting back and taking an accurate history even if it takes half an hour or more to do so.

Chapter 22

ATTACKS OF ALTERED CONSCIOUSNESS

This deliberately all-embracing title has been used to emphasise the fact that loss of consciousness is not synonymous with epilepsy. From the patient's point of view the diagnosis of epilepsy has far-reaching implications both for employment and social activities and in some instances the inability to drive a motor vehicle may lead to loss of employment. In some countries there are still laws denying an epileptic patient the right to marry and have children, based on Victorian concepts as to the cause and nature of epilepsy. While the protection of the patient and the public implicit in the restrictions placed on an epileptic have to be accepted by an epileptic patient, the tragic consequences of an incorrect diagnosis are obvious. Many patients are on anti-convulsant drugs quite unnecessarily because of misinterpretation of the history or the significance of an E.E.G. Too often the E.E.G. has been allowed to act as a final arbiter in cases of clinical uncertainty, with diagnostic errors in both directions. The diagnosis *must* be firmly based on the history and in this particular instance on any eye-witness accounts that are available. It is worth going to any lengths to get such an account if there is any chance of locating the eye witness to an attack. A long-distance phone call or even a detailed letter answering specific points can often completely alter the diagnosis.

As epilepsy is such an enormous subject coverage will be confined to fairly classical identifiable attacks, and a neurological opinion is suggested for borderline cases rather than an E.E.G. The alternative possibilities will be covered in greater detail than is usual in a textbook of neurology—as the alternatives lie in the field of general medicine and should be diagnosed without recourse to neurological advice.

EPILEPTIC PHENOMENA

Epileptic phenomena fall into three main groups, petit-mal attacks, temporal lobe attacks and grand-mal epilepsy. There are considerable misconceptions about the meanings of these terms and serious therapeutic errors may result from this problem (see drug therapy of epilepsy, Chapter 24). The single most important error is an almost universal belief that "petit-mal" is a literal translation and merely means *any* short-lived attack or any attack in which the patient falls, but does not actually jerk or become incontinent.

Petit Mal

Petit mal describes the single most easily identifiable and constant variant of epilepsy. Attacks usually begin in childhood between five and ten years of age. It is *very* unusual for attacks to start after twenty years of age. Episodes last three to twenty seconds and consist of a brief suspension of awareness. The only motor activity may consist of some fluttering of the eyelids or a jerk of the hands. The facial expression may remain quite normal and the colour does not alter. At the end of the episode there is no confusion and conversation or play will resume as if nothing had happened. The patient is usually unaware that an attack has occurred. If there is awareness it is normally because of the reaction of bystanders, and the child learns to sense that something has happened. An E.E.G. is usually diagnostic as a run of 2–3 c.p.s. spike wave activity during an observed attack confirms the diagnosis. The reverse is *not* true and this is the second serious cause of misdiagnosis. In any epileptic patient the most frequent epileptic event seen on an E.E.G. is a short run of spike-wave activity. This does *not* mean that the patient has petit mal *unless* the E.E.G. technician noted a clinical attack of petit mal *at the same time*. Non-neurologists reading an E.E.G. report frequently make this serious mistake; serious because of the therapeutic problems that follow (see Chapter 24).

Temporal Lobe Attacks

A wide range of epileptic phenomena arise in the temporal lobe. Brief episodes of this type are those most often mistakenly diagnosed as "petit mal". There are many features to distinguish these "minor" temporal lobe attacks.

In a child the differentiation presents some difficulty, but a careful history will usually elicit the following pointers. The child will become pale and distressed. He may complain of abdominal pain, or just run and hold on to his mother's legs in a frightened way, but cannot describe what is happening to him. The episode may last several minutes and is often followed by drowsiness. In older patients an epigastric rising sensation may be followed by pallor, lip-smacking or chewing movements, and more complex "zombie-like" activity. Recurrent irrelevant sentences may be uttered but no formal conversation can be carried on with the patient. Afterwards the patient is usually aware that an attack has occurred as he feels confused, "washed out" or sleepy, but he is amnesic for events that occurred while his consciousness was impaired. Because of the amnesia and the complex motor activity, the patient may come to, to find himself in a different room, or if the attack occurs in the street, several hundred yards from his intended route. Occasionally, what starts as a temporal lobe or "psychomotor" attack ends in a major convulsion.

Major Seizures

Major episodes are those most generally recognised. One of the variants that is difficult to distinguish from a "faint" is the type known as an "akinetic seizure". In these episodes the patient falls suddenly and heavily, often seriously injuring his head or face, and then after a brief period of rigidity, comes round. The absence of prodromal symptoms and the injury are useful pointers to the diagnosis of epilepsy. More classical major attacks with tonic-clonic movements leave little doubt as to their nature, lasting two to five minutes with post-ictal confusion, drowsiness and headache. Fortunately, relatively few attacks occur in the street, as the majority of patients have their attacks in bed on awakening or shortly thereafter. For this reason even neurologists see surprisingly few actual seizures so much so that when a patient has a convenient attack in the clinic one immediately wonders whether it is organic!

Although incontinence of urine and injury are thought to be diagnostic of epilepsy, both can occur in other types of unconsciousness including "simple faints". These symptoms should always be very carefully assessed. Less than half the patients with epilepsy have ever been incontinent in an attack, and relatively few have ever sustained a serious injury.

When a patient is referred to a neurologist with the diagnosis of epilepsy the chance that it indicates that the patient has a cerebral tumour is *not* high. This does not indicate a lack of awareness but merely the appreciation that of all patients with epilepsy less than one per cent have a cerebral tumour. Even in the peak decade for cerebral tumours (45–55 years of age) prospective studies have shown that only ten per cent of this highly selected group— presenting with a first epileptic seizure in this decade— eventually prove to have a cerebral tumour.

In general cerebral tumours can present as epilepsy in all age groups and the writer has seen two children under 15 with gliomas in this category but the order of risk ranges from 0·02 per cent below 15 years of age to ten per cent at 50 years of age. Careful history taking and physical examination is important in selecting tumour suspects. In any age group a focal onset, residual weakness or numbness after an attack or

a focal abnormality on E.E.G. should certainly be taken into consideration. In children, however, focal attacks, focal E.E.G.s and a post-ictal (or Todd's paralysis) occur so often that these findings have minimal significance in this age group. In the adult *any* residual weakness after an attack has very ominous implications and it is perhaps wrong to use the expression "Todd's paralysis" with its benign connotation, in this group. If a focal E.E.G. abnormality is also found, full investigation is indicated. At this stage non-neurologists are usually quite happy if cerebral scanning and angiography reveal no abnormality. The neurologist is not—"once a tumour suspect, always a tumour suspect" is a useful rule. Quite often the patient develops permanent neurological signs some five to fifteen years later and re-investigation then reveals the tumour that has been there throughout. Some would regard this as a serious diagnostic failure, but when one considers the possible consequences of cerebral surgery if a patient can conceal his tumour for fifteen years, it is very much to his advantage! It is surgical accessibility and the potential physical defects resulting from surgery that govern operation in these situations, *not* the mere demonstration of a tumour. There is also a view not based on any published data that uncontrolled epilepsy indicates the presence of a tumour. This is certainly not so and one of the disarming features of epilepsy associated with cerebral tumours is that it is often easy to control. The only exception to this is the tendency for frontal tumours to cause status epilepticus (see Chapter 9).

SYNCOPAL ATTACKS

Syncopal attacks, vasovagal attacks or simple faints are the main differential diagnosis in a patient who has had an attack of unconsciousness, or more colloquially a "black-out". A careful history will readily reveal the diagnosis. The attack is often postural and indeed it is very unusual for a faint to occur in any position other than standing. Hot, stuffy rooms, a hot bath, or severe abdominal pain may all predispose to a sudden drop in blood pressure, Syncopal attacks seem to occur more frequently in young females and often in association with their periods. In Victorian times, "swooning" was an everyday part of female life to judge from contemporary novels. In males at any age "fainting" is almost invariably associated with emotional pressures, such as examinations, pending divorce, etc. In a few cases, when the circumstances are appropriate, a faint may occur almost instantaneously. These situations would include the sight of blood, severe emotional shock, or extreme fear and the circumstances would lead to an automatic presumption that a faint had occurred. In a more typical faint there is quite a long prodromal period described as "feeling faint". This consists of a feeling of hunger, coldness with "goose-pimples", light-headedness, pallor and sweating. A dizzy feeling with noises seeming to become louder and louder is usually the prelude to the loss of consciousness. This often happens when the patient unwisely gets to his feet to "get some fresh air". Almost as soon as the patient falls to the ground he becomes conscious as cerebral blood flow is restored. If he attempts to get up immediately, a further period of unconsciousness may occur. Fainting can only occur in the supine position in a few rare pathological states. These include, diabetic autonomic neuropathy, tabes dorsalis, Shy–Drager syndrome (autonomic neuropathy and parkinsonism), late pregnancy and during severe blood loss. Occasionally cerebral anoxia during a faint may lead to an epileptic seizure, especially if the patient is held in the upright position and not allowed to fall. There is no doubt that with increasing age there is a greater risk of a simple syncopal attack terminating in an epileptic seizure. This is presumably because the brain is less able to tolerate the period of cerebral anoxia that is the cause of loss of consciousness. In this situation it is best to defer diagnosis and the use of anti-convulsants as such attacks usually prove to be isolated episodes. During a faint, even though the prolonged warning usually allows a fairly graceful fall, the patient will sometimes injure himself. Similarly if the patient has a full bladder at the time, incontinence may occur.

An E.E.G. is rarely of help in this situation. Many neurologists, if they are certain that a faint occurred, do not order an E.E.G. This is because some twenty per cent of non-epileptic patients have abnormal E.E.G.s and such a finding may lead to diagnostic confusion. It is best to rely on clinical judgement in this situation and await further developments. Whenever a patient, either a child or adult has a series of syncopal attacks the commonest underlying cause is a stress situation, and this possibility should always be explored.

Specific Types of Syncopal Attack

There are three special varieties of syncopal attack, all likely to occur in elderly males. These are carotid sinus hypersensitivity (also known as vasodepressor syncope), cough syncope and micturition syncope. Carotid sinus hypersensitivity causes abrupt fainting whenever the patient touches the side of the neck. This may occur when he turns his head, wears a tight collar or while shaving. It may easily be mistaken for arterial diseases such as carotid artery thrombosis or vertebral-basilar ischaemic attacks. Cough syncope occurs at the end of a protracted bout of coughing, which is in effect a prolonged Valsava manœuvre, impairing venous return and reducing the cardiac output. Micturition

syncope is an unpleasant and dangerous syndrome. The attacks mainly occur when the patient has had to get up from a warm bed to pass urine. While standing and straining against a hypertrophied prostate gland the patient inadvertently performs the Valsava manœuvre. There is also speculation that the sudden emptying of the bladder has a reflex effect. In any event, syncope is the result, and in a toilet or bathroom this can be disastrous. What started as a faint may end up as a serious head injury, with the additional concern that the patient may have seizured or suffered a cerebral vascular accident. Elderly males with nocturia are well advised to pass urine in a sitting position!

HYPERVENTILATION ATTACKS

These episodes are also called hyperventilation syncope, although it is unusual for the patients actually to lose consciousness. Vision is blurred and may "blackout" but actual loss of consciousness is rare. These episodes are well recognised in the U.S.A. but are very underdiagnosed in Britain. Many anxious patients referred with "dizziness" are suffering from this condition. The patient is usually anxious and in a great many cases a phobic situation exists that provokes episodes. One patient had an attack every time she had to cross the road where her mother had been knocked down and killed.

The condition occurs almost exclusively in females and attacks occurring in supermarkets are such a constant feature that the writer now calls this the "supermarket syndrome". The patient typically develops the episode while queueing at the checkout desk. Many relate either placing everything back on the shelves or just leaving their basket and hurrying from the shop. Many patients suffering from various phobic situations seem to respond well once the mechanism of their "phobic" attacks are explained to them, often after long periods of ineffectual psychotherapy. Although the attacks are determined by anxiety the severity and frightening nature of the physical symptoms should not be underestimated.

The fully developed picture can only develop in a state of anxiety with elevated blood catecholamines. It is impossible to reproduce a full attack merely by hyperventilating. The patient feels hot and stuffy and finds the surroundings oppressive. Friends advise taking deep breaths. This gradually causes a lightheaded feeling, increasing the patient's fear of passing out. As the blood becomes alkalotic the ionised calcium falls producing fine tingling sensations in the limbs and around the mouth. The muscles become weak and the patients nearly always use the expression "my legs turn to jelly". By this stage the chest muscles become tired and ache and a fear that respiration is failing compounds the problem. The patients complain that they feel as if the chest were in a vice and that "deep enough breaths" cannot be taken. By this time the fall in serum CO_2 tension causes cerebral vasospasm leading to further lightheadedness (but *not* vertigo) and flickering of vision, sometimes culminating in everything going black.

The classical tetanic posture of the hands is usually illustrated as a diagnostic feature of the condition. In fact surprisingly few patients develop tetany and typical carpal-pedal spasm is rare. This may be one of the reasons why this diagnosis is so often missed.

In some cases of chronic mild anxiety a steady state is reached in which the patient always feels slightly light-headed and gets "dizzy" whenever his or her anxiety increases. The importance of excluding this group of patients from those with vertigo has been discussed in Chapter 7. If this symptom is coupled with peripheral parasthesiae a misdiagnosis of multiple sclerosis can be easily made. A recent newspaper article described a patient's experiences of multiple sclerosis and his symptoms. Within the next six weeks twelve patients were seen with typical hyper-ventilation syndrome, all had read the article and were convinced they had multiple sclerosis. Considerable re-assurance was necessary before all the patients' symptoms completely subsided.

A very dangerous and well-known schoolboy trick (also known in the Navy as the "mess lark") is to combine forced hyperventilation with a Valsava manœuvre in a squatting position. This leads to loss of consciousness, and oc-casionally the combined metabolic and anoxic insult causes an epileptic seizure.

Furthermore, during E.E.G. recorded one of the best ways of accentuating an abnormality is to ask the patient to hyperventilate for two to three minutes. This will oc-casionally produce an epileptic attack. This may be a pre-disposing factor in some epileptic patients who insist that their attacks are related to stress situations.

DROP ATTACKS

This is another condition that occurs almost exclusively in females. Attacks may occur at any age but mainly in the elderly. The aetiology is not understood and the evidence that it is caused by brain stem vascular disease is far from convincing. Typically the attacks always occur without warning, and almost invariably while the patient is actually walking along. The patient will often liken the sensation to that experienced when someone "chops you behind the knees with the heel of the hand". There is no dizziness or

confusion and no impairment of consciousness. The knees and nose are invariably grazed or bruised, but the patient can get up immediately with no risk of a repeat attack. The feeling is one of considerable embarrassment. The attacks may occur fairly frequently for a few weeks or months and then stop, or may occur as infrequently as once a year for several years. There is no effective treatment. However, reassurance that the attacks appear to be without ominous significance and will eventually clear up is wholly justified by the natural history of this peculiar disorder. Although similar episodes have been described by patients with pineal tumours and intraventricular cysts the writer has yet to see a patient with the condition who proved to have an underlying cerebral lesion.

CEREBRAL VASCULAR DISEASE

Although little "strokes" are popularly supposed to cause brief episodes of unconsciousness in the elderly the evid-ence for this is sparse. In fact, other than in massive cerebral haemorrhage or cerebral embolism, loss of consciousness during a cerebral vascular accident is unusual. Therefore, it seems unlikely that a "little stroke" without observable sequalae would be capable of causing unconsciousness. The majority of patients who have had a stroke and are not rendered dysphasic are able to describe in great detail the sequence of events that occurred. Therefore one must always be alert to the other causes of loss of consciousness in the elderly and avoid the "ragbag" diagnosis of a "small stroke".

TRANSIENT GLOBAL AMNESIA

This is another rare and intriguing condition that occurs in the middle-aged of either sex. It consists of episodes of total amnesia lasting minutes to many hours during which time the patient may appear to behave perfectly normally.

CASE REPORT

One patient seen by the author, a 56-year-old male, completed spraying his car a different colour during the attack. The next day he could not recognise his car because of the colour change.

CASE REPORT

A physician's wife, aged 52, met her husband at the door, prepared his evening meal and spent a normal evening with him. The next morning she had no recollection of events beyond going to open the front door. The husband noticed no abnormality in her be-haviour during the entire period. She was severely hypertensive.

The majority of patients reported have had no detectable disease process. Bilateral ischaemia of the temporal lobes has been suggested as an explanation, and two patients have been reported who came to autopsy in whom evidence of bilateral medial temporal lobe infarction was found. Some of the early reported cases developed the syndrome while seabathing, but many other attacks have occurred under normal circumstances. The majority of patients reported have had only one attack.

An important differential diagnosis of this condition is a temporal lobe epileptic attack. As noted earlier, patients may continue semi-purposeful activity during an epileptic attack. One patient seen by the author collected her children from school by car with no recollection of events over a two-hour period. Subsequent attacks and investigation left no doubt that this was a prolonged temporal lobe attack.

MIGRAINE AND LOSS OF CONSCIOUSNESS

There is considerable and renewed interest in the occurrence of attacks of altered consciousness occurring in association with migraine. There are three varieties: a pathological drowsy state resembling narcolepsy, prolonged syncopal episodes possibly due to spasm of the basilar artery with brain stem ischaemia, and epilepsy. Although migraine and epilepsy are common conditions, some series show a ten per cent incidence of epilepsy in migraine sufferers as opposed to 0·8 per cent in the general population. One certainly sees many patients with migraine who have fainted at the height of an attack without there being any suspicion that this was an epileptic attack. The possibility of epilepsy occurring in association with migraine should always be considered in those patients who have both headaches and attacks of loss of consciousness. Occasional epileptic patients are seen who have only ever had a fit at the height of a migraine attack.

MÉNIÈRE'S DISEASE AND LOSS OF CONSCIOUSNESS

In the original description of the syndrome that bears his name, Ménière included "a fainting state" as part of a typical attack. Certainly the tendency to fall during the severe vertigo is understandable, but some patients do appear to lose consciousness during the attack. Differentiation from a temporal lobe epileptic attack preceded by a vertigo (a rare but well-recognised variant) or migraine affecting the basilar artery, with vertigo and unconsciousness, must be made. The typical auditory phenomena of Ménière's Disease are an important clue to the diagnosis (see Chapter 6).

NARCOLEPSY AND CATAPLEXY

Both these conditions are related and are rare disorders. They are sometimes associated with two other symptoms, sleep paralysis and hypnagogic hallucinations in the full-blown syndrome of narcolepsy. Narcolepsy is most often seen as an isolated event. The patient is overcome by an irresistible desire to go to sleep, and does so. This may even happen while driving a car. It may occur at any time but is exaggerated in circumstances that induce a drowsy state in normal persons such as a stuffy room, a boring lecture, or a heavy meal. In fact the condition appears to be an exaggeration of normal rather than a disease state. Cataplexy can occur alone or in association with narcolepsy. Sudden noise, laughter or a shock may result in the patient going limp and falling to the floor without loss of consciousness. Sleep paralysis, which can also happen to normal people, consists of awakening and being quite unable to move. Although this lasts only seconds it may seem like an eternity at the time. Hypnagogic hallucinations are very vivid frightening dreams occurring when the patient is not sure if he is awake or still asleep. These may happen several times a week and are extremely disturbing to the patient, but this part of the history is often concealed unless a specific enquiry is made about "dreaming".

CARDIAC DISEASE

If the heart beat ceases for longer than a few seconds, consciousness is lost. The most frequent cause is a Stokes-Adams attack occurring in patients who have complete heart block. The slowly beating denervated ventricle may stop beating for five to thirty seconds leading to an abrupt loss of consciousness, without warning, the patient often being unaware that anything has happened.

CASE REPORT

A middle-aged extremely obese man was admitted following a fall from a ladder; he had no idea why he had fallen. While the history was being taken he had six Stokes-Adams attacks, at the end of each apologising for "dropping off". He had complete heart block caused by a recent silent myocardial infarction.

In these attacks the patient becomes abruptly unconscious and extremely pale. As the attack continues there is rapidly increasing cyanosis until the heart starts beating again when the patient suddenly flushes and abruptly regains consciousness.

Patients with valvular disease, especially aortic stenosis, are prone to have syncopal attacks. Paroxysmal arrhythmias are responsible in some cases and careful cardiac evaluation is indicated in all cases of syncope, even in those cases that at first sight would appear to be straightforward vasovagal episodes.

HYPOGLYCAEMIA

Although special charts distinguishing between diabetic and hypoglycaemic coma are included in many texts the differentiation is usually easy. The patient going into diabetic coma becomes progressively obtunded over a period of hours, whereas hypoglycaemia can be truly "syncopal" in onset. The cause is usually excess insulin or an inadequate diet in a known diabetic. Primary hypoglycaemia is extremely rare, although frequently suspected. In the patient who is becoming hypoglycaemic the prodomal symptoms are very similar to the prodrome of a syncopal attack. (In both cases these symptoms are produced by adrenaline release in response to falling blood pressure and falling blood sugar respectively.) However, in the premonitory phase of hypoglycaemia there is often a personality alteration with aggression as a common feature which may be homicidal in degree. Increasing pallor and sweating and finally yawning are the physical clues to the diagnosis. In fact, any pathologically drowsy patient who yawns continually should be quickly checked for hypoglycaemia. Once consciousness is lost, there is a real risk of the patient having an epileptic fit. Immediate intravenous injection of glucose is indicated. There is a considerable risk of brain damage and every minute counts. In spite of adequate replacement if the coma has been prolonged and particularly if a fit has occurred, the patient may take several hours to regain consciousness. If the diagnosis is suspected and there is likely to be delay in getting the patient to hospital, it is essential to give intravenous glucose or glucagon even though pathological confirmation may be prevented. The considerable danger of prolonged hypoglycaemia cannot be over-emphasised.

CASE REPORT

A girl of 22 was referred because of frequent syncopal attacks and had been admitted in coma to several hospitals over four years. She had gradually developed a spastic dysarthria and a spastic tetraparesis. Her blood sugar during an attack was 8 mgm per cent. She was subsequently shown to have an islet cell tumour. Her blood sugar had not been estimated on any of her previous admissions.

In any unconscious patient the blood sugar and serum drug levels should be estimated immediately however obvious the clinical diagnosis may seem to be.

CASE REPORT

A 30-year-old Civil Servant collapsed by a post-box. When the ambulance arrived he was dead. He was rescusitated in the ambulance and extensive investigations were performed to try to determine the cause of his collapse. Three days later the suicide note that he had posted to his brother, just as he died, arrived. At no stage had the possibility of a drug overdose been considered. Unfortunately, in spite of intensive care the patient subsequently died from irreversible brain damage.

One of the most frequent reasons for referring a patient to the neurological clinic is for the investigation of an attack of altered consciousness. Almost invariably there are no physical signs between the episodes and the E.E.G. does not always give diagnostic information. The diagnosis depends on the history and the eyewitness account. Too often the patient attends without the eyewitness. The referring doctor could make a very helpful contribution if whenever he referred such a patient, he could advise him to find, question and if possible bring the eyewitness to the clinic with him.

Table 12   DIFFERENTIAL DIAGNOSIS OF EPILEPTIC VARIANTS

	PETIT MAL	TEMPORAL LOBE EPILEPSY	GRAND MAL	AKINETIC GRAND MAL
Age	5–15 years	Any age	Any age	Any age
Onset	Instantaneous	Prolonged prodrome	Very brief warning, if any	None at all
Duration	5–20 seconds	5 seconds to hours or days	2–5 minutes	1–2 minutes
Type of attack	Brief suspension of awareness	Prolonged altered behaviour may culminate in major attack	Period of rigidity with cyanosis (the tonic phase) then generalised jerking (the clonic phase) and then sleep	Unheralded sudden fall. Very brief attack—little or no jerking but injury risk high
Facial features	Eyelids may flutter—"day-dreaming"	Pallor, anxious bewildered expression—lip smacking or chewing movements	Unconsciousness—eyes may roll upwards or to the sides	No particular features
Limbs	Slight jerking movements of arms—this is unusual	Rather ponderous "Zombie like" activity or fiddling with clothing	Generalised jerking—(look for *focal* jerking at onset)	Initially rigid then quite still
End of attack	Abrupt—no confusion	Confused and amnesic	Confused, drowsy, headache	Often severe headache
Continence	Very rarely incontinent	Rarely incontinent	Occasionally incontinent	Occasionally incontinent
E.E.G.	Invariably abnormal and diagnostic	Often normal—sphenoidal recording may increase value	Normal in 40 per cent patients	Often normal

Table 13   DIFFERENTIAL DIAGNOSIS OF NON-EPILEPTIC ATTACKS

	VASOVAGAL	HYPERVENTILATION	DROP ATTACKS	STOKES-ADAMS ATTACKS	HYPOGLYCAEMIA
Age/sex	Young males/females	Females>males	Elderly females	Any age or sex	Any age or sex
Prodromal symptoms	Feeling "faint", hot, stuffy, "swimmy", sweaty, vision blurred, noises distant	Prolonged "dizziness", tingling, paraesthesiae in limbs and around mouth, legs feel like "jelly"	None—typically very sudden	None	Personality change confusion, aggressive hunger, sweating, yawning
Consciousness	Briefly unconscious	Rarely unconscious	Conscious throughout	Unconscious	Unconscious
Duration of attack	Seconds	Prolonged symptoms often hours *but* rarely unconscious	Seconds only	Up to thirty seconds or fatal arrest	Minutes to hours if diagnosis not established
Colour change	Very pale	Pale	Normal	Pale initially. Cyanosed during attack. Flushed on recovery	Pale and sweating
Recovery	Abrupt but often sick	Slow, ? from exhaustion	Abrupt and complete	Abrupt and complete	Slow and confused
Precipitating features	Anxiety, pain especially visceral pain. Blood loss. Heat	Anxiety and phobic states	Unknown—almost invariably occur while walking along	Complete heart block with ventricular standstill	Excess insulin dose Hypoglycaemic drugs Islet cell tumour Retroperitoneal sarcoma
Risk of seizure	Small, but occasionally does lead to a fit, especially in the elderly	Slight risk if patient is epileptic	No risk	High risk due to cerebral anoxia	High risk and often prolonged recovery phase
Special types	Micturition Syncope Cough Syncope Carotid sinus hypersensitivity	"Supermarket" syndrome			

Chapter 23

TRAUMA AND THE NERVOUS SYSTEM

HEAD INJURIES AND THEIR COMPLICATIONS

Accidents accompanied by head injuries are an increasingly significant cause of death and morbidity in children and young adults. The complications and sequelae of head injuries present many problems of management, some of which may require lifelong medical supervision.

As many of the accidents occur while the patient is on holiday, indulging in dangerous pastimes, or in road traffic accidents, the primary evaluation of the situation may become the responsibility of a doctor who has no special experience in the management of head injuries. The need to get the patient to specialist care may result in the continued observation of the patient being performed by a series of doctors. This makes for poor continuity of assessment, which is so vital for early detection of impending disaster in head injury management. Finally, the patient may return home to his general practitioner's care many hundreds of miles away. Subsequently, if an event such as an epileptic seizure occurs the full significance or importance of this is hard to assess unless a full report of the original injury is available. If the injury occurred abroad it may prove impossible to obtain such details.

In this chapter we will discuss head injuries in the child and adult separately as there are important differences in the clinical features and the outcome. In all age groups the single most important factor in the management of a head injury is the maintenance of an adequate airway and the prevention of hypoxia. Even slight hypoxia greatly increases the risk of cerebral swelling and may lead to unnecessary neurosurgical intervention.

Careful monitoring of fluid intake and salt metabolism are essential. Hypernatraemia, and less commonly hyponatraemia, may cause metabolic problems aggravating cerebral oedema. In patients with extensive injuries elsewhere, particularly long bone fractures, any cerebral deterioration may indicate fat embolism. Fat released into the blood from the fracture may block both pulmonary and cerebral vessels causing hypoxia or direct cerebral damage. In the conscious patient confusion, incontinence of urine, and occasionally petechiae over the conjunctivae or skin of the upper chest are important diagnostic clues. The syndrome usually occurs within three days of the injury and is of dramatic suddenness. The only useful treatment is prevention of hypoxia using hyperbaric oxygen if available. If the patient becomes comatose there is an eighty per cent death rate, if the patient only becomes confused the death rate is fifteen per cent.

HEAD INJURIES IN CHILDHOOD

Head injuries account for some fifteen per cent of childhood admissions to surgical wards. There are two important features of head injury in childhood.

1. Children may initially appear to be more ill than an adult. Even quite minor trauma may cause drowsiness, confusion and vomiting without there necessarily being serious implications. The rules for observation still apply.

2. The potential for recovery from serious craniocerebral injury is very much greater in the child than in the adult.

In addition to the usual causes of head injury at any age there are certain special risks to children. Falls from balconies of high rise flats, injuries from swings and roundabouts, and increasingly recognised the trauma inflicted on the child by the parents. Another form of potentially lethal injury that may be overlooked is the penetrating type of lesion around the orbit, from knitting needles, sharp sticks or pencils. A small skin laceration or perhaps a wood splinter may mark the entrance of a track leading through the skull and dura into the brain. This type of injury often occurs without loss of consciousness, and it is not until meningitis or brain abscess occurs a few days later that the seriousness of the original injury is apparent.

Following head trauma children develop cerebral swelling very easily, rapidly leading to confusion and drowsiness. This must be carefully distinguished from an intracranial collection of blood and appropriate contrast studies may be indicated, if there is any suspicion of a developing focal abnormality.

Epileptic seizures occur very easily in the child and a fit may occur within minutes of any injury severe enough to produce loss of consciousness. In this situation there is a double danger. Either the head injury will be thought to be more severe than it really is, the post-ictal state being mistaken for cerebral swelling, or, the whole situation may be thought to be a fit and its sequelae, and the developing complications of the unrecognised head injury missed. The child who is apparently "sleeping it off" may be going into coma.

The apparent severity of the injury (judged from the height of fall, etc.) does not bear a reliable relationship to the risk of complications. The elastic skull of the child is less easily fractured than that of the adult, and basal fractures occur much less frequently in the child. But, even a mild knock without loss of consciousness may cause a skull fracture and a fatal extradural haematoma, whereas the same injury in another child may cause alarm because of drowsiness and vomiting but be followed by full recovery in a few days. The admission and observation rules are as in the adult.

All children who have lost consciousness must be admitted. A skull fracture (x-rays should always be performed following any injury that appears to be of any severity), or the possibility of a puncture type of injury both require admission whether or not the child has been unconscious. Other serious injuries to the cervical spine, thorax or abdominal contents should also be excluded. It is very important to remember that even in childhood head injuries *rarely* cause surgical shock. The presence of a fast pulse, falling blood pressure and rapid respiration indicate the presence of a lesion elsewhere and rupture of the liver, spleen or kidney should be excluded. The only exception to this rule is when massive blood loss has occurred from serious scalp lacerations. The child whose clinical condition is worsening due to the head injury will have a slowing pulse, a rising blood pressure and slow respiration.

In any case of head injury it is essential that the first doctor to see the child establishes the conscious level. This can include the ability to answer questions but the age and emotional state of the child may render this criterion invalid. The alertness of the child, the response to voice, the response to pain, unresponsiveness to either stimulus or the level of unconsciousness (lash reflexes, corneal response) should be clearly recorded. The terms "stuporose", "semicomatose", "obtunded" or "unconscious" mean different things to different people and are unreliable if several other doctors are subsequently going to be evaluating the patient. As alteration in the responsiveness of the child is the most important sign of an impending emergency, the importance of clear notes on this aspect cannot be overemphasised. If the child is drowsy he should be awakened every fifteen minutes or so to establish that he is not becoming comatose. Some children go though a period of confusion and irritability just before becoming unconscious, and this should be regarded as an ominous sign even if the child appears to be more active than previously.

The size, symmetry and reactivity of the pupils and the ability of the child to move all his limbs are the next most important set of objective signs. Although a slowing pulse, a rising blood pressure and periodic respiration are the classical signs of rising intracranial pressure they indicate a very serious pre-terminal stage rather than a remediable situation. Increasing drowsiness, or relapse into unconsciousness, a dilating pupil on one side or a developing hemiparesis all require immediate action. (Pathophysiological details discussed later.) If the child had regained consciousness before the deterioration the most likely cause of the condition is an acute extradural haematoma (Figure 23.1). If x-rays reveal a fracture line across the temporal fossa the diagnosis is almost certain. Early recognition and treatment should allow a full uncomplicated recovery. If the child has failed to recover consciousness and then developed these signs the situation is not quite so hopeful. He may well have a serious laceration of the brain with an acute subdural haematoma. The serious underlying brain damage in these cases makes the outcome, even following successful evacuation of the clot, much less certain.

Assuming no complications have occurred, following any injury with a prolonged period of unconsciousness the child will go through a period of confusion. The presence of the parents at this time will hasten full recovery. Strange faces in a strange building will tend to worsen the confusion and make this period more distressing for the child.

Later Sequelae

1. *Chronic Subdural Haematoma* (Figure 23.2)

Just as in the adult, chronic subdural haematoma may occur in the weeks following head injury. Any deterioration of school performance, headaches, drowsiness, unsteadiness of gait, double vision or vomiting should raise suspicion. In the infant, vomiting is a notable early sign and tense fontanelles are usually found. In the older child the symptoms are more subtle, especially as children do not seem to notice or complain of headache in the way that adults do. In these cases, although there are no fontanelles to bulge, the head can expand and either the skull sutures separate or a bulge may appear on the skull, usually in the temporal fossa overlying the haematoma.

CASE REPORT

A boy, 12 years of age, fell twelve feet on to concrete. He did not recall losing consciousness but remembers striking his head. He did not tell his parents. Several weeks later he complained of failing vision and some mild headache. He denied drowsiness and there had been no decline in his schoolwork. On examination there was a bulge in the skull above the left ear, severe bilateral papilloedema

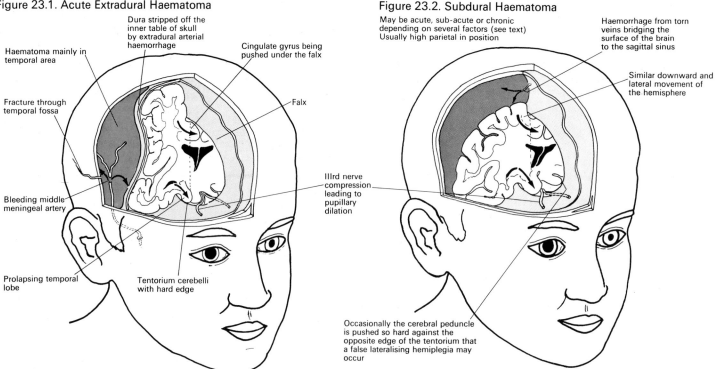

Figure 23.1. Acute Extradural Haematoma

Dura stripped off the inner table of skull by extradural arterial haemorrhage

Cingulate gyrus being pushed under the falx

Haematoma mainly in temporal area

Fracture through temporal fossa

Falx

Bleeding middle meningeal artery

Prolapsing temporal lobe

Tentorium cerebelli with hard edge

Figure 23.2. Subdural Haematoma

May be acute, sub-acute or chronic depending on several factors (see text) Usually high parietal in position

Haemorrhage from torn veins bridging the surface of the brain to the sagittal sinus

Similar downward and lateral movement of the hemisphere

IIIrd nerve compression leading to pupillary dilation

Occasionally the cerebral peduncle is pushed so hard against the opposite edge of the tentorium that a false lateralising hemiplegia may occur

and increased reflexes on the right side. He had a very large subdural haematoma in the left temporal fossa.

2. *Post-Traumatic Epilepsy*

Although seizures occurring immediately following trauma are more common in the child, the ultimate risk of post-traumatic epilepsy is no greater than in the adult and indeed appears to be rather less in some reported series. Immediate seizures may imply an increased risk of further seizures, but in many cases early fits are of no long-term significance. In general the longer after the injury the first attack occurs the more likely it is that the child *will* have further attacks. The first attack will usually occur within the first eighteen months after the injury. The risk of seizures occurring even if none occur during the acute phase of the injury, is greatly increased if there has been a depressed fracture, a haematoma requiring evacuation (especially an acute subdural haematoma), or infection following a penetrating injury. There is probably a case for putting children in these categories on prophylactic anticonvulsants for the first two years after the injury.

3. *Post-Concussional Syndrome and Behaviour Disturbances*

The well-known post-concussional syndrome of adults is fortunately not a feature of childhood head injuries. How-

ever, there is some similarity, in that children who suffer from behavioural problems following a head injury usually do so after a relatively mild injury. Furthermore, careful evaluation often reveals that their pre-morbid behaviour was poor. Very often the incident that led to the head injury occurred under circumstances that raise suspicion of the child's "normal" behaviour. Usually the home circumstances are unsatisfactory and the difficulties presented by the treatment of such a child are formidable. At the other end of the scale are over-protective parents and teachers who create a difficult situation for the child by prolonging the period away from school, making special concessions and preventing the child from resuming normal activities, especially games. As the latter provide the only light relief in a week at school this restriction is rarely appreciated by the child. It is essential to allow the child to resume normal activities as soon as possible. Even if the head injury has been a serious one, the potential for recovery is very high and will not be fully realised if the child is unnecessarily restricted.

HEAD INJURIES IN THE ADULT

As the majority of adult head injuries occur in road traffic accidents or industrial accidents it is essential that very complete and accurate medical records are kept for medico-legal purposes. If the patient is conscious the first examination should include evaluation of the sense of smell, the visual acuity and fields (to confrontation) and the hearing. Loss of one or other of these senses occurs sufficiently frequently to make immediate evaluation worth while. So often the initial notes do not include specific statements to the fact that these functions were tested and found to be normal. If a patient has been drinking, it is very dangerous to assume that drowsiness, confusion or ataxia are purely due to alcohol.

CASE REPORT

A man, 38 years of age, who was a known epileptic went drinking every Friday evening. He usually became mildly drunk and this often brought on an epileptic seizure. One evening, as he returned home with his brother, he had a fit on the stairs and fell some eight feet back into the hall. His brother, following his usual practice, put him into bed to sleep it off. He became alarmed when he could not rouse him the following morning. The patient's pupils were widely dilated, asymmetrical and fixed to light. Both legs were spastic with bilateral Babinski responses. There was a palpable fracture across the vertex. He was not post-ictal or post-alcoholic but had large bilateral extradural haematomas.

It is also very important to remember that because of impaired clotting mechanisms, the heavy drinker has a greatly increased risk of developing subacute or chronic subdural haematomas following head trauma.

The evaluation of an adult who has suffered a head injury is identical to that of the child. As more serious trauma is usually involved, the exclusion of co-existent injuries to the cervical spine, thorax and the abdominal contents is exceptionally important. As in the child, the presence of surgical shock can rarely be ascribed to a head injury alone unless massive scalp bleeding has occurred.

A great deal of emphasis is usually given to the presence of retrograde amnesia in assessing the severity of the injury (if the patient has recovered consciousness). If the patient is befuddled by alcohol or has had a fit prior to the injury clearly his judgement and memory prior to the event will be poor. Furthermore, it is not widely appreciated that even following severe head injury it is exceptional for the retrograde amnesia to have a duration of more than a few seconds or a few minutes. If a patient claims very prolonged retrograde amnesia it is likely to be non-organic. The duration of post-traumatic amnesia gives a better guide to the severity of the injury. There is complete amnesia for the period of unconsciousness, then relative amnesia during the confusional stage after recovery. Post-traumatic amnesia ends when the patient establishes continual memory. The duration of this period, which may run into several weeks, gives some indication of the severity of the injury.

If the patient has recovered consciousness by the time he reaches hospital he may be fully alert or confused, restless and extremely irritable. This latter condition may be caused by alcohol, the post-ictal state, painful injuries elsewhere or a full bladder. Handling patients in this stage can be extremely trying for everyone but pressure to sedate the patient must be resisted. No drugs should be given that will alter the conscious level or alter the pupillary reactions. In the latter respect it is essential that mydriatic drops are not used to facilitate a search for papilloedema. Not only is it extremely unlikely that the patient will have papilloedema but the use of drops will prevent the recognition of the pupillary dilatation that indicates a developing tentorial pressure cone and will occasionally lead to unnecessary surgical action if the use of drops has not been recorded in the notes. In Figures 23.1 and 23.2 the right pupil is shown dilated. In both instances a unilateral clot is pushing the hemisphere across to the other side and then downwards. As the medial part of the temporal lobe slips down between the brain stem and the edge of the tentorium cerebelli it will distort the third nerve. This leads to pupillary dilation on the *same* side as the clot in the majority of cases.

At the same time the brain stem is pushed across to the other side and comes up against the hard edge of the tentorium cerebelli. This tends to damage the cerebral peduncle which leads to a hemiparesis on the wrong side, i.e. on the *same* side as the clot. If the patient is dying and there are no facilities for angiography a burr hole is most likely to encounter the clot on the side of the dilated pupil. This re-emphasises the unique importance of the pupil reactions in the observation of a patient with a head injury.

Of less immediate importance, but very important to the future management of the patient, is the inspection of the ear drum for evidence of a tear of the drum, leakage of blood and/or C.S.F., or blood behind the intact drum. C.S.F. leaking from the nose is less easy to demonstrate if the nose is bleeding. The finding of a sub-conjunctival haemorrhage in either eye that extends back behind the visible limit of the conjunctiva is also important, as is bruising over the mastoid which may take several days to appear. All these signs indicate the presence of fractures involving the base of the skull. Radiological evidence of such fractures may be difficult to obtain but particular attention should be paid to the skull films looking for (a) fluid levels in the sinuses, particularly the ethmoid and sphenoid sinuses, or (b) air inside the skull. Either finding indicates a basal fracture with a dural tear. The greatest risk in this situation is that of infection entering the head through the fracture line via the sinuses or the middle ear.

Epileptic fits may occur in the first few hours following

Figure 23.3. Longitudinal fractures of the Petrous Temporal Bone
(Right half of skull base seen from behind)

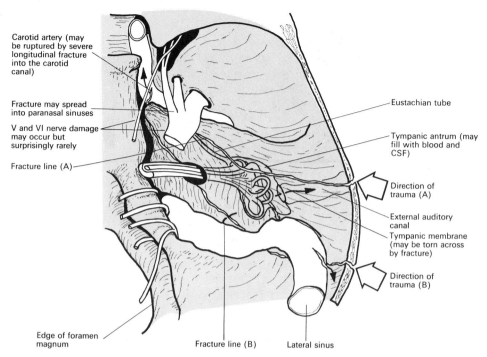

Carotid artery (may be ruptured by severe longitudinal fracture into the carotid canal)

Fracture may spread into paranasal sinuses

V and VI nerve damage may occur but surprisingly rarely

Fracture line (A)

Eustachian tube

Tympanic antrum (may fill with blood and CSF)

Direction of trauma (A)

External auditory canal

Tympanic membrane (may be torn across by fracture)

Direction of trauma (B)

Edge of foramen magnum

Fracture line (B)

Lateral sinus

head injury. This need not necessarily indicate that the patient will suffer from post-traumatic epilepsy (see later).

In the first forty-eight hours following injury the main risk to the patient is the development of an acute extradural haematoma. This risk is virtually confined to those patients with a demonstrable fracture of the temporal bone crossing the middle meningeal artery. A fracture across the vertex may tear the superior sagittal sinus, and the haemorrhage can strip up the dura and lead to an acute extradural haematoma over the vertex. In either instance the diagnosis is not difficult if the patient recovers consciousness and then becomes drowsy again, the so-called "lucid" interval. Problems arise when the patient does *not* recover consciousness and goes steadily downhill. This may be caused by serious brain laceration and oedema, but exploratory burr holes should be made in such a situation.

A special group of complications and problems are based on the fractures of the skull base that traverse the petrous temporal bone. These fractures complicate some thirty per cent of all head injuries. Even in patients without a demonstrable fracture of the bone, damage to the contained structures may occur. The organ or Corti may be affected by blunt trauma to the petrous temporal bone, causing a transient perceptive deafness. The vestibular apparatus is less easily damaged, but many cases of the condition known as benign positional vertigo appear to be related to mild head

trauma. This causes transient giddiness whenever the position of the head is altered, especially as the head is put back on to a pillow. This symptom may persist up to eighteen months after the injury but eventually subsides.

Fractures of the petrous temporal bone occur in two directions. Blows from the temporoparietal or frontotemporal direction, tend to cause longitudinal fractures which may extend across the midline into the opposite middle cranial fossa, occasionally causing fatal laceration of the carotid artery (Figure 23.3). These fractures often tear the tympanic membrane and dislocate the auditory ossicles. Although the fracture line extends to the petrous tip it is very unusual for the fifth or sixth nerve to be clinically involved. However, in some twenty per cent of patients with this type of fracture a seventh nerve palsy appears. Even without therapy of any sort seventy-five to ninety per cent of these will recover fully. Recently, evidence has been presented that the use of ACTH improves the prognosis further. If the onset is delayed until a few days after the injury, the prognosis is excellent in any event. The acute damage to the ossicles and the blood and C.S.F. in the middle ear cavity causes conductive deafness that should improve. The degree of perceptive loss caused by concussion of the organ of Corti will be apparent later.

Blows to the posterior pole of the head tend to lead to fractures that traverse the occipital bone, continue across the foramen magnum and then extend up transversely across the

Figure 23.4. Transverse fractures of the Petrous Temporal Bone

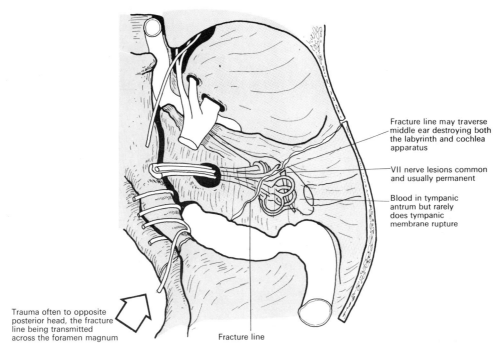

Fracture line may traverse middle ear destroying both the labyrinth and cochlea apparatus

VII nerve lesions common and usually permanent

Blood in tympanic antrum but rarely does tympanic membrane rupture

Trauma often to opposite posterior head, the fracture line being transmitted across the foramen magnum

Fracture line

petrous temporal bone (Figure 23.4). The fracture usually destroys both the cochlea and the vestibular apparatus. Occasionally one or other of these functions is spared. The severe vertigo produced by this injury disappears over a period of three to twelve weeks. The facial nerve is also frequently damaged by these fractures and with this type of fracture the nerve rarely recovers. The ear drum is usually intact. Occasionally lower cranial nerve palsies occur due to damage to the jugular foramen. This is relatively unusual as such fractures are almost invariably fatal.

The long-term implications of fractures that traverse the skull base is that whatever the immediate problems, i.e. loss of sense of smell, deafness or vertigo, the main risk to the patient is meningitis. In the days before antibiotics seven per cent of patients died of meningitis. The risk continues over many years and is a recurrent one. If the dural tear can be identified surgical closure is indicated.

Late Sequelae

1. Chronic Subdural Haematoma

This subject is dealt with first, *not* because it *is* the most frequent complication, but because it is the most frequently *suspected* complication of head injury. Subdural haematomas may be acute, subacute or chronic. Acute subdural haematomas occur over an area of lacerated brain and are

associated with a very bad prognosis for both serious residual disability or survival. Subacute subdural haematomas occur within a few weeks of the original injury and usually follow a fairly typical progression of symptoms. These include headaches, increasing drowsiness, confusion and finally the signs of tentorial herniation. Usually the history of recent trauma and the clinical course make the diagnosis obvious even if the clinical picture is not classical. The problem really arises when we consider the chronic subdural haematoma. Although this may follow head trauma the exact relationship is rather tenuous. As the patients are often elderly or alcoholic it may be difficult to elicit a clear history of trauma at all. A mild confusional state may develop over weeks and when a mild hemiparesis becomes apparent the picture is easily labelled "cerebral vascular disease" or "a small stroke". There is no typical clinical picture. Any patient with progressive intellectual impairment or a slow evolution of signs suggesting a stroke should be considered a subdural haematoma suspect.

CASE REPORT

A man, 67 years of age, was in hospital for the investigation of a gastric ulcer. On the day following a barium meal he was noticed to have a right facial weakness, and further examination revealed a mild right hemiparesis. This had appeared overnight. His C.S.F. was examined and showed an elevated protein. He gave a history of having been unconscious after being run over by a car seven years before. Investigation showed an enormous left-sided chronic subdural haematoma. At operation the capsule of the haematoma was nearly half an inch thick.

The reason for the sudden onset of physical signs, with a lesion that had clearly been the same size for many years, is not apparent. If this had not occurred while he was in hospital it would undoubtedly have been regarded as a mild stroke.

The typical site for these haematomas is shown in Figure 23.2. The leak is a low pressure venous ooze resulting from tearing of the veins bridging the veins of the cortex to the sagittal sinus. Why there is such a variation in the rate of development of the various types and the exact mechanism by which the contents change from blood to a thin yellow fluid in the chronic type is unknown. The latter are often called "subdural hygromas" as the evidence of previous bleeding is minimal or absent.

2. The Post-Concussional Syndrome

This is the most frequent complication of head injury leading to referral to the neurological clinic, and invariably the question is raised: Has the patient got a subdural haematoma?

The syndrome consists of a triad of symptoms— headache, dizziness and difficulty in concentration. The headache is described as a continual burning pain or a tight band or pressure on top of the head. This is similar to a patient's description of tension headache. It is exacerbated by noise, fatigue, mental stress and attempts to resume work. The dizziness is not accompanied by a sense of rotation but is more a feeling of lightheadedness. It is provoked by standing up, turning suddenly or indeed by any sudden movement. The difficulty in concentration prevents the patient working and is often ascribed to the headache.

As mentioned previously the syndrome is not encountered in children and occurs infrequently after serious head injuries. It usually follows very mild head trauma without loss of consciousness. Studies on service personnel have shown that an early return to full activities is the best way of improving the symptoms. Unfortunately as many civilian cases involve litigation the patient is very unwilling to return to work and is often aided and abetted in this by relatives and other advisers. Most studies reveal that the pre-morbid personality of the patient is critical to the development of the syndrome with hypochondriacal and depressive personality traits being of major importance. Hysterical features may also occur in some cases. The condition has no known pathological basis but constitutes a disabling complex of symptoms in persons of a certain pre-morbid personality.

3. Post-traumatic Epilepsy

When a patient has suffered injuries involving the dura of the skull (penetrating trauma), the risk of post-traumatic epilepsy is between thirty per cent and fifty per cent. The risk is much higher if the injury is to the central part of the brain in the frontotemporal area. In closed head injuries (no fracture demonstrated) the risk is about five per cent. If there is evidence of laceration of the brain with focal neurological deficit the risk is also about fifty per cent. In all cases there is a tendency for the attacks to become less frequent with the passage of time, although the longer the period after the injury when the first attack occurs the less likelihood there is of eventual remission. If the patient has not had a seizure by the end of the second year after the injury it is increasingly unlikely that he will do so. Standard anti-convulsant drugs are effective, but effective control may be difficult if the post-traumatic epileptic state is complicated by personality disorder. These patients are likely to be irregular attenders and do not take their medication regularly.

Patients with personality problems following head trauma are usually aggressive and paranoid and very difficult to manage. As in the case of children, in many cases, there is considerable evidence that the pre-morbid personality was abnormal and that their drinking and fighting and outbreaks of aggression towards their family are exaggerations of previous habits. As this situation and post-traumatic epilepsy often co-exist in the same patient much of the bad behaviour is incorrectly held to be caused by post-epileptic confusion or even part of the actual seizure. When closely questioned most patients will admit that they are not having an epileptic attack when these outbursts occur.

TRAUMATIC LESIONS OF THE SPINAL CORD

Although the cervical and lumbar spine are the least supported parts of the spinal column their mobility to some extent protects them from damage. The majority of serious spinal injuries occur in the dorsal area particularly between D6 and D12. In the absence of any pathological abnormality of the vertebra (osteoporosis due to steroids, metastatic cancer), considerable force is needed to fracture the spine. This may be either compressive i.e. falling from a height on to the feet or due to hyperflexion, when a weight falls on to the back. The force needed is so great that these fractures are frequently accompanied by cord transection. Cervical cord injuries, although less frequent, account for the majority of early deaths, due to respiratory paralysis.

Cervical Spine Injuries

1. The mechanism and results of fractures of the cervical

Figure 23.5. Diagram to show the Mechanism of Cervical Spine Injuries

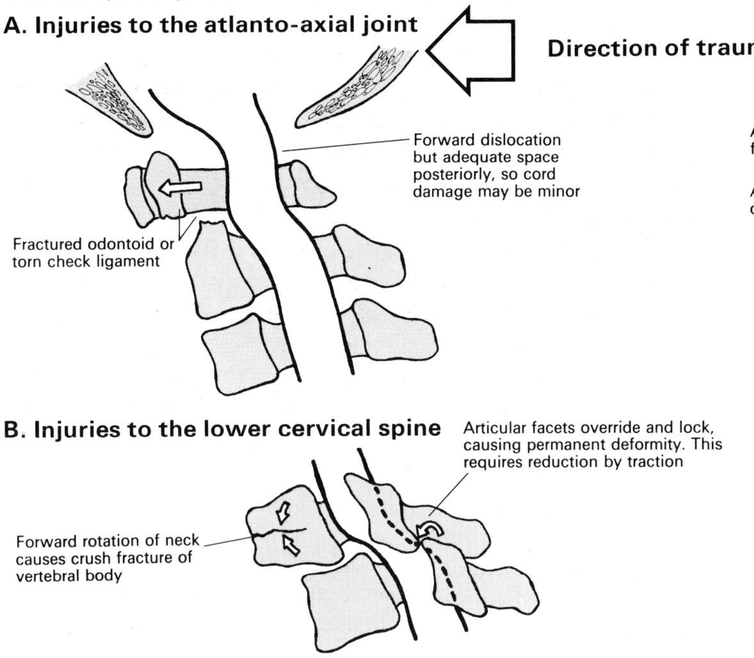

A. Injuries to the atlanto-axial joint

Direction of trauma

Forward dislocation but adequate space posteriorly, so cord damage may be minor

Fractured odontoid or torn check ligament

B. Injuries to the lower cervical spine

Articular facets override and lock, causing permanent deformity. This requires reduction by traction

Forward rotation of neck causes crush fracture of vertebral body

Figure 23.6

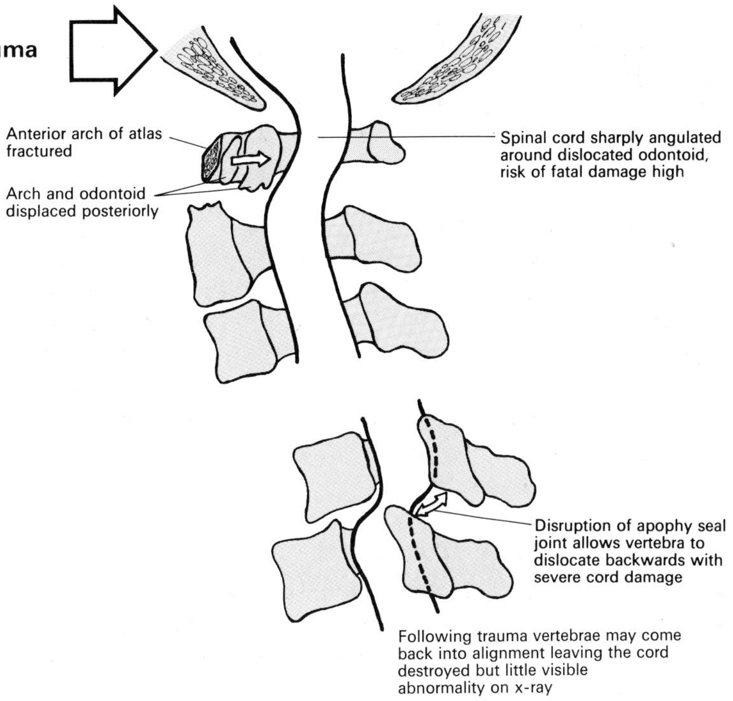

Anterior arch of atlas fractured

Arch and odontoid displaced posteriorly

Spinal cord sharply angulated around dislocated odontoid, risk of fatal damage high

Disruption of apophyseal joint allows vertebra to dislocate backwards with severe cord damage

Following trauma vertebrae may come back into alignment leaving the cord destroyed but little visible abnormality on x-ray

spine are indicated in Figures 23.5, 23.6. These may result from trauma to the front or back of the head as shown.

2. Atlanto-axial dislocation may also occur in patients with rheumatoid arthritis due to ligamentous degeneration or absorption of the odontoid peg. This usually but not always occurs in patients on steroids.

3. Atlanto-axial dislocations occurring in childhood may produce an unusual delayed myelopathy. The injury often results from a fall on to the back of the head from a swing. An acute transient tetraparesis lasting less than thirty minutes may occur with complete recovery. Some twenty years later the patient develops a progressive tetraparesis punctuated by acute episodes of tetraparesis while flexing the neck, sneezing or when slapped on the back. This is presumably due to repeated mild trauma inflicted by the sliding dislocation on neck flexion. (The anatomical features of the foramen magnum region are shown in Figure 23.7).

CASE REPORT

A 38-year-old man was referred because of increasing clumsiness of gait. He was partially sighted due to retrolental fibroplasia. At the age of 4 he fell from a swing. He was unconscious and totally paralysed for about twenty minutes. Following recovery he was completely deaf, suggesting bilateral temporal bone fractures. He was otherwise well until four years before referral. Over that period he had developed stiffness of the limbs and clumsiness. He

frequently played touch football (the American Game) and his friends found that if he was running with the ball he could best be stopped by a sharp push into the middle of his back. This made him drop the ball and fall to the ground, temporarily tetraplegic! It was these repeated insults that probably led to his spastic tetraparesis. He was found to have a sliding atlanto-axial dislocation.

4. Mid cervical fractures at C3/4 level are potentially more serious as there is less room for the spinal cord to ride the blow and the risk of respiratory paralysis is maximal at this level. Fragments of vertebra are more likely to break off and compress the cord; and fractures of the transverse process may damage the vertebral artery. This may cause brainstem signs or further vascular damage to the cord below the level of the fracture (see cord blood supply, Chapter 14).

Clinical Features

The clinical features of damage at any level are dominated initially by the stage of spinal shock with a total flaccid paralysis below the level of the lesion. At this stage the sensory findings provide the best evidence of the extent and severity of the damage. As soon as the cord settles down (the nature of spinal shock is *not* understood) tone returns to the limbs below the level of the injury and the extent of local damage becomes obvious, as the residual weakness and wasting of the supplied muscles becomes apparent.

Figure 23.7. **(a)** Foramen Magnum—bony structure (anterior)

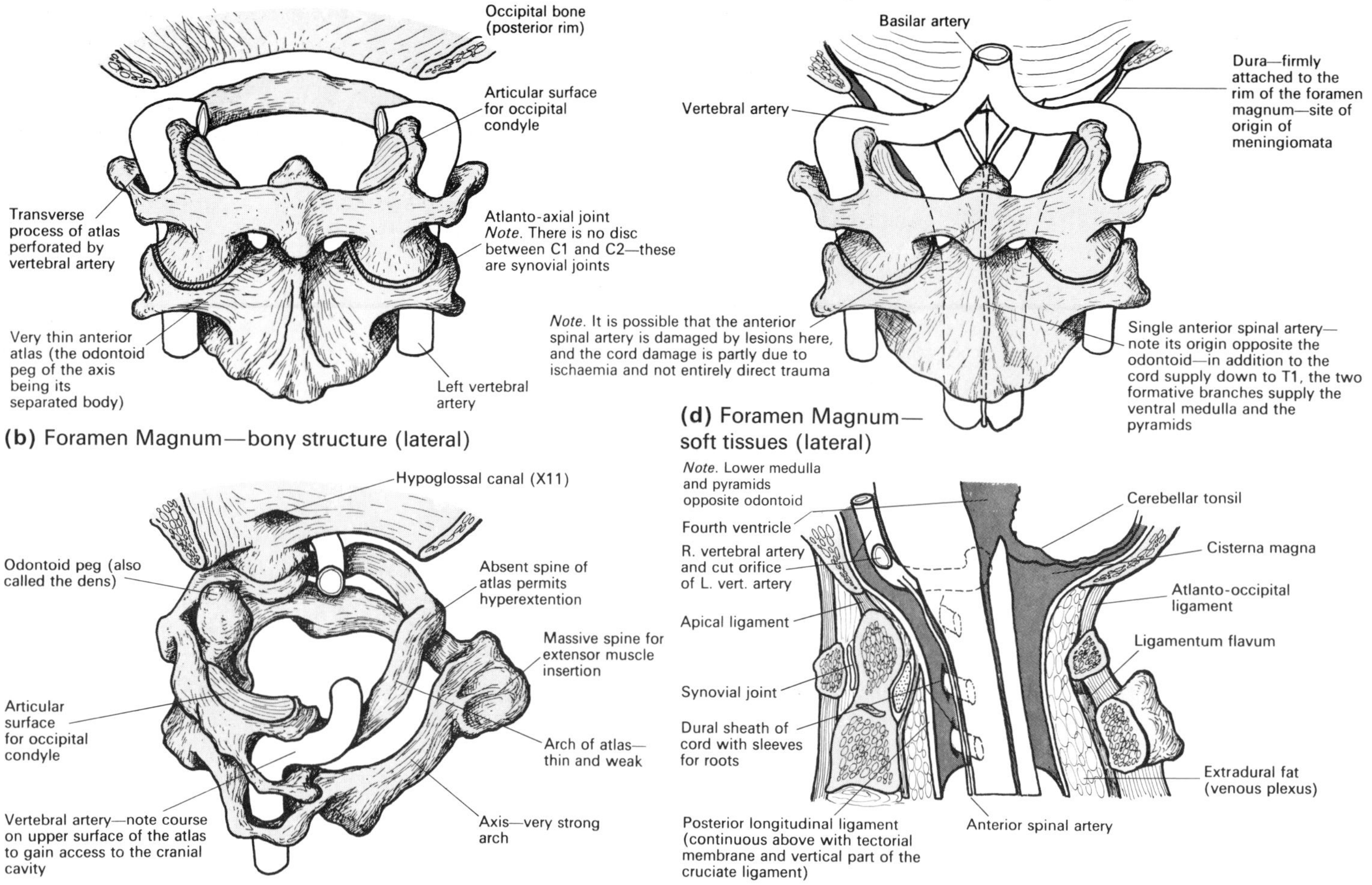

Occipital bone (posterior rim)

Articular surface for occipital condyle

Transverse process of atlas perforated by vertebral artery

Atlanto-axial joint
Note. There is no disc between C1 and C2—these are synovial joints

Very thin anterior atlas (the odontoid peg of the axis being its separated body)

Left vertebral artery

(b) Foramen Magnum—bony structure (lateral)

Hypoglossal canal (X11)

Odontoid peg (also called the dens)

Absent spine of atlas permits hyperextention

Massive spine for extensor muscle insertion

Articular surface for occipital condyle

Arch of atlas—thin and weak

Vertebral artery—note course on upper surface of the atlas to gain access to the cranial cavity

Axis—very strong arch

(c) Foramen Magnum—soft tissues (anterior)

Basilar artery

Vertebral artery

Dura—firmly attached to the rim of the foramen magnum—site of origin of meningiomata

Note. It is possible that the anterior spinal artery is damaged by lesions here, and the cord damage is partly due to ischaemia and not entirely direct trauma

Single anterior spinal artery—note its origin opposite the odontoid—in addition to the cord supply down to T1, the two formative branches supply the ventral medulla and the pyramids

(d) Foramen Magnum—soft tissues (lateral)

Note. Lower medulla and pyramids opposite odontoid

Fourth ventricle

R. vertebral artery and cut orifice of L. vert. artery

Apical ligament

Synovial joint

Dural sheath of cord with sleeves for roots

Cerebellar tonsil

Cisterna magna

Atlanto-occipital ligament

Ligamentum flavum

Extradural fat (venous plexus)

Posterior longitudinal ligament (continuous above with tectorial membrane and vertical part of the cruciate ligament)

Anterior spinal artery

Taking a mid-cervical fracture as an example; a flaccid tetraparesis occurs acutely but the patient may show a flicker of movement in the feet and have some preservation of pinprick sensation in the sacral dermatomes. This picture is typical of the so-called "central cord syndrome", the signs being rather similar to an advanced case of syringomyelia. As time passes power in the legs will improve in the extensor groups and the reflexes become brisk. Some finger movement may reappear but wasting and weakness will remain in muscles supplied by C4, C5 and C6. Sensation tends to improve but some slight loss of joint position sense in the feet usually remains.

Management

As long as the neurological state is static or improving, treatment is aimed at maintaining reduction of the fracture dislocation using skull calipers and whatever weight is necessary to maintain reduction. If the reduction remains unstable after six weeks, fixation may be required.

The main indications for surgical intervention are progression of neurological signs or radiological evidence of a fragment of the vertebral body or the arch still compressing the cord after reduction.

Thoraco-Lumbar Injuries

Simple crush fractures of the upper lumbar vertebrae are quite common in the elderly patient, and a crush fracture with cord compression may be the presenting symptom of metastatic malignant disease, particularly of the prostate gland. Crush fractures may also occur during the tonic phase of a major epileptic seizure. In the majority of instances the spinal cord is not damaged and symptomatic treatment is all that is required.

In severe fracture dislocation of the vertebra with complete shearing of the ligaments and fractures of the articular facets, total cord destruction occurs. The very unstable fracture will often reduce spontaneously by the time the patient reaches hospital. In these cases cord damage is complete and irreversible and the immediate aim must be the prevention of urinary tract infection and bed sores while one awaits the recovery of reflex tone. The position in which the patient is nursed can be critical in determining whether the patient develops a paraplegia in flexion or a paraplegia in extension. From a rehabilitation point of view the latter is more desirable.

Fracture dislocations below L1 level damage the cauda equina and as these are peripheral nerves there is considerable potential for recovery. Complete reduction is necessary and operative fixation may be required to prevent further damage to the cauda equina.

Delayed Complications

In recent years it has been increasingly recognised that a syringomyelic syndrome may complicate spinal cord trauma. Typically after a period varying from one to fifteen years the previously static neurological state alters. The first symptom is usually pain above the level of the lesion followed by the development of further lower motor neurone signs in the same area. Myelography and surgical exploration has confirmed that this syndrome is due to a syringomyelic cavity developing in and extending from the damaged area. It has now been shown that a similar syndrome may follow apparently trivial trauma, particularly to the cervical spinal cord.

Chapter 24

DRUG INTERACTIONS AND SIDE-EFFECTS IN NEUROLOGY

As might be anticipated, many of the drugs used in the treatment of neurological disorders are liable to produce neurological side-effects. Sometimes these side-effects are merely extensions of the therapeutic effect but in other cases serious new neurological phenomena are produced.

Many drugs in use for non-neurological diseases may also produce neurological side-effects which may be mistaken for neurological complications of the underlying disease. Drugs may occasionally worsen the situation for which they are being administered. For example, it is not widely appreciated that all anticonvulsant drugs can produce seizures in toxic doses and even in therapeutic dosage if used inappropriately.

To avoid the risk of the text becoming a bewildering list of complications we will consider the special problems encountered in the treament of various neurological disorders and then the neurological complications of drugs with similar therapeutic indications.

Two tables are included, one showing the drug groups and the side-effects likely to be encountered (Table 15) and the other specific neurological complications with a list of drugs that could be responsible (Table 14).

Although these lists are fairly comprehensive other drugs may be found to have similar side effects and a constant awareness of the possibility that drugs may be responsible for a patient's symptoms should always be maintained. A complete list of *all* drugs taken by the patient in the previous year is an essential part of the history, and it should be remembered that some patients who have taken a drug for years may completely fail to consider it a drug as it has become part of their daily routine!

One never ceases to be amazed at the attitude of the patient who is reluctant to take a prescribed "drug" and yet has been happily taking eight or more aspirins or compound analgesic tablets daily for many years, on the dubious premise that anything one can buy cannot be a "drug". The press publicity of the "drug problem" has also led to considerable difficulty in persuading elderly patients to take any medication for fear of becoming an addict, and a belief that all doctors are totally ignorant of drug side-effects.

There have been many papers and sociological surveys on the frequency with which patients fail to take the medication as prescribed or dispose of it down the drain as soon as they arrive home! This is *not* a failing of the patient but the responsibility of the doctor who has failed to explain to the patient the reason for prescribing the drug, its anticipated effect on the symptoms and the potential side effects. The latter feature is rather disputed but in an anxious patient the onset of even quite minor and predictable side-effects may lead to their stopping treatment. It seems sensible for the patient, who after all is the person using the medication, to be fully aware of these possibilities. It must be admitted that even the most painstaking explanation may fall on deaf ears and the writer will never forget the expression on the face of a Mexican-American patient as he left the clinic, after an explanation, including mime because of the language barrier, as to the correct use of an ergotamine suppository!

Occasionally the patient must be asked specifically to tolerate quite unpleasant side-effects in order to get the benefit of the drug. Perhaps the best example of this was in the early days of L-Dopa therapy when the patient had to tolerate nausea, vomiting, constipation and postural hypotension for several weeks before any improvement in the parkinsonian symptoms was apparent. The sedative effects of anticonvulsants are another very good example as the initial sedation wears off if the patient can be persuaded to persevere and this is best achieved if he is completely aware of the necessity to do this and the fact that eventually the side-effects will lessen or disappear.

GENERAL CONSIDERATIONS OF MECHANISMS OF DRUG TOXICITY

1. Every drug has inherent toxic potential. This is quantitative and varies from patient to patient in the exact dose required to produce the toxic effect.

2. The age of the patient influences the risk of an unanticipated toxic effect. The dangers of chloramphenicol in infancy, and the increasing risk of eighth nerve damage by streptomycin with increasing age are well known.

3. Toxic blood levels of a drug may be achieved with normal doses in the presence of renal failure. This risk is a particular problem of antibiotic therapy.

4. Similar side-effects of two drugs may summate if the drugs are used in combination. This is a problem of

Table 14
NEUROLOGICAL SYMPTOMS AND CAUSATIVE DRUGS

PERIPHERAL NEUROPATHY:	Thalidomide Nitrofurantoin Isoniazid Vincristine/Vinblastine Imiprimine Amitriptyline		Birth control pill Hypervitaminosis A

ACUTE MUSCLE WEAKNESS:	Diuretics—Potassium loss
	Carbenoxolone—Potassium
	  loss
	Neomycin—muscle blocking
	  effect
	Penicillamine—
	  myasthenic syndrome
		DEPRESSION:	Diazepam
			Chlordiazepoxide
			Reserpine
			Birth control pill
			Clonidine hydrochloride

*CHRONIC MUSCLE
WEAKNESS:*
	Steroids (especially fluorinated
	  steroids)
	Chloroquine
		*CONFUSION AND
		HYPOMANIA:*
			Antiparkinsonian drugs
			Steroids
			Excessive penicillin/cephalo-
			  sporins (prior to encephalo-
			  pathy and coma)

EPILEPTIC SEIZURES:	Anticonvulsants
	Sedatives (especially
	  meprobamate)
	Triptylines
	Phenothiazines
	Amphetamines
	Mono-amine oxidase inhibitors
	Amantadine hydrochloride
	Cycloserine
		PARKINSONISM:
		
		DYSTONIC REACTIONS:
			Reserpine
			Phenothiazines
			Tricyclic antidepressants (rare)
			Lithium carbonate
			Phenothiazines (especially
			  anti-emetic group)
			Metoclopromide (Maxalon)
			L-Dopa

HEADACHES:	Indomethacin Mono-amine oxidase inhibitors Excessive doses of ergotamine	*VISUAL DISTURBANCES:*	Tricyclic antidepressants Mono-amine oxidase inhibitors Streptomycin Chloramphenicol Isoniazid Chloroquine Ethambutol Birth control pill

anticonvulsant combinations where excessive sedation often becomes a major problem.

5. The possibility that the metabolic effect of one drug alters the action of another should always be considered. The onset of digitalis toxicity caused by hypokalaemia produced by diuretics is an example.

6. Individual variations in the ability of the patient to metabolise some drugs can occur and is based on inherited enzymic defects. Sensitivity to isoniazed and diphenylhydantoin (Epanutin or Dilantin U.S.P.) can occur on this basis.

7. One drug may interfere with the metabolic degradation of another. Phenylbutazone (Butazolidine) can block the metabolism of Tolbutamide (Rastinon) leading to hypoglycaemic reactions. Coumarin anticoagulants and sulthiam (Ospolot) block metabolism of diphenylhydantoin (Epanutin or Dilantin U.S.P.) and may lead to toxic blood levels.

8. Conversely some drugs may facilitate their own metabolism and that of other drugs by the process known as enzyme induction. Phenobarbital, glutethimide (Doriden) and meprobamate (Equanil) share this property and all can speed the metabolism of diphenylhydantoin—reducing the expected blood levels of this drug.

9. A drug may sensitise the body to otherwise innocuous endogenous substances. The potentially fatal rise in blood pressure or subarachnoid haemorrhage produced by dietary tyramine in patients receiving monoamine-oxidase inhibitors is well known.

10. Drugs may unmask a latent enzyme defect in the patient. This is an important factor in the precipitation of attacks of acute porphyria by a series of drugs listed in Chapter 16.

It is clear that in such a complex setting of possible mechanisms of drug toxicity that the simultaneous use of even innocuous and unrelated drugs requires careful consideration. As will be pointed out later, one of the dangers of drugs in combined capsules is that one of the agents in the combination may not be familiar to the user and could lead to

Table 15
NEUROLOGICAL SIDE-EFFECTS OF DRUG GROUPS

ANTICONVULSANTS:	*Cause* seizures in toxic doses		Choreiform movements
	Grand mal drugs worsen petit mal, (especially diphenyl-hydantoin)		Amantadine causes ankle oedema and a scaly red skin rash on the legs called livedo reticularis
	Cerebellar disturbances in acute or chronic overdose; (which may be permanent in the case of diphenylhydantoin)	*ANTIBIOTICS:*	Nitrofurantoin—peripheral neuropathy
	Recurrent confusional episodes		Penicillin and cephalosporins
SEDATIVES:	Addiction		—encephalopathy
	Withdrawal seizures (especially meprobamate)		—epileptic seizures
	Recurrent confusional episodes	Streptomycin Neomycin Colomycin	Eighth nerve damage, Retro-bulbar neuritis Neuromuscular blockade
ANTIDEPRESSANTS:	*Triptylines*		
	Blurred vision/glaucoma/ urinary retention		
	Hypertonicity/hyperpyrexia/ cardiac arrythmias/seizures in acute overdose		*Antituberculous drugs:*
	Peripheral neuropathy		Ethambutol —visual disturbance to green
	Mono-amine Oxidase Inhibitors		Isoniazid —retrobulbar neuritis peripheral neuropathy epileptic seizures
	Headaches		
	Confusional state		
	Epileptic seizures		
	Retrobulbar neuritis		
	Subarachnoid haemorrhage (if tyramine containing food taken)	*ANTI-ARTHRITIC DRUGS:*	*Steroids:*
TRANQUILLISERS:	Parkinsonian syndrome (in prolonged high doses)		Toxic psychosis Raised intracranial pressure
	Acute dystonic and dyskinetic reactions (acute allergic response)		Proximal myopathy Vertebral collapse with cord compression
	Chronic facial dyskinesias		Dislocation of Odontoid peg
	Oculogyric crises		*Indomethacin:*
	Epileptic seizures		Headache
ANTI-PARKINSONIAN AGENTS:	Dry mouth/blurred vision/ urinary retention		*Chloroquine:* Retinal damage
	Acute confusional state with visual hallucinations		Lens changes Proximal myopathy
	Paranoid psychosis		*Penicillamine* Myasthenic syndrome Polymyositis

a drug interaction. Even the "inert" constituents in capsules may have unrecognised significance. In 1968 the manufacturers of Epanutin (Dilantin U.S.P.) capsules in Australia changed the excipient in the capsules from calcium sulphate to lactose. This led to an epidemic of Epanutin toxicity. Experimental work suggested that calcium lactate was depressing the drug activity in some way and its removal from the capsules led to toxic blood levels!

ANTICONVULSANT THERAPY

All anticonvulsants have convulsant properties in toxic doses. Barbiturates tend to provoke seizures as the blood level is falling. When a recently admitted patient has a first seizure in hospital it is worth giving serious consideration to the possibility that the patient is habituated to barbiturates, meprobamate or alcohol, and that the seizure was caused by withdrawal of one of these agents. Conversely, the attack may be the result of the patient's first experience of barbiturate as a night sedative or as part of anaesthesia. This is such a frequent event that an intravenous dose of a short-acting barbiturate has become the method of choice for provoking seizure activity during E.E.G. recording.

Anticonvulsants are designed to be effective in three types of epilepsy; grand mal, temporal lobe or psychomotor seizures and petit mal. Although there is some overlap of activity it is incorrect to assume that any drug may be safely tried in any type of epilepsy. It is not sufficiently appreciated that diphenylhydantoin (very useful in grand mal) may make petit mal attacks much worse, and that anti-petit mal drugs all tend to provoke grand mal seizures. As a broad generalisation diphenylhydantoin (Epanutin or Dilantin U.S.P.) is the drug of choice for grand mal (even though there are some case reports of patients who had episodes of grand mal made worse by this drug). Primidone (Mysoline) appears to have some degree of specificity for temporal lobe attacks, is effective in grand mal and does not share the tendency to provoke petit mal. Ethosuximide (Zarontin) is the drug of choice for petit mal. When a child with petit mal is put on ethosuximide, a first attack of grand mal may be provoked. The addition of diphenylhydantoin may then worsen control of the petit mal leading to a vicious spiral of increasing dosage of both drugs. Either phenobarbitone or Primidone are probably the best drugs to use to prevent or control co-existent grand mal seizures in children with petit mal.

Diphenylhydantoin (Epanutin) (Dilantin U.S.P.)

The side-effects of diphenylhydantoin are predictable and usually dose related. Giddiness, nystagmus, ataxia, drowsiness and diplopia occur in a sequence closely related to the blood level. Unusually high blood levels may result from deliberate overdosage, genetic metabolic problems or the introduction of other drugs. Coumarin anticoagulants, PAS, INAH, sulphaphenazole (Orisulf), Phenylbutazone (Butazolidine) and sulthiame (Ospolot) may all elevate diphenylhydantoin blood levels. The latter drug, sulthiame, is an anticonvulsant and serious cerebellar damage has been reported after the accidental elevation of diphenylhydantoin levels following its introduction into an epileptic drug regime.

In children diphenylhydantoin tends to cause gross gum hypertrophy, hairiness and acneform skin rashes. Osteomalacia due to diphenylhydantoin has been recognised in recent years. There is considerable controversy about the role of reduced serum folate levels in patients on diphenylhydantoin which may cause a frank megaloblastic anaemia in some instances. Transient internuclear ophthalmoplegia, and rarely permanent cerebellar damage, are other rare but serious side effects that may be mistaken for evidence of progressive neurological disease.

In spite of this alarming list of side effects, and there are many others, diphenylhydantoin remains the single most reliable anticonvulsant drug available. The value of diphenylhydantoin in the control of pain has been discussed in previous chapters. It has a useful action in spinothalamic pain disorders and trigeminal neuralgia.

Primidone (Mysoline)

The side-effects of this drug are unpredictable. A proportion of patients are quite unable to tolerate it. The author gives a test dose of 64 mg. (One quarter of a 250 mg. tablet) taken at 6 p.m. If the patient becomes severely "drunk" on this dose it is extremely unlikely that he will be able to tolerate the drug. This appears to be a true hypersensitivity reaction in some patients. Others will tolerate up to 2 gms. daily with minimal side effects. In acute overdosage cerebellar ataxia and nystagmus occurs but permanent cerebellar damage has *not* been reported.

The best indication for the use of this drug is temporal lobe epilepsy and in many cases it is the only effective drug. Due to an almost identical chemical structure it is considered inappropriate to combine it with phenobarbitone and yet in some patients this does appear to be a useful combination and although theoretically unsound it is worth considering in a difficult situation. It is also useful in combination with diphenylhydantoin, particularly in patients with focal epilepsy when quite a small dose may dramatically improve the epileptic control. Such a regime could be diphenylhydantoin 100 mg t.d.s. and Primidone 125 mg. t.d.s. If Primidone is used alone a dose of 125 mg. t.d.s. to 250 mg. t.d.s. is usually required.

Phenobarbitone

Phenobarbitone is not a strong anticonvulsant and produces drowsiness. Although it is traditionally used in combination with diphenylhydantoin this is by no means an obligatory combination and the writer prefers to use diphenylhydantoin alone when initiating anticonvulsant therapy. There is, however, a very useful feature of phenobarbitone, and that is its use as a 64 mgm, or 100 mg, spansule. The majority of epileptic attacks occur between 6 and 9 a.m., as the patient is waking up or shortly thereafter. Yet most patients are on a t.d.s. drug regime and taken their last dose of drugs at six o'clock in the evening. This leaves the most vulnerable time of the day poorly covered by the medication. If taking the evening drugs as late as possible before going to bed fails to prevent attacks, a phenobarbitone spansule may dramatically improve the situation. Often the daytime dosage of medication can be reduced if the diurnal variation of the patient's epilepsy is treated by a regime "tailored" to his needs.

Although there is much experimental evidence that once a patient is stabilised on diphenylhydantoin or mysoline the blood levels do not alter diurnally, in clinical practice changes in the pattern of medication, i.e. shifting the evening dose of diphenylhydantoin from 6 p.m. to 10 p.m., *does* influence the degree of control achieved. A typical and effective regime for a patient who is having "nocturnal" attachs between 5 a.m. and 9 a.m. would be diphenylhydantoin 100 mg. at 8 a.m. and 10 p.m. and a phenobarbitone spansule 60 mg. at 10 p.m. There is rarely any need for additional drug cover during the day.

Sulthiame (Ospolot)

This is a second-line drug for use in intractable epilepsy, and may produce special problems if used with diphenylhydantoin. It blocks the liver enzymes involved in diphenylhydantoin degradation and may suddenly increase the serum diphenylhydantoin level by 100—150 per cent with serious cerebellar toxicity.

It has been specially recommended for the treatment of temporal lobe epilepsy, but many patients complain that they feel "vague", "detached" or "strange" on this drug and often stop taking it because of these side effects. Even if the patient is unaware of any change, if the relatives of a patient on sulthiame complain that the patient's personality has changed, the first move should be to stop the drug. The patient then often volunteers that he feels quite different psychologically. When sulthiame is withdrawn the dose should be decreased slowly over a two-week period. Of all anticonvulsant drugs sulthiame is the one most likely to precipitate an attack of status epilepticus if suddenly discontinued.

Ethosuximide (Zarontin)

This is the drug of choice in petit mal. It is much less toxic than its forerunners (Tridione and Paradione) although a few cases of aplastic anaemia have been reported. It is important to remember the tendency of Zarontin to provoke grand mal. It should not be given on a "let's see if it helps" basis in patients with grand mal. It is also essential to keep reviewing the need for the drug as the patient becomes older. It is unusual for petit mal to persist beyond 18 or 19 years of age. The author has seen several patients in their early 20's with poorly controlled seizures who were still taking Zarontin unnecessarily. Stopping the drug led to complete control of the major epilepsy without recurrence of petit mal.

Carbamazepine (Tegretol)

Although this drug is usually used for treating trigeminal neuralgia, it was originally synthesised as an anticonvulsant and is occasionally of value in temporal lobe epilepsy. It produces acute cerebellar dysfunction which is reversible, and cases of aplastic anaemia have been reported.

Methsuximide (Celontin)

Methsuximide is a succinimide synthesised for use in petit mal. The considerable effectiveness of ethosuximide has reduced its use in this type of epilepsy but in the writer's experience it has an extremely useful action in epilepsy, complicated by myoclonic jerking.

In some patients the entire epileptic problem consists of sudden jerks which may throw them to the ground without loss of consciousness. In other patients with grand mal epilepsy, myoclonic jerking particularly at breakfast time may cause considerable problems with a tendency to lead to the destruction of breakfast crockery. A single dose of methsuximide 300 mg. on retiring may completely control these morning jerks and in the writer's opinion methsuximide is the drug of choice in this situation. Overdosage may cause a reversible internuclear ophthalmoplegia, cerebellar ataxia and drowsiness.

These are just a few of the drugs available for the control of epilepsy and some recently introduced drugs that are still under evaluation may gain an important place in the treatment of epilepsy. The drugs discussed are those used by the writer or those that seem to cause particular management problems. It is better to have a good knowledge of the best use and side effects of a few effective and tried drugs than to be continually using the latest drug in the all too often vain hope that it will prove more effective.

Whenever a patient with epilepsy goes out of control the following possibilities should be carefully considered.

1. Has the patient really got epilepsy? At first sight this may seem an extraordinary question, but in general anticonvulsant drugs *do* have some beneficial effect even if not entirely successful. A complete failure to respond to anticonvulsants should prompt re-appraisal of the diagnosis.

2. Is the patient deliberately faking fits for attention? Again this is a surprisingly frequent problem; when an epileptic discovers that he or she can bring unpleasant confrontations to an end by having a seizure, the temptation to do so is great. Even the most expert observer may have difficulty in distinguishing genuine and non-organic fits in this situation.

3. Are the drugs used appropriate to the type of epilepsy? Is there any chance that the anticonvulsants are triggering

attacks? Have any other drugs been given to the patient that could trigger attacks; i.e. phenothiazines, short-acting barbiturates or is the patient taking excessive alcohol?

Status Epilepticus

Status epilepticus is the situation that exists when one seizure follows another *without* the patient regaining consciousness between attacks. The main danger to the patient is the inhalation of vomit or secretions, repeated cerebral anoxia and exhaustion. Management should aim to protect the airway, prevent anoxia and the physical dangers of seizures such as vertebral crush fractures. Diazepam 10 mg. I.V.I. repeated as often as necessary is the treatment of choice, but the risks of causing respiratory depression, particularly in children, should be remembered. Paraldehyde 5–10 ccs. by deep I.M.I. is the second line of treatment. Short-acting barbiturates should not be used. Although they may have an immediate beneficial effect there is a risk of further seizures being provoked as the blood level rapidly falls a few hours later.

Although it is important to get the seizures under control as quickly as possible it is essential *not* to worsen the situation by using too many drugs simultaneously. The majority of cases respond to diazepam and this should be regarded as the mainstay of management. The patient's normal medication should be re-introduced by nasogastric tube or parenterally in an adjusted dose if a suitable preparation is available, as soon as it is apparent that the episode is under control.

DRUG TREATMENT IN PARKINSONISM

The drug treatment of parkinsonism is one of the most significant therapeutic advances of recent years.

Until 1968 the only drugs available were anti-cholinergic drugs based on atropine derivatives. These agents had some effect on tremor but did very little for the more disabling symptoms of rigidity and bradykinesia. Dosage, particularly in the older patient, was often limited by the risks of precipitating glaucoma, urinary retention and severe confusional states with vivid visual hallucinosis. These drugs still have a minor role in treatment, particularly in patients with severe tremor which may not respond to L-Dopa therapy.

At the same time as the discovery of L-Dopa a chance observation made in the U.S.A. indicated that Amantadine hydrochloride, a drug synthesised as an antiviral agent, had a beneficial effect on parkinsonism. Although overshadowed ever since by L-Dopa, Amantadine is still a useful drug in some patients. It is given as a twice daily dose of 100 mg. A higher dose may precipitate epileptic seizures and it is contraindicated in epileptic patients. Its main advantage is an almost immediate response. In general if there is no response within forty-eight hours it is unlikely that it will prove effective. Its disadvantage is that in many cases the beneficial effect wears off in a period of three to six months. In common with all effective anti-parkinsonism drugs, it may precipitate a confusional state with vivid visual hallucinations.

L-Dopa was introduced in 1968 and in the first few years an enormous range of side effects were reported. These were acceptable only because of the dramatic alleviation of symptoms in the majority of cases.

These side effects included involuntary movement disorders of choreiform type in some fifty per cent of patients treated with 3 gm. or more daily. In the author's own experience this problem does not occur if the total dose can be kept below 2·5 gm. daily. Every described variety of dyskinesia, akathisia, ballistic, myoclonic and facial movement has been reported. Nausea and vomiting, particularly after the morning dose, hypotension, constipation and palpitations are more common and more often disabling side effects. These are primarily due to peripheral effects of L-Dopa, and a search was made to find ways of blocking these effects. The introduction of agents that block Dopa-decarboxylase has allowed much lower doses of L-Dopa to be used with a great reduction in peripheral side effects and a more immediate response. L-Dopa alone could take up to three months before any improvement was noted. The newer combined agents usually produce an identifiable improvement within the first two weeks with minimal peripheral side effects and represent a very major advance in treatment.

However, the central side-effects—the movement disorders, confusion, hallucinations, paranoid delusions, depression and sleepiness which marred L-Dopa treatment—may also occur and in view of the greatly increased potency of the Dopa-decarboxylase inhibitor drugs the risks of producing these effects are just as great if not greater and considerable caution should be exercised in initiating treatment and increasing the dosage.

The treatment of associated psychotic reactions can be difficult and clearly many phenothiazines would have an adverse effect on the parkinsonism. Thioridazine (Melleril) seems to be particularly useful in this situation with the least risk of producing side effects.

Depression is best treated by Tofranil. The use of amine-oxidase inhibitors is absolutely contraindicated in the presence of L-Dopa. Particular care should be taken *not* to use composite capsules containing an anti-depressant and a phenothiazine tranquilliser. The risk of the latter constituent worsening the parkinsonism is obvious. Severe depression is a frequent complication of parkinsonism and although in many cases L-Dopa relieves the depression in a few patients the depression gets worse. This presents a formidable therapeutic problem.

ANTIDEPRESSANT DRUGS

The use of antidepressant therapy forms a significant part of neurological practice. A vast number of patients are seen with neurological symptoms caused by underlying depression, and many patients with intractable neurological disease become depressed. There are two main groups, the weakly "atropinic" agents, closely related to the phenothiazines (imiprimine and the tryptiline group), and the monoamine-oxidase inhibitors.

Imiprimine (Tofranil), and Amitriptyline (Tryptizol)

In spite of close structural similarity there are differences in both therapeutic actions and side-effects of these drugs. One unusual shared property is that both have been shown to cause peripheral neuropathy. No other antidepressants or closely related phenothiazines have been shown to have this side-effect. The atropine-like action leads to predictable symptoms; dry mouth, blurred vision, tachycardia, postural hypotension and urinary retention. Glaucoma may be caused by both acute and chronic administration. Imiprimine has caused a parkinsonian syndrome, but before the use of L-Dopa this drug was frequently used in depressed parkinsonian patients, as the anticholinergic effect helped the parkinsonian part of the illness as well as the depression. Overdosage of these drugs leads to hypertonia, restlessness, convulsions, hyperpyrexia and fatal cardiac arrhythmias. This picture is readily provoked by the administration of a MAO inhibitor to patients on either of these drugs. The triptyline drugs tend to potentiate barbiturates and may provoke epileptic seizures. They should therefore only be used in a depressed epileptic with great care.

Monoamine-Oxidase Inhibitors

This series includes Isocarboxazid (Marplan), iproniazid (Marsalid), phenelzine (Nardil), nialamide (Niamid) and tranylcypromine (Parnate). (The latter is also combined with tri-fluo-perazine (Stelazine) in Parstelin Capsules.) The use of these drugs is seriously limited by their side-effects. Liver and marrow toxicity occurs, but from a neurological point of view we must include headaches, confusional states, hallucinosis and epileptic seizures. They should never be used with imipramine, triptylines, barbiturates, sympathomimetic amines and anti-hypertensive drugs. In fact it is generally advisable not to use any other drug while a patient is on MAO inhibitors. Several cases of visual impairment due to drug induced retrobulbar neuritis have been described. Perhaps the most dramatic neurological side-effect is sub-arachnoid haemorrhage caused by acute hypertension when a patient on MAO inhibitors eats cheese or other foods with a high tyramine content. From the author's experience tranylcypromine seems to be particularly dangerous in this respect.

Lithium Carbonate

This is used in the treatment of patients with manic depressive psychosis. Its main neurological side effects range from a fine tremor to severe extrapyramidal movement disorders including parkinsonism. The serum level should be estimated regularly and not allowed to exceed 1·5 mEq/L.

TRANQUILLISERS

There are three main groups; the reserpine derivatives, the minor (non-phenothiazine) tranquillisers and the major phenothiazine tranquillisers.

Reserpine Derivatives

These agents are used in psychiatric disease and in the treatment of hypertension. Reserpine causes a parkinsonian syndrome in lower dosage than any other drug. It may also provoke a serious depressive reaction even in the small doses used in the treatment of hypertension.

Minor Tranquillisers

The most widely used members of this group are chlordiazepoxide (Librium) and diazepam (Valium). Both appear to be extremely safe in combination with other drugs. Although seizures have occurred on Librium withdrawal, this was after very high dosage. Valium is the drug of choice for the management of status epilepticus, and often appears to have a potentiating effect on other anticonvulsants in long-term management. It is an effective antispastic agent in paraplegic patients and the only limiting factor with either drug appears to be excessive sedation.

Major Tranquillisers

These are the phenothiazine drugs and unlike the drugs discussed above, these agents are responsible for a wide range of serious neurological side effects. There are two main groups of phenothiazines with different toxic effects. The dimethylamino substituted compounds include chlorpromazine (Largactil) and promazine (Sparine), and the propylpiperazine substituted group include perphenazine (Fentazine), trifluoperazine (Stelazine), thioridazine

(Melleril), fluphenazine (Modecate and Moditen), pericyazine (Neulactil), chlorprothixene (Taractan) and thiopropazate (Dartalan).

All these drugs can produce parkinsonian syndromes, but chlorpromazine in prolonged high dosage is the drug most likely to do so. The piperazine side chained drugs on the other hand are more likely to produce the acute dyskinetic or dystonic syndromes, even following a single dose in susceptible patients. Personal experience suggests that perphenazine is the most frequent offender in this respect. The acute dyskinetic reactions include torticollis, retrocollis, tongue protrusion, facial grimacing, uncontrolled chewing movements and oculogyric crises. Such reactions are easily and frequently misdiagnosed as hysteria, tetanus or a seizure phenomenon. Paradoxically chlorpromazine, 25 mg I.M.I. is an extremely effective antidote to such a reaction producing a response within a few minutes.

All the phenothiazines are epileptogenic and their use in epileptics should be carefully considered. Seizures have followed single injections of chlorpromazine given as an anti-emetic.

When the drug is stopped there is usually a considerable, if not complete, improvement in the drug-induced parkinsonian condition. However, the more distressing facial dyskinesias (not the acute reactions discussed above) that follow prolonged administration are often permanent, and sometimes appear after the drug has been discontinued. There is no consistently useful drug in treating these side-effects, although haloperidol may help at first only to later add a parkinsonian syndrome of its own.

There are many other complications associated with phenothiazines, but we will confine ourselves to this brief discussion of the special neurological problems.

Sedative Drugs

The commonly used sedative drugs include barbiturates, meprobamate (Equanil), glutethimide (Doriden), dichlorophenazone (Welldorm) and nitrazepam (Mogadon). The first three drugs may cause problems. Many people are addicted to these agents; especially to barbiturates in Great Britain and meprobamate in the U.S.A. We have already mentioned the risk of withdrawal seizures if any of these drugs is stopped suddenly. The possibility of children having access to these drugs should always be considered.

CASE REPORT

An American boy, 13 years of age, repeatedly came home from school drowsy and ataxic. He was extensively investigated for a cerebellar tumour before referral. A careful history revealed that he was like this only in the evenings and his pupils were always widely dilated when he was in this state. He finally revealed under intensive questioning that he was taking a combination of barbiturates and amphetamine at school.

Even in the elderly, episodic or even progressive confusional states should always raise the possibility of drug intoxication. Bromides are still available in proprietary medicines and are an important constituent of several old nerve "tonics" or cough medicines. Every year a few cases of dementia caused by bromide poisoning are discovered, but only by maintaining a high index of suspicion. Glutethimide overdosage produces dilated pupils and brisk reflexes. Barbiturate overdosage causes ataxia, nystagmus and depressed reflexes, but the pupil reactions are always normal.

THE TREATMENT OF MIGRAINE

We have already discussed some aspects of the treatment of migraine applied to specific headache patterns. From a strictly pharmacological point of view the following side effects are important.

Clonidine hydrochloride (dixarit) in a dosage of 0·025–0·05 mg. is occasionally of value in prophylaxis. The only significant side effect is a depressive reaction in some patients.

A proprietary preparation containing ergotamine 0·3 mg., a barbiturate and belladonna alkaloids (Bellergal®) is of value in prophylaxis but has side effects produced by each constituent. The daily dose of ergotamine is only 0·9 mg. but occasionally elderly patients develop ergotism with peripheral paraesthesiae and numbness and occasionally angina may be provoked. The belladonna alkaloids cause blurring of vision due to their mydriatic effect on the pupil, a dry mouth and occasionally urinary retention. The sedative effect is usually mild, but a proportion of patients develop a barbiturate skin rash.

Methysergide maleate used in a dosage of 1 to 3 mg. t.d.s. is the most effective anti-migraine prophylactic drug and also the most dangerous. It may produce acute vertigo, nausea, vomiting and ataxia. In prolonged high dosage reversible retroperitoneal or mediastinal fibrosis may occur. Occasionally, anginal attacks or myocardial infarction may follow its use in elderly patients.

The treatment of an acute attack of migraine usually involves the use of ergotamine in some form. The therapeutic problems result from the devastating speed of onset of a headache and the nausea and occasionally vomiting that occurs.

To obtain speed of action various preparations have been tried. Tablets that are chewed and absorbed in the mouth have great theoretical advantage but ergot tastes so vile that a genuine migraine sufferer can rarely tolerate this mode of administration. A spray inhaler is dangerous because of the ease of overdose. Preparations containing 2 mg. of ergotamine seem to provoke more vomiting. An ergotamine suppository can be used in the acute attack, but is rarely successful. Used at night a suppository occasionally helps to prevent nocturnal attacks of the cluster type. In the writer's experience if one or two standard tablets of 1 mg. ergotamine fails to help a higher dose is *not* effective, and very high doses, i.e. up to 6 mg. in an attack, may cause ergotism and often *provoke* headaches. Some patients' headaches get better if all ergot preparations are withdrawn. Once a headache is established 50 mg. promethazine (Phenergan) relieves vomiting and enables the patient to get to sleep which usually terminates the attack. Narcotic drugs do not relieve the headache; often provoke further vomiting and the addiction risk is high.

THE TREATMENT OF MYASTHENIA GRAVIS

It is widely thought that myasthenia is easy to diagnose and treat. Few realise the ominous significance of the term "gravis" which applies to this extremely unpleasant and potentially lethal disease. The dangers are greatly compounded by the fact that it is just as easy to harm the patient by over-medication as by under-medication and that "cholinergic crisis"—the effect of over-medication—is a much greater danger.

The basic defect is a failure of neuromuscular transmission, usually affecting the extra-ocular and bulbar musculature. Most of the other muscles are *normal* and therefore in treating the abnormal muscles there is a risk of overdose effects appearing in the normal muscles. In a critical situation it is best to aim to treat the most dangerous weakness (usually swallowing or breathing difficulty). Most overdose disasters result from attempts to restore the entire patient to normal.

The standard drugs block cholinesterase so that the side-effects are those of parasympathetic overactivity. These include excessive salivation, bronchial secretion, increased sweating, pupilloconstriction, increased gut motility and cramping abdominal pains. These side-effects can be partially blocked by the use of atropine but this increases the ease with which an overdose can be given. The dangerous side effect is on the neuromuscular junction. Complete inhibition of cholinesterase allows acetylcholine to persist at the end plate producing a depolarising or "cholinergic blockade".

Further anticholinesterase drugs or cholinergic drugs such as edrophonium (tensilon) can only make the situation worse; with increasing paralysis—often of previously unaffected muscles. The correct management consists of airway protection, assisted respiration if necessary and complete withdrawal of anticholinergic drugs.

Returning sensitivity to edrophonium (tensilon) is the best way to monitor the situation. This test is not without dangers and may precipitate acute paralysis if the patient is in cholinergic blockade. It should never be performed unless rescusitative equipment is available. 10 mgm. are drawn up. 2 mgm. are given I.V. having selected a suitable muscle to test—i.e. a drooping eyelid or the ability to count out loud. If the patient does not feel faint or flushed the rest of the dose should be given over one to two minutes. The effect should be apparent within this period and on occasions may persist for several minutes.

The standard oral drugs are neostigmine (prostigmine), pyridostigmine (mestinon) and ambenonium (mytelase). The writer prefers to use prostigmine in difficult patients. It has the advantage of an action within fifteen to thirty minutes and wears off in four hours. This means the dose can be tailored to suit meals with little risk of cumulative overdose. Although pyridostigmine provides good background activity it takes longer to act (four to six hours) and has a variable duration of action that increases the risk of cumulative overdosage.

The management of myasthenia gravis requires considerable expertise and experience and an adequate back-up respiratory unit for acute emergencies. The role of thymectomy in these patients is beyond the scope of the present discussion.

ANTIBIOTIC THERAPY

Because of widely differing side-effects we will discuss each group separately. It is worth emphasising that many of these problems occur only when due allowance for impaired renal excretion of the drug has not been made.

Nitrofurantoin (Furadantin)

This drug used to be widely suspected as one of the most frequent causes of drug-induced peripheral neuropathy. It is hard to be certain of its exact role as it was mainly used in patients with chronic renal failure who are liable to develop a neuropathy because of uraemia.

Penicillins

An acute anaphylactic reaction is the most serious problem encountered with penicillin. For many years it has been known that intrathecal and intraventricular use of penicillin could cause seizures. Only relatively recently has it been realised that the use of high doses of penicillin in elderly people with renal failure can lead to confusion, coma, myoclonic twitching and finally generalised seizures and very often death. An identical syndrome has been reported following the use of cephaloridine.

Streptomycin, Gentamycin, Kanamycin, Colomycin and Polymyxin-B

Impaired renal function underlies the majority of problems caused by these drugs. Streptomycin and gentamycin cause severe vestibular damage but have little effect on hearing. The risk is greatly increased in the elderly patient. Streptomycin may also cause retrobulbar neuritis. Neomycin and kanamycin cause deafness, which in the case of kanamycin may continue to deteriorate even after the drug is discontinued.

All the drugs under discussion are administered by intramuscular injection, and many patients complain of tingling around the mouth and in the limbs, occurring some fifteen to thirty minutes after injection. This may be mistaken for a developing neuropathy, although a neuropathy as such has never been reported. Colomycin may produce an acute transient syndrome like myasthenia gravis after an intramuscular injection. All these drugs are capable of producing neuromuscular blockade and this may lead to serious problems.

CASE REPORT

A woman, 56 years of age, had an episode of apnoea followed by an epileptic fit and required assisted respiration following surgery for a perforated viscus. She was referred for a neurological opinion as a suspected "stroke". A careful history revealed that neomycin had been instilled into the peritoneal cavity during surgery. This had paralysed the diaphragm by neuromuscular blockade and led to an anoxic seizure. She made a full recovery several days later.

All these drugs can be absorbed from open wounds and cavities and the dosage instilled should be carefully monitored, especially if the patient has renal failure.

ANTITUBERCULOUS DRUGS

INAH is the prime offender from a neurological point of view. The drug interferes with pyridoxine metabolism, and the side-effects can be avoided by giving supplementary pyridoxine. There are three major problems—a confusional state with epileptic seizures, a peripheral neuropathy, and retrobulbar neuritis. Evidence has recently been presented that patients on this drug have impaired memory function although the extent and significance of this finding is not yet apparent.

Cycloserine causes a confusional state and seizures. This risk is so high that the drug is contraindicated in patients with a history of epilepsy.

Viomycin causes vestibular damage and hearing loss.

Ethambutol causes blurred vision and in particular loss of green vision.

DRUGS USED IN ARTHRITIC CONDITIONS

Steroids

Long-term steroid therapy for rheumatoid arthritis may lead to several complications of neurological interest. Toxic confusional states and hypomania occur, usually following prolonged high dosage. Raised intracranial pressure may occur following sudden withdrawal; this is especially likely to happen in children.

A limb girdle myopathy is particularly likely to complicate long-term therapy with fluorinated steroids such as triamcinolone. A localised myopathy, underlying the area of local application of fluorinated steroid cream, has been reported in an infant. Significant amounts of steroid are absorbed through the skin and can produce evidence of depression of the pituitary-adrenal axis. Demineralisation of the vertebrae may lead to vertebral collapse, with paraplegia or cauda equina compression. When the odontoid peg is affected, it may break off, causing a sliding dislocation of the atlas on the axis, with potentially fatal compression of the upper spinal cord and medulla.

Indomethacin

This drug often causes quite severe headache. In some series as many as thirty per cent of patients had this symptom. The author has seen several cases of intractable headache caused by this drug, and yet it is a side-effect that few doctors seem to recognise.

Chloroquine

In addition to the side-effects of this drug on the retina and lens, that can cause serious visual problems, much less frequently a proximal myopathy is produced. A patient seen by the author died of aspiration pneumonia caused by this complication. The myopathy is severe and may affect the bulbar muscles. Recovery may take several months following withdrawal of the drug.

Penicillamine

Recently reported side-effects of this drug include polymyositis and myasthenia gravis (see Chapter 17).

Patients with chronic rheumatoid arthritis are subject to a bewildering array of complications caused by the disease itself. It is essential that doctors looking after patients on these drugs are aware of the side-effects so that new symptoms are not dismissed as yet another manifestation of the underlying disease.

Miscellaneous drug side-effects

Diuretics

Any diuretic that causes potassium loss may cause generalised muscle weakness. In a patient with periodic paralysis of the hypokalaemic variety a serious attack may be precipitated. In the hyperkalaemic variety, diuretics may have a beneficial effect. Ethacrynic acid (Edecrin) and lasix (Frusemide) have been shown to cause impairment of hearing and this should be considered in the long-term use of either agent.

Carbenoxolone (Biogastrone)

The liquorice extract drugs used in the treatment of peptic ulceration may cause severe potassium loss, and several cases of acute generalised paralysis caused by this drug have been reported. The clinical picture is a very severe one and resembles Guillain–Barré syndrome. Assisted respiration may be necessary.

Vincristine

This antimitotic drug used in the treatment of lymphomas and leukaemias causes severe motor and sensory neuropathy in some fifty per cent of patients who are receiving it.

THE BIRTH CONTROL PILL

1. Headaches (usually of migrainous type)

Headaches and quite severe depressive illness may be provoked by the birth control pill. In the author's opinion changing the pill to one of a different type or one containing different compounds does not influence these symptoms. It is preferable to stop the medication altogether if the patient really requires relief from her symptoms.

2. Cerebral Vascular Accidents

It is now generally accepted that the pill can cause cerebral vascular disease with cerebral infarction. It is only the magnitude of the risk that is disputed.

3. Retro-Bulbar Neuritis

One of the first recognised side effects of the pill to be reported was acute retro-bulbar neuritis.

4. Choreiform Syndromes

A clinical picture identical to Sydenham's chorea has been recognised as being provoked by the pill. In two patients seen by the author the movements stopped after withdrawal of the pill.

Conclusion

A wide range of neurological complications of drug therapy have been described. The particular problems created by the need for polypharmacy in many neurological disorders has been highlighted. A full history of all drugs taken by the patient within the last twelve months is now an essential part of any clinical history.

Chapter 25

NEUROLOGICAL INVESTIGATION

Neurological investigations are potentially dangerous. The decision to embark on full neurological investigation must be based on a firm clinical diagnosis and a full appreciation of the potential hazards.

In Chapters 8 and 9 some of the applications of the various tests were indicated. Unfortunately the simple and harmless tests are widely abused because of their safety. Faced with a seriously ill patient it can be very difficult to arrange an immediate E.E.G. or scan due to a queue of patients having routine exclusory investigations for "headaches" or "faints". In fact, in both situations the main investigation should be the history and very few patients should require further investigation.

With the exception of a few neurotics, most patients are interested only in a reasonable explanation of their symptoms and symptomatic treatment or reassurance. Very few patients demand or welcome extensive investigation to prove that there is nothing wrong. Overinvestigation is a product of inadequate clinical ability, *not* evidence of diagnostic skill.

The chances of doing a patient serious harm are greatest in neurology. The whole aim of this book has been to attempt to provide the necessary clinical framework to enable the neurological beginner to approach neurological diagnosis and investigation in a rational way.

The most easily performed, and possibly the only special investigation undertaken by the majority of doctors is a lumbar puncture. A considerable portion of this chapter will therefore be devoted to a discussion of this much abused investigation.

LUMBAR PUNCTURE

Few lumbar punctures as such are performed in neurological units. Lumbar puncture and cerebrospinal fluid (C.S.F.) examination are usually incidental to the performance of a myelogram or an air encephalogram. In spite of repeated pleas from neurologists and neurosurgeons, general physicians in hospitals that lack neurological facilities continue to regard lumbar puncture as an alternative to more precise diagnostic procedures such as angiography. Used in this way the test may be extremly hazardous and far from helping to clarify the situation the neurological unit may have to

accept a moribund patient requiring life-saving procedures instead of diagnosis.

On one occasion a general medical firm borrowed a bed on the neurological service during their "take" day. Unknown to the neurologists a lumbar puncture was performed on a teenage girl with a short history of headache, vomiting and ataxia. Not only was a pressure into the bulb of the manometer recorded but a second manometer was mounted in the first so that the rise in pressure when the Queckenstedt test was performed could be seen. Fortunately this patient, with a cerebellar tumour, survived this potentially lethal investigation and the C.S.F. was quite normal apart from the grossly raised pressure, so that no useful information was gained.

Apparently the reason for embarking on the lumbar puncture was, "because there was no papilloedema". This is a perennial fallacy. Often a whole series of doctors will take a vote on whether or not a patient has papilloedema and then require a neurologist to give a casting vote. The writer would refuse to do so. If the history is such that there seems to be a possibility that the intracranial pressure is rising, *whether or not* there is papilloedema is of no consequence—lumbar puncture should not be attempted. It would seem likely that the risk of coning is greater in the very acute situation where papilloedema has not had time to develop than where a long slow pressure rise has already led to some compensatory brain shifts and some sort of equilibrium has been established.

Although this may seem a strange way to introduce a description intended to make lumbar puncture easier to perform, it would be unforgivable not to include these reservations and I would suggest that whenever a lumbar puncture is contemplated the following questions should be asked:

1. Why am I doing this—is it because it is the only test available to me?
2. What positive information will it give me? Just to see that it is normal is a dubious indication.
3. Is this a potentially hazardous situation, is there anything in the history to suggest that the patient has raised intracranial pressure?

Some may ask, "Why not do a careful lumbar puncture?"

This implies that the majority of lumbar punctures are *careless*. When one hears patients relate details of previous lumbar punctures, this is possibly true! Quite often when one suggests admitting a patient to hospital they say, "Yes, but promise not to do a lumbar 'punch'." This generally used malapropism has quite a strong basis in fact in many patients' experience! The answer to the "careful" lumbar puncture question is that there can be no such thing. Either the subarachnoid space is entered by a needle or it is not. Once a hole is made the fluid will continue to leak out after the needle is withdrawn. Although a smaller needle may slow the rate of coning the risk is still present.

Indications for the Examination of the C.S.F.

1. *Peripheral Nerve Diseases*

Suspected Guillain–Barré syndrome (acute infective poly-neuritis).
Diabetic polyneuropathy, especially the proximal variety affecting the leg.
Suspected hypertrophic polyneuritis (Dejerine–Sottas disease).

In fact, lumbar puncture is a useful investigation in all cases of peripheral neuropathy.

2. *Suspected C.N.S. Infection*

Suspected meningitis—viral or bacterial.
Suspected fungal meningitis.
Neural involvement by syphilis.

3. *Suspected Intracranial Bleeding*

Suspected subarachnoid haemorrhage. (Remember that an intracerebral clot may act as a space-occupying lesion and if focal signs are present it is as well to take neurological advice before doing an L.P. An hour or so delay in confirming subarachnoid haemorrhage is not going to affect the outcome.)

4. *Suspected Multiple Sclerosis*

In some patients, raised C.S.F. protein, a positive Pandy test, a paretic Lange curve and raised gamma globulin may be found. At least half the patients have normal C.S.F. so that the examination is not exclusory.

Contraindications to Lumbar Puncture

1. *Local Sepsis*

Severe pustular acne on the back, or infected bedsores greatly increase the risk of C.S.F. examination, and may possibly result in iatrogenic meningitis.

2. *Unconsciousness*

Over sixty per cent of unconscious patients do *not* have neurological disease, so that the C.S.F. will be normal. The forty per cent who do have neurological problems are likely to be unconscious because of an intracranial catastrophe, and the chances of a lumbar puncture making the situation worse are considerable. Unless infection seems likely, lumbar puncture should await neurological advice.

3. *Headache*

With the exception of infection or subarachnoid haemorrhage (with their associated signs of meningeal irritation) lumbar puncture is obviously the most dangerous way of investigating headache!

4. *Suspected Raised Intracranial Pressure*

Any patient with headaches who has definite signs of an intracerebral lesion in the hemisphere or in the posterior fossa should not have a lumbar puncture.

5. *Suspected Spinal Cord Compression*

If a lumbar puncture is done in this situation the acute alteration of the C.S.F. dynamics, especially during the Queckenstedt test may lead to abrupt worsening of the cord compression. Furthermore, it is extremely difficult to perform a myelogram within a week of a lumbar puncture as the contrast medium easily enters the subdural space under these circumstances. Therefore, not only may the patient be acutely worsened clinically but the necessary test may be made impossible. A planned myelogram with the neurosurgeons alerted is the correct way to handle the situation in which the patient appears to have rapidly developing cord compression.

6. *Neck Stiffness*

Finally, we must consider neck stiffness. This is widely recognised as the prime indication that the patient has a subarachnoid haemorrhage or meningeal infection. But it must also be pointed out that the physical sign that accompanies herniation of the cerebellar tonsils through the foramen magnum is neck stiffness. Usually the clinical course of a patient with infection or haemorrhage will be a fairly acute one. If a patient becomes drowsy with a stiff neck after several weeks of illness it is as well to consider the possibility of coning and withhold lumbar puncture while urgent neurological advice is obtained.

The Technique of Lumbar Puncture

Notwithstanding the reservations and contraindications to the performance of a lumbar puncture, once the decision has been taken, it is worth doing properly. Many patients have been investigated for iatrogenic "subarachnoid haemorrhage", and once there is blood in the C.S.F. from a traumatic tap there is nothing that can be done about it. The morbidity of lumbar puncture; i.e. backache and headache are greater in tense individuals whose worst fears are realised when they experience a really badly performed lumbar puncture. This is not to say that these symptoms never occur after technically perfect lumbar punctures. The problem is that many doctors qualify without the advantage of performing a lumbar puncture under supervision. Once qualified they teach themselves, to the patient's discomfort!

Positioning the Patient

The single most important factor in performing an easy, atraumatic tap is the positioning of the patient. Yet, very often the most junior nurse is left to put the patient on their side while the doctor washes his hands. If you are right-handed always have the patient on his left side as shown in the diagrams; even if you have to move the bed out from a wall to do so.

1. Get the patient right on to the edge of the bed—this provides firm support and helps keep the back straight.

2. Put one or two pillows between the legs—this provides support for the top leg and prevents the patient rolling forwards. By providing support for the upper arm it also prevents the shoulders rolling over.

3. There is no need forcibly to flex the neck, or for a strapping nurse to suffocate the patient in a fully flexed position—if the patient is in a comfortable position his co-operation is encouraged.

Note in Figure 25.1 the incorrect, rolled over "Rokeby

Figure 25.1. Incorrect ("Rokeby Venus") position

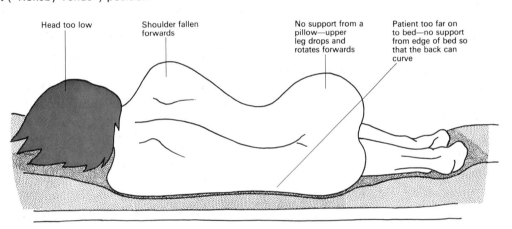

Head too low

Shoulder fallen forwards

No support from a pillow—upper leg drops and rotates forwards

Patient too far on to bed—no support from edge of bed so that the back can curve

Vertebral position with patient in incorrect position

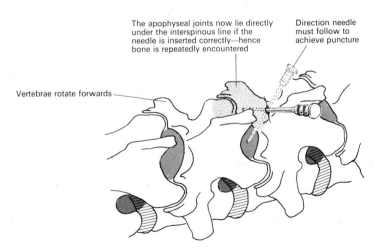

The apophyseal joints now lie directly under the interspinous line if the needle is inserted correctly—hence bone is repeatedly encountered

Direction needle must follow to achieve puncture

Vertebrae rotate forwards

Figure 25.2. Correct position

Head in comfortable neutral position need not be forcibly flexed

Top shoulder square

Supporting pillows hold top leg up in the air

Back is straight and vertical

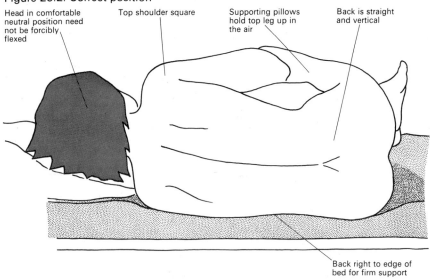

Back right to edge of bed for firm support

Vertebral position with patient correctly positioned

L3/4 disc

Target area lies in midline beneath spinous process

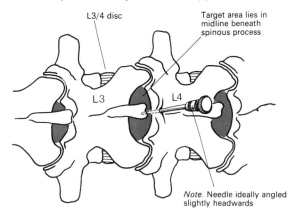

Note. Needle ideally angled slightly headwards

Figure 25.3. Correct position from above

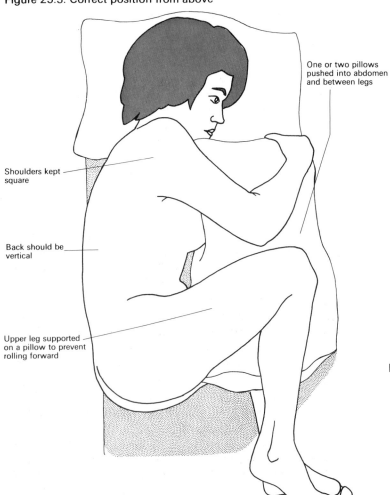

One or two pillows pushed into abdomen and between legs

Shoulders kept square

Back should be vertical

Upper leg supported on a pillow to prevent rolling forward

Figure 25.4. Some common stilette problems

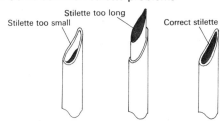

Stilette too small

Stilette too long

Correct stilette

Venus" posture and the effect this has on the target area between the laminae of the two vertebrae and compare this with the correct position shown on Figures 25.2 and 25.3. The importance of repeatedly checking that the back is vertical (which keeps the target area directly beneath the spines) must be stressed.

Sterile Procedures

Meningitis after lumbar puncture is exceptionally rare. The author knows only of one example in the last fifteen years in hospitals with which he has been associated. Nevertheless, sterile precautions should be observed. The author prefers not to wear rubber gloves as they spoil the feel. This would seem to be quite safe provided the hands are correctly scrubbed and the shaft of the needle is not touched during the procedure.

Equipment

The equipment provided varies so much from hospital to hospital that no specific advice can be given. However, the most important thing is to check that all the needles, stopcocks and manometers fit each other. One may have to "cannibalise" several packs to get a suitable kit, but it is worth the effort. Then check that the stilette on the needle chosen fits flush to the end of the needle (Figure 25.4), if it does not, it becomes a very traumatic weapon. Check that the stilette is not stuck, check that the stopcock rotates freely, and check the flow direction in the different stopcock positions. Finally make sure that the manometer is not broken inside its pack. Having established that there are not going to be any holdups caused by equipment failure, the actual lumbar puncture can begin.

1. Select a sharp, medium-sized needle. (Needle sizes are 18, 19, 20 and 21—the higher the number the smaller the bore and length.) A number 19 is best for general use, a number 21 for small people and children other than infants.

2. Select the interspace between the spines of L3 and L4. This lies just below the line joining the anterior superior iliac spines. Mark the postion of the spines with a ball pen for further reference if needed.

3. Clean the area with whatever skin cleansing agent is available, and finally with alcohol. Allow to dry. Then finally prepare the skin over an area about six inches square, centred on the chosen space, with either mercurochrome or iodine (Figure 25.5).

4. Arrange three towels as shown in Figure 25.6. The upper one should not hang down on to the needle, but it is very useful for moving the patient about and checking the position of the anterior superior iliac spine if the landmarks

are lost. The writer prefers not to use the towel with a window in it that is sometimes provided. It makes it difficult to see where you are, is hard to keep in position and tends to fall down on to the needle.

5. While the skin preparation is drying, drawn up 1–2 cc. of two per cent lignocaine in a small syringe. There is no need to infiltrate the area with 5–10 cc. as some do. This usually causes a lot of bleeding and turns the entry route into a bloody mush that destroys the "feel". Warn the patient that the local anaesthetic will "sting" for about ten seconds. Raise a skin bleb about 1 cm. across as shown in Figure 25.7 and then inject another 0·5 ml just below the skin. Massage it in with a finger. If the skin is not held taut as in the diagram, you may find that the area you have anaesthetised is about one inch from the midline.

Check that the skin is anaesthetised with a small needle. Then check that the patient has not altered position and warn him that he will feel a pushing sensation against the back. Ask him to tell you immediately if he feels any sharp pain. Holding the skin as shown in Figure 25.7, push the needle through the skin. This may be difficult but do not lunge at it or you will suddenly plunge in too deeply. As soon as you are through the skin check that the position is correct and then penetrate the dense supraspinous ligament (Figure 25.8). Once you have done so, stop, let go of the needle and see that it is at 90 degrees to the back. A correct line through this ligament is vital; if the needle has been deflected off line start again.

7. Once the needle is correctly aligned push it gently inwards and slightly towards the head. Usually the interspinous ligament is quite easily penetrated and little effort is needed.

8. If the line is correct at about $1\frac{1}{2}$–2 inches deep a slight resistance will be felt. Check the needle line, and if it is in the correct position, give the needle a little push quite firmly but only for about $\frac{1}{8}$ inch. This will penetrate the ligamentum flavum with a slight "pop". As the same push often also penetrates the dura *do not* advance the needle any further without withdrawing the stilette from the needle. If no fluid emerges it is always worth rotating the needle slightly as a nerve root may be lying across the end. If no fluid emerges replace the stilette (*never* advance the needle without the stilette in position) and advance the needle another $\frac{1}{8}$ inch and repeat. Continue advancing in this way until fluid emerges, firm resistance is encountered or the patient complains of pain down either leg.

9. If firm resistance is encountered *do not* force the needle, it may be against the opposite intervertebral disc and this can be damaged. If a nerve root is hit, find out which leg was affected. If the pain was in the right leg, withdraw the

Figure 25.5. Preparing the area for the lumbar puncture

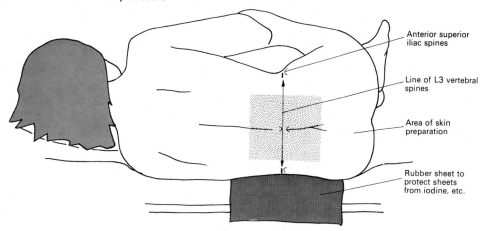

Anterior superior iliac spines

Line of L3 vertebral spines

Area of skin preparation

Rubber sheet to protect sheets from iodine, etc.

Figure 25.6. Towelling up for the procedure

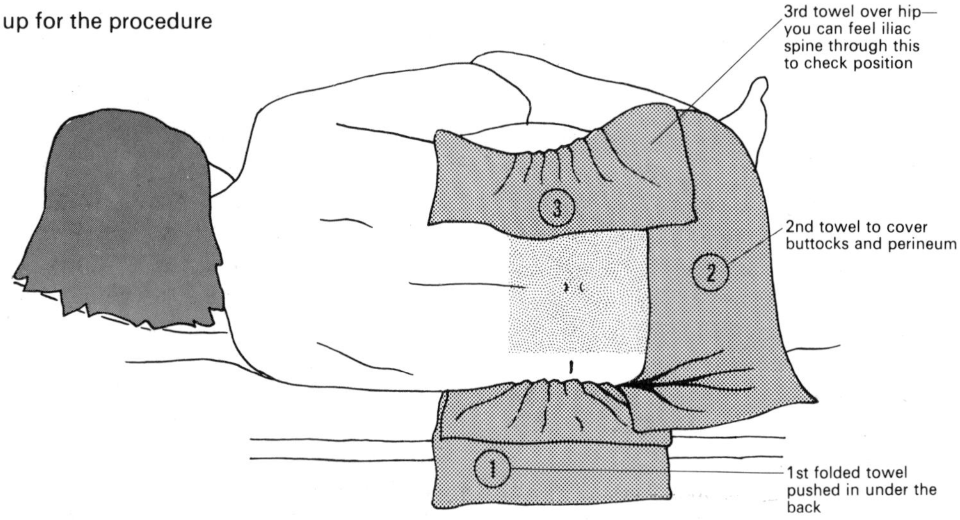

3rd towel over hip—you can feel iliac spine through this to check position

2nd towel to cover buttocks and perineum

1st folded towel pushed in under the back

Figure 25.7. Injecting the skin

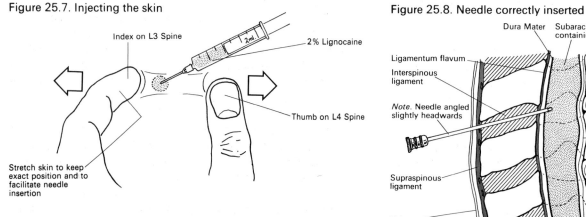

Index on L3 Spine

2% Lignocaine

Thumb on L4 Spine

Stretch skin to keep exact position and to facilitate needle insertion

Figure 25.8. Needle correctly inserted

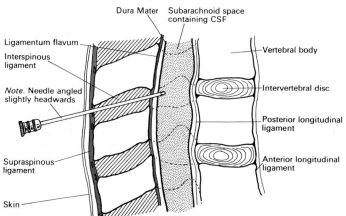

Dura Mater

Subarachnoid space containing CSF

Ligamentum flavum

Interspinous ligament

Note. Needle angled slightly headwards

Vertebral body

Intervertebral disc

Posterior longitudinal ligament

Anterior longitudinal ligament

Supraspinous ligament

Skin

needle almost to the skin and then re-insert it angled slightly towards the left side, i.e. hopefully nearer to the midline than on the previous needle track. To pull back only half an inch or so is not sufficient. The needle will usually go straight back down the same track and hit the same root again!

10. Do not have more than three attempts in an interspace and do not be afraid to ask someone more senior to try at another interspace (usually L2–3). One may have a failure after a hundred or more successful punctures and you will not be thanked for traumatising three interspaces before you seek advice. Remember that a bloody tap often creates more problems than it solves. Never attempt a tap above L2–3 or the spinal cord may be damaged.

11. Assuming you are in the subarachnoid space—as soon as fluid appears re-insert the stilette. You *cannot* estimate the pressure from the rate of flow from the needle and the pressure should be checked with the manometer as the first part of the test. If the pressure goes very high (i.e. above 250 mm. H_2O) do not panic and pull the needle out and spill the fluid. Collect the fluid from the manometer but do not take any more fluid off. (At 300 mm H_2O the manometer contains 7–8 ml. of fluid which is adequate for all tests, and having run the risk to get the fluid it is silly to waste the specimen.) If the pressure is normal—as it should be if the case was properly evaluated—take the manometer contents and then two further specimens of about 5 ml. each (about half an inch of fluid in the standard bottles that are usually provided). A 2 cc. specimen should also be taken into a fluoride bottle for glucose estimation.

12. Remove the needle with a gentle pull—there is no need for a dramatic flourish, with a thumb placed immediately on the exit hole. The hole in the dura is the one that needs plugging and that is impossible! Place a sterile gauze square over the hole held on with Nobecutane spray or plaster. The traditional collodion has no special significance and the lid is usually stuck. The author once ruined a pair of trousers as a result of the sudden freeing of the lid by the assisting nurse.

Following the puncture the nurses will traditionally confine the patient to bed for twenty-four hours with all the minor discomforts that implies. It is advisable for the patient to lie almost flat (one pillow) for four hours. He may then get up. If he subsequently gets a headache there will be no difficulty persuading him to stay in bed, but relatively few patients get a headache if they have not developed one within four hours. Occasionally the onset is delayed to twelve or twenty-four hours and the headache may then take several days to clear.

Never use a syringe to aspirate C.S.F. during a lumbar puncture. The reason for low C.S.F. pressure may be a serious one, such as tonsillar impaction or spinal block, and active aspiration may cause a disaster. At a less dangerous level, if the needle is blocked by a root lying across the end, severe damage and prolonged sciatica may occur if the root is "aspirated". If turning the needle fails to produce a good flow retap the patient in another interspace.

Finally, make sure that the bottles have been labelled 1, 2 and 3 correctly (in order collected) especially if the tap was a traumatic one so that the red cells can be counted in sequential specimens. This is not foolproof. Even with a clean tap a major vein may be hit while penetrating the dura and continual severe bloodstaining may occur and mimic a subarachnoid haemorrhage, which, of course, it is. A clue to this situation is a tendency for the blood to swirl in the C.S.F. as it emerges from the needle, whereas with a true subarachnoid haemorrhage the blood is completely admixed. Furthermore, if the fluid is centrifuged immediately, xanthochromia of the supernatant indicates contamination by blood prior to the lumbar puncture.

What to do if the Pressure is Abnormally High

A pressure over 200 mm H_2O is technically abnormal. However, in a very tense patient, especially if a difficult tap was performed, the pressure may easily exceed this level. Allow the patient to relax for a few minutes and recheck the pressure. If the patient is extremely obese and has been held fully flexed the intracranial pressure will be elevated by increased venous pressure in the head. Gently straighten the patient out and allow him to breathe fairly deeply for a few minutes before rechecking the pressure.

If the pressure is genuinely elevated and especially if it is in excess of 300 mm. H_2O take the manometer specimen and pull the needle out. Examine the patient's pupils immediately and record their size and symmetry. Take the patient's pulse rate and blood pressure and chart them on a head-injury observation chart.

Raise the bottom of the bed and lie the patient face down without a pillow. If neurosurgical help is available advise them of the situation at once. If no neurosurgical help is available either mix up a bottle of "Urevert" or obtain a bottle of ten per cent Mannitol solution. These should be given by intravenous infusion over twenty minutes if the pupils become irregular, the conscious level alters, the pulse slows or the blood pressure starts to rise. Arrangements for transfer to a neurosurgical unit should be made without delay. Often no specific measures are necessary but one should never under-estimate the lethal potential of this situation.

There is no evidence that attempts to replace the C.S.F. with saline before removing the needle are of value. Raising the pressure may encourage further leaking, and during the unavoidable movements of the needle while fitting the syringe the dura may be torn and this will increase the rate of C.S.F. leakage.

What to do if the Pressure is Abnormally Low

It is not generally realised that a low pressure may also carry considerable danger for the patient. A pressure of less than 80 mm. H_2O can be regarded as below the normal range. As previously noted never use a syringe to aspirate C.S.F. This will usually apply to the situation where the pressure is lower than usual. When lumbar puncture was the only neurological investigation available, one of the well recognised causes of low C.S.F. pressure in a patient who had a cerebral disturbance was a subdural haematoma. Nobody would recommend lumbar puncture to diagnose this condition today. When the outflow of the C.S.F. into the spinal canal is impaired, because the cerebellar tonsils are impacted in the foramen magnum, the pressure is not transmitted to the spinal theca. Similarly, with a complete spinal block the pressure may fall, and the difficulty in obtaining C.S.F. may be magnified by the very viscous fluid due to the raised C.S.F. protein (the Froin syndrome). Attempts to aspirate fluid may cause irreversible cord damage.

CASE REPORT

A young man was admitted with several days history of headaches, dizziness, unsteady gait, a stiff neck and a slight temperature. His C.S.F. was examined. The pressure was 85 mm. H_2O. The fluid contained thirty-five lymphocytes. No firm diagnosis was made but the possible significance of the low pressure was not appreciated. He was found dead in his bed two hours later. He had a cerebellar abscess with a tonsillar pressure cone.

This example also points out the other risk, that of mistaking neck stiffness caused by tonsillar coning for meningitis. The management of low pressure is the same as for raised pressure.

Although details of a technique for performing lumbar puncture have been given, considerable stress has been laid on the importance of carefully assessing the need for the test, and the potential hazards of the procedure. Because occasionally well-intentioned and carefully planned lumbar punctures may reveal raised pressure or low pressure the management of these complications has been included.

Some may wonder why the Queckenstedt test has not been discussed. It is another time-honoured part of the ritual without special or reliable significance. In the presence of a cerebral lesion the performance of the test may prove lethal; with spinal cord compression it may complete the cord transection, and if cord compression was suspected the patient should be having a myelogram and not a simple lumbar puncture. A quick cough by the patient while recording the pressure will reveal a brisk 10 mm. rise and fall of the pressure and this is all that is needed. It was the thoughtless following of the ritual that led to the Queckenstedt test being performed on the patient quoted in the first part of this discussion.

ELECTROENCEPHALOGRAPHY (E.E.G.)

The E.E.G. has the considerable advantages of being harmless, inexpensive and easily repeatable. Unfortunately E.E.G. findings are relatively non-specific and their value depends on the careful correlation of E.E.G. findings with the history and physical findings in the patient. For this reason the physician ordering the E.E.G. should have a clear idea as to what information he expects it to provide. The E.E.G. can give both false negative and false positive results and serious errors can only be avoided if this is recognised.

Technique

The patient sits in a comfortable chair in a quiet room and either saline soaked pads or stick-on electrodes are applied to the scalp in internationally agreed positions.

Considerable skill is involved in assuring good electrical contact to avoid artefacts. Recordings are made on a multi-channel machine using special arrangements of electrodes (montages) in anterior-posterior and transverse positions to provide a grid of information. This enables the technician to isolate an abnormality in two planes.

A resting record is taken with the patient sitting quietly and opening and closing his eyes to command. This reveals the basic alpha rhythm which normally "blocks" (i.e. attentuates or disappears) on eye opening. The resting record may be normal.

Then the first provocative procedure begins. The patient is asked to hyperventilate for three minutes. This normally causes a slowing in rhythms and increase in amplitude. This accentuates abnormalities and often provokes epileptic discharges in epileptic patients.

Finally a flickering strobe light is placed in front of the patient and the flicker rate varied. Many normal people show a following response; phasic potentials over the occipital pole at the same rate as the flicker. In photic-sensitive epilepsy epileptic discharges and even an epileptic fit may be provoked.

When the clinical suspicion of epilepsy or an intracerebral lesion is high and a routine E.E.G. is normal further provocative measures can be used coupled with special electrodes. The inner and inferior surfaces of the temporal lobe are inaccessible to normal electrodes. An electrode in the pharynx or more commonly a wire inserted under the base of the skull through a special needle (called a sphenoidal electrode) are used to pick up abnormalities in this area.

This special recording technique may be coupled with a sleep recording, or provoked by a sleep dose of short acting barbiturate drugs given intravenously. This greatly increases the detection of abnormalities in the temporal lobes in particular.

Interpretation

A full discussion of E.E.G. abnormalities would require several chapters; only a brief mention of the most significant wave forms is possible.

α Rhythm: The alpha rhythm consists of cyclic activity at a rate of 8–12 Hz maximal in the posterior leads and most easily seen when the eyes are closed. The voltage is normally slightly lower over the dominant hemisphere. Unilateral absence of the alpha rhythm indicates a lesion in the appropriate hemisphere.

β Rhythm: The beta rhythm consists of fast activity at rates of 20–22 Hz usually seen in the frontal leads. It is increased in anxious patients and markedly increased by all sedative drugs and tranquillisers. Asymmetry of beta activity may indicate an underlying lesion on the side of the reduction.

θ Rhythm: Theta waves occur at rates of 4–7 Hz and cause the most diagnostic confusion. They are normally present in childhood but diminish with maturation of the E.E.G. in adolescence. They often reappear during overbreathing and a symmetrical "increase in theta activity" in the temporal leads is often of dubious significance. As with other rhythms marked asymmetry is significant and suggests a lesion in the temporal lobe on the side of the theta activity.

δ Rhythm: Delta waves are the most significant and ominous abnormalities seen in the E.E.G. They consist of slow waves of very low to extremely high voltage at rates of 1–3 Hz. In children delta activity is often seen in the resting record, and is greatly accentuated by overbreathing. This is not pathological in children but is grossly abnormal in the adult. A focal delta wave abnormality nearly always indicates a serious lesion in the underlying brain.

Clinical Applications

The use of the E.E.G. in the investigation of attacks of unconsciousness is discussed in Chapter 22. The importance of careful clinical evaluation of the attack must be emphasised. The E.E.G. cannot say whether someone is epileptic or not, and if a syncopal attack is diagnosed an E.E.G. is unnecessary. Conversely, if the patient had an unequivocal epileptic convulsion a normal E.E.G. cannot alter the diagnosis. Overinterpretation of minor abnorma-

lities may condemn a patient who has fainted to years of unnecessary restrictions and anticonvulsant drugs. Even worse, an epileptic patient may remain untreated and be allowed to continue normal activities because the E.E.G. was normal. The potential value varies in different types of epilepsy. In petit mal the E.E.G. is invariably diagnostically abnormal. In grand mal epilepsy in forty per cent patients the E.E.G. is normal and this "false negative" rate may be even higher in patients with nocturnal epilepsy and akinetic grand mal. When akinetic grand mal or grand mal is preceded by myoclonic jerking a characteristic "poly-spike and wave" pattern may be found. The E.E.G. is of limited value in the follow-up of epileptic patients unless an underlying lesion is suspected. The E.E.G. may become normal as children with epilepsy mature in spite of continuing attacks. Conversely a grossly abnormal E.E.G. may persist in patients who have been attack-free for years.

In the investigation of a suspected intracranial lesion there are several problems. Quite substantial extracerebral lesions may fail to produce any E.E.G. abnormality, whereas small intrinsic tumours may produce subtle E.E.G. abnormalities years before investigation confirms the presence of a tumour. When there are obvious clinical findings the E.E.G. usually merely confirms the location of the lesion but cannot provide conclusive evidence as to the nature of the lesion—it cannot distinguish a recent cerebral vascular accident from a tumour for example. In the investigation of headache there are difficulties due to the wide range of abnormalities that have been reported in association with migraine, abnormalities that might suggest a neoplastic lesion in "non-migrainous" subjects.

Having stressed the limitations of E.E.G. in diagnostic neurology it is only fair to reiterate the immense value of the test as a screening procedure. It is an extremely useful investigation in patients with atypical psychiatric disorders and dementia even in the absence of physical signs.

Other E.E.G. Related Investigations

Many other investigations have been developed utilising surface electrode recording over the head. Somato-sensory evoked potentials have limited clinical value at present but improved recording techniques may increase their use and significance in the future.

One of these techniques has rapidly become established as a valuable addition to investigational techniques. This is the visual evoked response (V.E.R.). The technique is a useful measure of optic nerve function. Recording electrodes are placed on the occipital poles and the patient sits in front of a screen. A continually flickering chequerboard pattern is projected on the screen while the patient fixes his eye on a central target light. Numerous sweeps triggered by the pattern changer are averaged and a slow biphasic potential is produced. The latency of this response is calculated and has to be standardised for each apparatus.

A prolonged latency indicates damage to the optic nerve of the eye being tested. The test has particular value in suspected multiple sclerosis; prolonged latencies may be detected in clinically normal eyes in these patients.

RADIO-ISOTOPE SCANNING

Radio-isotope scanning depends on the uptake of radio-isotopes by highly vascular tumours, abscesses or oedematous cerebral infarcts. Originally radio-isotopes of mercury and arsenic were used but a long half-life and concentration in the kidneys were drawbacks. Currently radioactive technetium is used. This has a very fast pick-up rate and a short half-life allowing immediate scanning with little risk.

The isotope is administered intravenously and the whole head scanned in four positions AP, PA, right and left lateral. Either x-ray plates, a coloured print-out or screen display are possible.

The limitations of isotope scanning are:

1. The venous sinuses, scalp muscles and face all show as very dense areas on the scan due to the repeated circulation of isotope during the scanning. This leaves relatively small clear areas in which abnormal uptake can be detected.

2. The resolution of the technique is such that lesions less than 2 cm. in diameter are unlikely to be detected.

3. A small posterior fossa lesion lying adjacent to the normal areas of uptake can easily be missed. An isotope scan is not particularly helpful in excluding a posterior fossa lesion.

4. Slow growing tumours, avascular tumours and non-eodematous masses do not concentrate isotope.

These problems mean that a high percentage of false negative scans are possible in the most difficult clinical situations. Conversely, false positive scans may occur with asymmetrical uptake of isotope in normal tissues. This often happens when there is scalp bruising or a recent craniotomy limiting the use of the scan in these situations.

Isotope scanning is most likely to be helpful in patients with suspected intracranial metastases, cerebral abscess or arterio-venous malformations.

Isotope scanning cannot be regarded as an exclusory investigation and further investigation must be pursued even if the scan is negative. In spite of its limitations until E.M.I. Scanners are universally available isotope scanning is likely to remain a widely used procedure.

CEREBRAL ARTERIOGRAPHY

Cerebral angiography may be performed by direct needle puncture of the carotid or vertebral arteries or by catheterisation of the vessel origin via the aortic arch. Catheterisation is normally used to demonstrate the vertebral arterial circulation but selective puncture of the internal carotid artery is used in cerebral investigation. The use of arteriography in the investigation of cerebral vascular disease has been discussed in Chapter 9.

Angiography still has an important place in the investigation of cerebral lesions even when E.M.I. scanning is available.

Technique

Under general anaesthetic a needle or catheter is inserted into the required vessel. The contrast material is injected by hand as a single bolus and serial films are taken. The first film shows the arterial tree and should include the needle site to exclude sub-intimal injection of contrast which could occlude the vessel if further injections are made. The second film shows the capillary phase—outlining the parenchyma of the brain as a fine network of vessels. The final film shows the venous phase as the contrast enters the great veins. The timing of films varies depending on whether hand changing of the plates or a multiple series changer is available. Both antero-posterior series and lateral series are taken as routine. If cerebral arterial aneurysm or a subdural haematoma are suspected oblique views are taken.

Following the procedure finger pressure over the needle site is maintained for five minutes and the neck observed for several hours in case a haematoma develops.

Cerebral lesions may be detected in the following ways:

1. A tumour may displace known vessels by a direct or remote effect indicating the site and size of the lesion and adjacent brain swelling.

2. The tumour may have a pathological circulation. This may consist of a profuse arterial and capillary network producing what is known as a "tumour blush", an appearance very characteristic of meningiomas. Malignant gliomas may contain abnormal new vessels, sinusoidal in type often acting as an arterio-venous shunt. In this situation either the abnormal vessels may be detected or early filling of the veins may be noticed even during the arterial phase—both these findings usually indicate a malignant glioma.

3. Avascular or oedematous lesions may produce bare areas in the arterial and capillary phases. However the parietal area is usually relatively avascular and the best

evidence of a tumour in this region is displacement of the central vein on the late films.

In the posterior fossa, not only may tumours be demonstrated in the same way but also important surgical information as to the blood supply of the tumour and adjacent brain stem may be obtained.

The indications for carotid angiography may be summarised as:

1. Suspected carotid arterial disease (see Chapter 9).
2. Suspected arterial aneurysm or AV malformation
3. Suspected cerebral neoplasm.

In all these situations deterioration in the patient's condition may occur following the investigation and prompt treatment of cerebral oedema and if necessary neurosurgical intervention should be immediately considered when angiography has demonstrated a cerebral lesion.

PNEUMOENCEPHALOGRAPHY

This investigation is carried out by performing a lumbar puncture with the patient in a sitting position. The patient is usually anaesthetised and the head is suspended in a harness. Special tilting chairs have been developed but are not absolutely necessary for a successful examination. A sample of C.S.F. is taken and 10–15 mls. of air are introduced by syringe. Lateral films are taken of the posterior fossa and foramen magnum. These films demonstrate the position of the cerebellar tonsils (indicating that it is safe to proceed) and the fourth ventricle and aqueducts. More air, usually about 50–60 ccs. is introduced and by tilting the head the entire ventricular system and the surface architecture of the hemisphere and basal cisterns can be demonstrated. The technique is time consuming and may take up to one and a half hours so that the test should not be embarked upon casually. If in the first film the cerebellar tonsils are found to be herniated through the foramen magnum the test should be terminated immediately and neurosurgical advice obtained.

The main advantages of pneumoencephalography are:

1. Not only masses but atrophy of the cerebral hemispheres or cerebellum can be detected.
2. The size and shape of the brain stem can be seen — the best way to detect a brain stem glioma
3. Lesions in the prepontine cistern and cerebello-pontine angle are well demonstrated.
4. Lesions in the region of the optic chiasm, particularly extrasellar extensions of pituitary tumours are well demonstrated.

Pneumoencephalography is contraindicated if a cerebral hemisphere tumour is strongly suspected, a cerebellar tumour is suspected or if intracranial pressure is raised even if the clinical diagnosis is thought to be benign intracranial hypertension. The risk of fatal herniation is too great to perform the test in these circumstances.

The main indications for pneumoencephalography are dementia (a tumour having been already excluded), suspected cerebellar degeneration, suspected brain stem glioma and suprasellar neoplasms (provided intracranial pressure is not raised).

When investigating for suprasellar extension of pituitary tumours it is important to give 200 mgm. hydrocortisone I.V. before anaesthesia to prevent shock due to pituitary-adrenal failure.

One special advantage of the test is the demonstration of the dynamics of C.S.F. flow. Fifteen years ago a new syndrome originally called "low-pressure hydrocephalus" but now called "normal pressure hydrocephalus" was discovered. In this situation the encephalogram shows marked ballooning of the third and lateral ventricles but no air can be induced to go over the surface of the brain. Shunting procedures to reduce intraventricular pressure may allow dramatic restoration of cerebral function.

If this syndrome is suspected a further test may be useful. This is a Rhisa Scan (Radioactive human iodinised serum albumen). This is injected intrathecally and the brain is then scanned at intervals over the next twenty-four hours. In "normal pressure hydrocephalus" the isotope accumulates in the ventricular system and remains there. In a normal patient the isotope flows over the surface of the hemisphere and is reabsorbed into the venous circulation. This is an experimental procedure.

Following pneumoencephalography the patient invariably has a severe headache and may develop a high fever. A repeat C.S.F. examination at this stage usually reveals a high protein and a pleomorphic leucocytosis. This seems to be a response to the air. These symptoms settle within forty-eight hours with simple analgesics.

MYELOGRAPHY

Myelography consists of the introduction of a contrast material into the C.S.F. to demonstrate the spinal cord, the subarachnoid space and in some instances the foramen magnum, basal cisterns and cerebello-pontine angles.

There are three main techniques now in use in different clinical situations.

Myodil myelography (sodium iophendylate in oil): This

agent is heavier than C.S.F. and can be manoeuvred by gravity to outline the subarachnoid space. Lumbar disc lesions, spinal cord compressive lesions and cervical canal lesions can be demonstrated. The disadvantages are the limited amount of contrast (6–9 ccs. are usually used) and its density making spinal cord demonstration difficult. It is also difficult to examine the dorsal spinal cord anteriorly as the contrast quickly flows over the normal curvature of the thoracic spine. Nevertheless myodil myelography remains the investigation of choice for spinal canal lesions in most centres.

Water Miscible Myelography (Dimer X): Water miscible contrast material mixes with C.S.F. and is useful for demonstrating disc lesions in the lumbar/sacral area. The contrast is rapidly absorbed. Unfortunately, the medium is highly irritant and cannot be run up to cord level or severe painful spasms occur. This greatly limits its value in neurology.

Air and Gas Myelography: This is the best way of demonstrating the spinal cord itself but is extremely unpleasant for the patient. Almost 100 ccs. of C.S.F. are removed and replaced by air or CO_2. The cord is then suspended in air. For accurate visualisation tomography is necessary. The sequelae are the same as pneumoencephalography with severe headache and fever.

The main indications are the demonstration of intrinsic cord tumours, cord atrophy and hydromyelia—in which there is a dynamic sac of C.S.F. in the cervical cord which empties when the patient is tipped head down as in myodil myelography. In air myelography the cervical cord can be outlined with the patient erect and the swollen cord is detected.

COMPUTERISED AXIAL TOMOGRAPHY (E.M.I. SCANNING)

The E.M.I. Scanner, a computerised densitometry technique, is already established as an outstanding advance in the investigation of intracranial disease.

The only drawback is the enormous expense of the necessary x-ray equipment and computer to process the results. For this reason the techniques previously discussed will remain in use for many years to come; although in many instances an E.M.I. Scan could provide more information at less risk to the patient.

The current brain scanner does have some drawbacks. To reduce the skull-air density interface the head has to be inserted into a rubber bag filled with water. This to some extent limits the lower level that can be scanned and only permits horizontal slice scans to be obtained. The more recent whole body scanner does not require a rubber bag and allows better orbital and posterior fossa scans and coronal slice scans can be made.

When the patient is in position the x-ray apparatus rotates around the head. Two x-ray sources and two detectors allow two adjacent slices to be scanned simultaneously, i.e. three sweeps will complete six slices of either 8 or 13 mm. thickness.

The apparatus swings round 1° at a time through 180°. At each point a full traverse of the x-ray beam is taken before it moves on to the next position. Although the scanning only takes a few minutes the computer takes nearly twenty minutes to perform the necessary calculations which are printed out on Polaroid film.

Very subtle density differences are detectable showing bone, C.S.F., normal brain tissue, oedema and blood, enabling a clear distinction between oedema, haemorrhage, tumour and infarction to be made. A single E.M.I. Scan may provide more information about an intracerebral mass than all other techniques combined.

It is likely that angiography will continue to be used to demonstrate the vascular anatomy of tumours and the state of cerebral vessels but pneumoencephalography will become an uncommon investigation when E.M.I. Scanners are universally available.

In conclusion we can see that neurological investigation is being revolutionised by E.M.I. scanning, but even when universally available the expense and limited scan time available will require that patients are carefully screened by other techniques to justify the need for an E.M.I. Scan.

Hence the careful clinical evaluation detailed in this text and the appropriate use of ancillary investigations will still be necessary in the forseeable future.

Table 16 — THE USE OF SPECIAL TESTS IN NEUROLOGICAL DISORDERS

(It is assumed that routine x-rays of the suspected area have been taken, a chest film is normal and routine haematological and biochemical studies as indicated have been performed.)

TEST	MAIN APPLICATION
ELECTROPHYSIOLOGICAL TESTS	
ELECTROMYOGRAPHY	To distinguish muscle and nerve diseases
NERVE CONDUCTION STUDIES	Peripheral neuropathy and nerve lesions
VISUAL EVOKED RESPONSES	Optic nerve lesions
AUDIOMETRY	Cochlear and auditory nerve lesions
ELECTRONYSTAGMO-GRAPHY	Vestibular nerve and brain stem lesions
ELECTROENCEPHALO-GRAPHY	Suspected epilepsy
	Suspected intracranial pathology
	Routine screening in psychiatric disease
ECHOENCEPHALOGRAPHY	To detect midline shift
ANGIOGRAPHIC STUDIES	
CAROTID ANGIOGRAPHY	Suspected cerebral mass, AV malformations, aneurysm or vascular disease
VERTEBRAL ANGIOGRAPHY	Suspected posterior fossa tumour or AV malformations
ORBITAL VENOGRAPHY	Suspected intra-orbital mass
FLUROSCEIN ANGIOGRAPHY	Suspected papilloedema
OTHER CONTRAST STUDIES	
AIR ENCEPHALOGRAPHY	Suspected cerebral atrophy
	Normal pressure hydrocephalus
	Suprasellar tumour
MYODIL VENTRICULO-GRAPHY	Intraventricular neoplasms, pinealomas and aqueductal stenosis
MYODIL ENCEPHALO-GRAPHY	To demonstrate the basal cisterns and cerebello-pontine angles
MYODIL MYELOGRAPHY	Suspected disc lesions, spinal cord compression and cord tumours
WATER SOLUBLE CONTRAST MYELO-GRAPHY	Lumbar disc lesions
GAS MYELOGRAPHY	Cord atrophy, hydromyelia, intrinsic cord tumour
RADIO-ISOTOPE SCAN	Suspected vascular lesions, oedematous tumours and cerebral metastases
E.M.I. SCANNING	Any suspected intracranial or intra-orbital lesion

---

Table 17 — SPECIAL TESTS USED IN SPECIFIC CLINICAL SITUATIONS

CLINICAL PROBLEM	MOST USEFUL TEST
VISUAL PROBLEMS (depends on type of field defect)	Careful field plotting
	Optic foraminae/sella turcica x-rays
	Visual evoked responses
SUSPECTED PAPILLOEDEMA	Fluroscein angiography
DIPLOPIA	
If variable due to extraocular nerve palsy	Tensilon test / Thyroid function tests / W.R. and blood glucose / Carotid angiography
CEREBELLO-PONTINE ANGLE LESION	Audiometry / Electronystagmography / Myodil encephalography
SUSPECTED CEREBRAL LESION	E.E.G. / Gamma scan / Ultrasound / E.M.I. Scan / Carotid angiogram on appropriate side
SUSPECTED CEREBELLAR LESION	Gamma scan, E.M.I. Scan / Ventriculography / Myodil ventriculogram
CEREBRAL VASCULAR DISEASE	Low carotid angiogram / Aortic arch angiogram
SUSPECTED BRAIN STEM TUMOUR	Air encephalography / Otoneurological studies / Vertebral angiogram
SUSPECTED SPINAL CORD TUMOUR	Myodil myelogram / Air myelogram
PERIPHERAL NERVE DISEASE	Electromyography / Nerve conduction studies / Serum phosphocreatinine kinase
MUSCLE DISEASES	Metabolic studies / Electromyography / Muscle biopsy / Tensilon test
SUSPECTED ROOT SYNDROMES	Myodil myelography
SUSPECTED EPILEPSY	Electroencephalography (further investigation of focal abnormalities)
SUSPECTED MENINGITIS / SUSPECTED SUBARACHNOID HAEMORRHAGE	Lumbar puncture / C.S.F. microscopy and culture

Chapter 26

NEUROLOGICAL COMPLICATIONS OF SYSTEMIC DISORDERS

Throughout this book great emphasis has been placed on the importance of detecting systemic diseases that may present as a neurological illness.

In a general hospital setting the neurological department has an important role in the evaluation of patients already diagnosed as suffering from a specific condition who have subsequently developed a neurological problem.

The potential neurologist therefore requires an extremely good knowledge of general medical and surgical disorders and their potential for causing neurological problems.

Although many of these conditions have been mentioned elsewhere it was felt that a final chapter in which some of these problems were grouped together would be helpful.

The material is considered in seven main sections:

1. Pregnancy and labour.
2. Diabetes mellitus and glucose metabolism.
3. Collagen-vascular disease.
4. Endocrine and metabolic diseases including alcoholism.
5. Cardiovascular diseases.
6. Neoplastic diseases.
7. Infectious diseases.

1. NEUROLOGICAL COMPLICATIONS OF PREGNANCY AND LABOUR

Eclampsia

This is the most serious complication of pregnancy. It is the ultimate expression of uncontrolled hypertension in pregnancy. It is best avoided by skilled management of the pre-eclamptic states which is indicated by rapid weight gain, proteinuria and a rising blood pressure. It occurs most often in the first pregnancy, in hydramnios, in patients with a multiple pregnancy, and in patients with pre-existing diabetes mellitus or renal disease. Eclampsia is heralded by a sudden uncontrollable rise in blood pressure, chest pain, confusion, drowsiness and the onset of focal or generalised seizures. Following the seizures the patients may remain unconscious due to cerebral oedema or multiple petechial haemorrhages in the brain. In this situation the mortality rate is ten per cent.

In most patients the onset of eclampsia occurs immediately before or during labour and the danger rapidly diminishes as soon as the uterus is evacuated. In some women the onset may occur a few days *after* delivery so that continued observation is necessary in patients who have had pre-eclampsia.

Seizures should be controlled with intravenous valium or barbiturates, and in comatose patients cerebral oedema should be reduced with dexamethazone or mannitol given intravenously.

CASE REPORT

A 21-year-old primigravida with a twin pregnancy became eclamptic at the onset of labour; having three major seizures. Immediate caesarean section controlled the blood pressure but forty-eight hours later the patient had not recovered consciousness. An E.E.G. showed symmetrical delta activity of high voltage although the physical response to deep painful stimulation suggested that the patient had a right hemiparesis. She was treated with intravenous dexamethazone and recovered consciousness some seventy-two hours after delivery and left hospital without sequelae.

Cerebral Vascular Accidents

Less specific forms of cerebral vascular disease than eclampsia may be associated with the pregnant state. Cerebral aneurysms and cerebral angiomas may rupture during pregnancy due to changes in blood pressure or altered circulatory dynamics.

Cerebral venous thrombosis is a specific complication of pregnancy and is especially likely to occur in patients with sickle cell anaemia. The thrombosis usually occurs within two to three weeks of delivery. The clinical picture depends on the site and extent of thrombosis. Localised cortical vein thrombosis may produce focal deficits such as a flaccid monoplegia, but thrombosis of the sagittal or lateral sinus will produce drowsiness, coma and papilloedema and may prove fatal. Even in the milder cases considerable residual deficit occurs and there is a high incidence of epilepsy in later years.

Embolic cerebral vascular accidents may occur during labour; when either air or amniotic fluid may be forced into the uterine veins. This will usually result in pulmonary embolisation. Occasionally cerebral embolisation may occur from these sources but the route taken to the cerebral circulation has not been satisfactorily explained.

Cerebral and Spinal Tumours

Certain cerebral tumours tend to be aggravated by pregnancy probably due to either increased vascularity or hormonal changes. Vascular tumours such as meningiomas, and tumours of the pituitary gland, which has a natural tendency to increase in size during pregnancy, are usually affected.

CASE REPORT

A 26-year-old primigravida suffered a series of focal seizures affecting the right arm during the third trimester of pregnancy. Full investigation after delivery revealed a large left parasagittal meningioma.

CASE REPORT

A 30-year-old female had suffered a mild paraparesis during two previous pregnancies and multiple sclerosis had been suspected. During her third pregnancy the paraparesis was more severe and worsened following delivery. Investigation and exploration revealed an extensive mid-dorsal lipoma.

CASE REPORT

A 36-year-old female developed a partial right third nerve palsy during pregnancy and failed to establish lactation or menstrual periods following delivery. She was referred for a neurological opinion two years later when her vision became impaired. On examination in addition to the partial third nerve palsy there was a bitemporal hemianopia and optic atrophy. Investigation and exploration revealed a very large cystic pituitary adenoma.

Epilepsy

Epilepsy is not seriously affected by pregnancy although some patients may suffer a slight increase in attacks in the later stages. The main risk occurs in the few days following delivery when patients may suffer their first attack for months or years. It is therefore very important to continue medication during delivery. Recently comment has been caused by a reported increased incidence of minor congenital abnormalities in children whose mothers took diphenylhydantoin in pregnancy. Most neurologists regard the risk as negligible compared with the risk of *uncontrolled* epilepsy during pregnancy; to *both* the mother and foetus.

Multiple Sclerosis

Multiple sclerosis occurs in females in the child-bearing age and therefore a chance association with pregnancy is highly likely. Although the risk is generally accepted as a small one, relapses usually occur in the puerperium. There are few neurologists who cannot recall individual patients who worsened dramatically following pregnancy. There are even a few patients who have only suffered episodes during pregnancy. It is very difficult to advise patients in this situation and one must weigh the risk against the desire to have children and the future possibility that progress of the disease may render the mother unable to care for a young family.

Myasthenia Gravis

Myasthenia gravis also occurs in young females. In many patients the myasthenia tends to improve during pregnancy and relapse within three weeks of delivery. The child may be born with a transient myasthenic state or cholinergic blockade, either situation requiring considerable skill in management. The neonatal myasthenic state usually clears within a week.

Chorea Gravidarum

Chorea gravidarum has become an uncommon disorder with the decline of rheumatic fever as it usually represents a recrudescence of previous Sydenham's chorea during pregnancy. It responds fairly well to diazepam in the writer's limited experience.

Peripheral Nerve Lesions

Carpal tunnel syndrome and lumbar root compression are the commonest neurological complications of the pregnant state. Meralgia paraesthetica due to traction of the lateral cutaneous nerve of the thigh and damage to the obturator nerve during obstetrical procedures are the other less common peripheral nerve complications of pregnancy. These conditions are discussed in detail in Chapter 19.

2. NEUROLOGICAL COMPLICATIONS OF DIABETES MELLITUS AND GLUCOSE METABOLISM

There are a large number of neurological complications of diabetes, most based on the accompanying vascular disease; particularly the changes in the small arterioles.

Peripheral Nerve Lesions

Diabetic peripheral neuropathy occurs most frequently in patients with late onset diabetes rather than in juvenile diabetics. Whether this form of symmetrical damage is due to vessel disease is uncertain.

Mononeuritis multiplex is very common and is undoubtedly due to pressure on a nerve which is rendered vulnerable by impaired microcirculation. Included in this category is infarction of the femoral nerve or upper lumbar nerve roots; the condition known as "diabetic amyotrophy".

Evidence of diffuse autonomic dysfunction has been detected in ninety per cent of diabetic patients but fortunately significant clinical symptoms occur in relatively few patients. Disorders of potency and postural hypotension are the main problems. Although nocturnal diarrhoea is always quoted as a specific pointer to this diagnosis there is considerable doubt as to the validity of this observation and no theoretical basis for its occurrence.

Isolated extraocular nerve palsies are a common complication and have been shown to be due to infarction of the extraocular nerves. The following case history provides a good example of this condition:

CASE REPORT

A 50-year-old Mexican-American presented with a very painful right third nerve palsy. This was thought to be due to his known diabetes but diagnostic confidence was somewhat shaken when a fourth nerve palsy also occurred on the same side a week later. However, within days the *left* third and fourth nerves also became affected and the diagnosis seemed certain. This was confirmed by complete recovery of all affected nerves over the next six weeks.

Visual problems in diabetes are common and diabetes remains one of the major causes of blindness. This is usually due to retinal arterial or venous disease and cataracts. Optic neuritis is rare.

Cerebral Vascular Disease and Spinal Vascular Disease

Diabetics are particularly likely to suffer a wide range of cerebral vascular accidents with greater frequency than the general population.

The diabetic is also subject to some particular vascular problems due to small vessel disease affecting the internal capsule, basal ganglia and the spinal cord.

These include the pseudobulbar palsy syndrome (Chapter 9), the athero-sclerotic rigidity syndrome (Chapter 12), and anterior spinal artery thrombosis (Chapter 14).

Metabolic Syndromes

Diabetic Ketotic Coma

The management of diabetic coma is the province of the general physician and the present section will be confined to the recognition of the condition. Neurological units must be continually on the alert for patients in diabetic coma; occasionally the diagnosis is not made until the C.S.F. glucose is found to be grossly elevated!

In general the onset is sub-acute and usually complicates an intercurrent disorder such as a urinary tract infection or pneumonia, often present for days before the patient becomes comatose. A careful history of the mode of onset of the coma is essential. In spite of this the diagnosis can present enormous problems. The following case is a good example.

CASE REPORT

A 30-year-old man who had been diabetic for many years was in normal health when his wife left to visit her mother on a Friday evening. She returned on the following Sunday afternoon to find him comatose. On arrival in hospital he was pale, sweating and comatose with a low blood pressure. The clinical appearance was suggestive of hypoglycaemia and intravenous glucose was given as soon as blood had been taken for glucose and electrolyte determination. Shortly after admission he started having focal and generalised seizures. He was pyrexial but had no detectable neck stiffness. The blood sugar on arrival was 1200 mgm per cent. He died within twenty minutes of admission and at post mortem was found to have miliary tuberculosis and tuberculous meningitis; presumably the infective factors which triggered the diabetic coma.

Hyperglycaemic, Hyperosmolar Non-ketotic Coma

This relatively recently recognised condition is of greater neurological importance as the clinical presentations embrace a wide range of neurological phenomena. These include focal or generalised epileptic seizures, transient or progressive "stroke-like" pictures, a tumour-like course or simple coma.

The dominant metabolic features are gross hyperglycaemia, and hypernatraemia and a considerable increase in serum osmolarity. The ketosis that is *the* feature of diabetic coma does not occur, and the condition is not really a complication of overt or sub-clinical diabetes. In fact the primary cause is not understood; and following recovery there is usually no evidence of diabetes.

The main clinical clue to the diagnosis is considerable clinical dehydration in a patient who has been unwell only for a few hours.

CASE REPORT

A 68-year-old retired hospital matron was admitted to hospital in a comatose state. She had normally reactive pupils and bilateral extensor plantars and she was markedly dehydrated. She had been perfectly well earlier in the day but had been noted by relatives to be excessively thirsty and had been drinking large quantities of Coca Cola. She had then developed slurring of speech, some dysphasic difficulties and a mild right hemiparesis and lapsed into coma during the drive to the hospital. To complicate matters she was and had been in atrial fibrillation for some months and diabetes had been excluded by full investigation a few months previously. She continued to deteriorate and both pupils became dilated and fixed to light. At this stage a serum glucose of 860 mgm per cent and a serum sodium of 158 mEq/L were found. There was no ketosis. She was given 17L of hypotonic saline and five per cent dextrose in water intravenously overnight. She recovered consciousness the next day. The initial clinical diagnosis was a cerebral embolism with subsequent cerebral oedema. The main clue to the diagnosis was the severe dehydration on admission.

Hypoglycaemic States

Hypoglycaemia has many important neurological features:

1. It may produce altered or psychotic behaviour.
2. It can produce focal neurological signs mimicking a cerebral vascular accident.
3. It can cause focal or generalised seizures leading to coma.
4. It can produce progressive neurological disease if unrecognised.

Although hypoglycaemia coma is widely discussed the important clinical states short of coma are rarely given the attention they deserve.

1. Hypoglycaemic pre-coma may produce altered behaviour often resulting in aggressive or anti-social behaviour. In diabetics on insulin this usually results from an inadequate diet. In patients with autonomous insulin secreting tumours hypoglycaemia is most likely to occur during the night when dietary intake ceases.

2. In patients with impaired cerebral perfusion hypoglycaemia may cause focal signs such as transient hemiparesis, dysphasia or dyspraxia. Animal experiments have shown that if one carotid artery is ligated focal signs develop in the poorly perfused territory when hypoglycaemia is provoked.

3. In some patients focal or generalised seizures may occur. Hypoglycaemia should be urgently excluded in any child who has a seizure. Following restoration of the blood sugar to normal recovery of consciousness is not always as prompt as might be expected. It is not unusual for a patient who has had a hypoglycaemic fit to take twelve to twenty-four hours to make a full recovery.

4. Repeated episodes of hypoglycaemia may cause irreversible damage to the basal ganglia, cerebellum, cortex and hippocampus. Progressive dementia, spasticity with dysarthria, extra-pyramidal syndromes and ataxia may result. A syndrome resembling motor neurone disease has been reported in patients with chronic hypoglycaemia although this would seem to be exceptionally rare.

3. NEUROLOGICAL COMPLICATIONS OF COLLAGEN-VASCULAR DISEASES

Collagen vascular diseases include a diverse range of disorders which have a common pathological basis in diffuse inflammatory changes in the connective tissue and particularly in the connective tissue of the blood vessels. The aetiology of these disorders is unknown although altered tissue immunity is suspected but unproven. Quite commonly features of different conditions overlap and all tend to become more dangerous with the development of widespread arteritis. Usually the neurological complications of these disorders reflect the extent and severity of the vasculitis.

Systematic Lupus Erythematosus

This disorder usually affects females (eighty-five per cent of cases). Neurologists should be particularly aware that occasional cases are provoked by drugs used in the treatment of neurological disorders. These include hydrallazine (used to treat acute hypertensive cerebral vascular disease), procaineamide (used as a muscle relaxant), and trimethadione and diphenylhydantoin (anti-convulsants). The pathological lesion consists of fibrinoid degeneration of the walls of small arteries and arterioles. Involvement of the joints, skin, heart and kidneys are the main non-neurological problems.

Focal or generalised seizures or episodes of acute psychosis may complicate up to thirty per cent of cases. Fifty per cent of patients with S.L.E. have abnormal electroencephalograms. Microvascular lesions are responsible for these cerebral manifestations and also predispose the patient to cerebral vascular accidents, extra-ocular nerve palsies, peripheral neuropathy, mononeuritis multiplex, polymyositis and Guillain—Barré syndrome. Retinal vascular lesions may cause visual symptoms and fundal appearances resembling papilloedema.

Rheumatoid Arthritis

In this disorder the brunt of the connective tissue damage falls on the peri-articular tissues but in the majority of cases there is also evidence of a systemic disturbance. The commonest neurological complications are carpel tunnel syndrome due to the changes around the wrist joint and ulnar nerve compression palsies due to the use of elbow crutches or prolonged periods of bed rest with consequent weight bearing on the elbows.

In very severe cases a diffuse peripheral neuropathy or mononeuritis multiplex may occur. For some time it was suggested that the use of steroids caused the neuropathy but it is more likely that the use of steroids merely parallels the severity of the disease.

The recent introduction of penicillamine into the treatment of the disease has produced a new complication. There are a few case reports of myasthenia gravis and possibly polymyositis complicating the use of the drug with improvement on withdrawal.

Considerable muscle atrophy occurs in long-standing cases and although much of this results from disuse, in five per cent of cases pathological evidence of inflammatory muscle disease has been found.

The most serious neurological complication is due to avulsion or absorption of the odontoid peg. This may happen acutely during a sneeze or a fall or be found on routine x-ray in patients complaining of neck pain. An acute or progressive spastic tetraparesis results and may prove fatal.

Polyarteritis nodosa

This is the most lethal of the collagen-vascular diseases and unlike systemic lupus erythematosus and rheumatoid arthritis occurs more frequently in males (eighty per cent of cases). The age incidence is similar, the majority of cases occurring in the 20–40 age group. A very similar disorder has been described as a reaction to sulphonamides, penicillin and diphenylhydantoin.

The main pathological lesion is a pan-arteritis with destruction of all layers of the arterial wall with local thrombosis and occasionally rupture of the vessel and microhaemorrhages.

The common neurological manifestations are due to peripheral nerve and nerve root infarction. The disease is one of the commonest causes of mononeuritis multiplex, but equally often infarction of multiple nerve roots occurs particularly affecting nerve roots C5–C7 and L2–L4. Once the patient is disabled the risk of further compression palsies is extremely high.

Although cranial nerve palsies and cerebral vascular accidents may occur they are uncommon.

The lethal nature of the condition is due to renal arteriolar disease often leading to uncontrollable hypertension. A few patients also develop polymyositis and the use of high doses of steroids to control the underlying disease may cause a steroid myopathy, adding to the diagnostic problems.

CASE REPORT

A 48-year-old aeronautical draughtsman had suffered from unexplained asthma for several years. Over a period of a few weeks he lost weight and felt very ill. Over a period of days he developed bilateral ulnar and median nerve palsies. His E.S.R. and eosinophil count were elevated. He was given steroids with complete remission of the systemic systems and a slow recovery of the nerve lesions. A few weeks later he became unable to walk because of gross weakness of both hip flexor muscles and the quadriceps. E.M.G. evidence confirmed an acute inflammatory myopathy. The dose of steroids was increased with a rapid improvement in muscle strength.

An unusual form of this disorder occurs in young patients which is known as "Cogan's syndrome". This consists of an association of interstitial keratitis, bilateral vestibular symptoms and deafness.

CASE REPORT

A 26-year-old housewife developed right-sided headache, felt increasingly unwell and lost weight. The headache was associated with vertigo. These symptoms partially remitted and then recurred on the left side. The clinical findings and oto-neurological studies suggested a left-sided cerebello-pontine angle lesion and the systemic illness suggested this might be due to metastatic malignant disease. During neurosurgical investigations she developed bilateral keratitis, the E.S.R. rose to 140 mm. and the eosinophil count rose to forty per cent. High dose steroids led to a prompt remission of symptoms although she remained partially deaf.

Although the E.S.R. is widely regarded as an old-fashioned and unreliable test it remains an important investigation for the neurologist. The speed with which the result is obtained and the almost invariable gross elevation in patients with collagen vascular disease cannot be matched by any other test.

Polymyositis

This acute inflammatory disease of muscle may complicate any of the collagen-vascular diseases already discussed. It also occurs as a primary condition and is sometimes a remote complication of malignant disease. It is discussed in detail in Chapter 17.

Scleroderma

Scleroderma is characterised by thickening of the collagen in the skin producing the typical skin changes of the disorder and similar changes in the bowel which may result in malabsorption. The condition may also occur in association with systemic lupus erythematosus and dermatomyositis.

Clinical presentations include Raynaud's phenomenon and rarely muscle weakness and evidence of cutaneous nerve damage in the thickened skin. Steroids are not helpful in this condition.

Sjögren's Syndrome

Sjögren's syndrome is now regarded as a collagen-vascular disease. The main features are a dry kerato-conjunctivitis, xerostomia (dry mouth) and a rheumatoid-like arthritis. In recent years an association with a progressive proximal myopathy has been recognised. Pathological and electromyographic evidence indicates that this is an inflammatory muscle lesion but there is rarely any response to steroids.

Polymyalgia Rheumatica

This disorder is also discussed in Chapter 17. It occurs in the elderly and is characterised by severe muscle pain in the limbs and girdle regions and is usually associated with a systemic illness and a high E.S.R. Some of these patients later develop temporal arteritis. The response to steroids is dramatic and diagnostic.

Thrombotic Thrombocytopenic Purpura

This is an extremely rare and usually ultimately lethal condition dominated by acute haemolytic anaemia and thrombocytopenia. The onset is usually acute with abdominal pain, fever, vomiting, headache and jaundice, quickly complicated by confusion, delirium and coma, with seizures, hemiplegia and almost any other acute cerebral vascular event.

The main pathological lesions are due to severe acute inflammatory changes in arteriolar walls with thrombosis and multiple petechial haemorrhages; throughout the substance of the brain but particularly in the cortex.

Very rarely the disorder may run a relapsing course over several years but is almost invariably eventually fatal. Steroids may occasionally prove beneficial.

The frequency with which collagen-vascular diseases present as an acute neurological disorder places considerable responsibility on the neurologist to recognise this group of diseases.

4. NEUROLOGICAL COMPLICATIONS OF ENDOCRINE AND METABOLIC DISEASE

Although there are some specific complications associated with changes in hormonal levels per se, in many instances the neurological involvement in endocrine disorders is really a reflection of alterations in electrolyte metabolism. These problems are discussed in greater detail in the chapters on muscle and peripheral nerve disease. Discussion in the present section will therefore be extremely brief and references to more detailed discussions are given.

1. Thyrotoxicosis

In thyrotoxic exophthalmos with ophthalmoplegia (Chapter 5), the exophthalmos is probably due to excessive T.S.H. production but the diplopia is not purely due to displacement of the globe. Pathological studies have shown inflammatory changes in the affected extraocular muscles.

A similar situation exists in thyrotoxic myopathy (Chapter 17). The muscle weakness usually recovers surprisingly rapidly once the euthyroid state is restored. Thyrotoxicosis also occurs in some patients with periodic paralysis (particularly in the Japanese) and in ten per cent of patients with myasthenia gravis.

Acute thyroid crisis with fever, delirium, epileptic seizures and coma has become rare now that quick control of the peripheral effects of thyroid hormone can be gained with guanethidine.

In addition to the typical fine tremor of the hands, a rare complication is the acute onset of choreiform movements due to hormonal effects on the basal ganglia (Chapter 12).

In the elderly "masked thyrotoxicosis" may occur, in which the classical signs of the disease may be easily overlooked. This is quite common in patients presenting with thyrotoxic myopathy. The other important group to consider are those patients in whom auricular fibrillation secondary to thyrotoxicosis has caused cerebral embolism.

2. Myxoedema

Carpal tunnel syndrome is a frequent complication of myxoedema (Chapter 18). Proximal muscle weakness is quite common in cretinism and adult myxoedema (Chapter 17). Although a great deal is made of myxoedema madness this is an extremely rare complication; complete mental and physical inertia usually dominates the illness. Cerebellar degeneration may also complicate myxoedema (Chapter 12) but is also exceedingly rare.

3. Hyperparathyroidism

The complications of hyperparathyroidism directly reflect the elevation of serum calcium. This may produce a variable proximal muscle weakness (Chapter 17) or profound personality change occasionally amounting to an acute psychotic state (Chapter 10).

4. Hypoparathyroidism

The lowered serum calcium level causes the complications although the mechanism in some situations is unknown. In children hypocalcaemia may cause convulsions and papilloedema which may direct investigations along purely neurological lines unless this unusual presentation is recognised. Extrapyramidal disorders may occur usually taking the form of choreiform movements associated with the deposition of calcium in the basal ganglia. Tetany may be provoked by minor hyperventilation or occur spontaneously. Proximal muscle weakness may occur (Chapter 17). Psychotic changes in personality have been reported but are much less frequent than in hypercalcaemia. In adults, cataracts are a common complication of unrecognised chronic hypocalcaemia.

5. Cushing's Syndrome

In the active stages of this disease mental changes due to high endogenous steroid levels may precipitate a "steroid psychosis". For the same reason a proximal "steroid myopathy" occurs and in combination with the typical deposition of fat over the back contributes to the "Buffalo Hump" shape of the patient who has the fully developed syndrome.

After adrenalectomy, or in those patients in whom the disease is due to a functional tumour of the pituitary gland bitemporal field defects (Chapter 3) or extra-ocular nerve palsies (Chapter 5) may be found.

6. Addison's Disease

The physical symptoms of this disorder are dominated by mental and physical lethargy and inertia. A mild proximal myopathy with easy fatiguability occurs and exertion is often accompanied by muscle cramping. Syncope due to the associated hypotension may also lead to neurological referral.

7. Acromegaly

In the early stages of this disorder there is a considerable increase in muscle strength, paralleling the dramatic changes in facial appearance and the size of the hands and feet. Later, as the pituitary gland is replaced by the enlarging eosinophil adenoma, weakness ensues as panhypopituitarism develops. The tumour may then compress the optic chiasm causing a bitemporal hemianopia.

The overgrowth of the hands frequently leads to carpal tunnel syndrome and peroneal nerve entrapment has also been reported.

Diabetes mellitus with all its neurological consequences occurs in some twenty per cent of patients with acromegaly.

8. Hypopituitarism

The features of panhypopituitarism, including the visual problems caused by pituitary tumours, are described in Chapter 3. The problems presented by the tumour itself may be combined with features of both myxoedema and Addison's disease.

9. Inappropriate Secretion of Antidiuretic Hormone

Hyponatraemia may occur for many reasons, but a variety of special interest to the neurologist is due to inappropriate secretion of antidiuretic hormone. The term "inappropriate" has been applied because normally when serum sodium and osmolarity are falling a hypotonic urine is secreted as ADH production falls. If ADH continues to be secreted a hyperosmolar urine is produced and the renal excretion of sodium continues, further compounding the situation. This is a very simple and incomplete explanation of an extremely complicated metabolic situation.

The neurological importance of the condition stems from the fact that the well-established syndrome may produce symptoms and signs suggesting intracranial disease *and* intracranial disease may cause the syndrome.

The neurological manifestations are due to water intoxication and typically include confusion, headache, nausea and vomiting. Later the patient may become comatose and epileptic seizures can occur. There may be considerable fluctuation in the symptoms on a day-to-day basis.

Most cases are due to an underlying oat cell carcinoma of the lung and in many instances the tumour itself secretes ADH. The difficulty in distinguishing the clinical picture from that produced by multiple cerebral metastases is obvious.

Meningitis, subarachnoid haemorrhage, cerebral tumours and head injury have all been responsible for examples of the condition. Myxoedema and acute porphyria have also been implicated and the possibility of the cerebral symptoms being ascribed to the underlying disease rather than to the potentially fatal disturbance of salt metabolism is obvious.

The condition is relatively easily treated by fluid restriction to less than 1,000 mls. daily. Salt loading does not help and is only indicated in patients who are comatose or convulsing in an immediate attempt to reduce the water intoxication.

The importance of routine electrolyte studies in confusion, comatose or convulsing patients cannot be overestimated.

CASE REPORT

An 18-year-old university student was admitted to hospital after having an accident on his motor-cycle. He was conscious on arrival but was remarkably confused. He insisted he was drunk and that it was 10 p.m. He was quite sober and it was 4 p.m. in the afternoon. He was bleeding from both ears but no fracture could be seen on x-ray. Far from improving he became increasingly confused over the next thirty-six hours; and his serum sodium fell to 119 mEq/L. He was secreting a concentrated urine (specific gravity 1030). An E.E.G. showed an alarming slow wave disturbance over the left frontal region suggesting contrecoup bruising of the left frontal lobe. His fluids were restricted immediately and osmolarity studies revealed a low serum osmolarity of 252 m osmoles/L and a urine osmolarity of 723 m osm/L. Within twenty-four hours he became rational and the E.E.G. became completely normal. The remarkably rapid onset of confusion in this patient suggests that he had cerebral bruising with oedema rapidly compounded by the simultaneous development of inappropriate ADH secretion with water intoxication.

10. Alcoholism

The neurological complications of alcoholism are considered here because they basically represent metabolic effects rather than a direct toxic effect of alcohol. In Great Britain this problem presents a minor, but unfortunately increasing, part of neurological practice. In the U.S.A. these complications are extremely common.

Alcoholic peripheral neuropathy, the complication most directly related to altered niacin metabolism, is the most common complication. It is described in Chapter 16. Acute compression palsies also occur due to the inebriated patient lying on the vulnerable nerves. The radial and peroneal nerves are usually affected.

Acute and chronic muscle changes due to alcohol have been reported. The symptoms of the acute form resemble the effects of sudden exertion on untrained muscles with muscle pain and tenderness on movement usually following a period of high alcoholic intake. The chronic form consists of a mild generalised myopathy.

Cerebellar degeneration may also occur in an acute reversible form and a chronic irreversible form with massive degeneration of the anterior lobe of the cerebellum (Chapter 12).

Acute haemorrhagic polio-encephalitis or Wernicke's encephalopathy is invariably associated with damage to the hippocampal-mamillary body complex, causing the abrupt memory deficit known as Korsakoff's psychosis. The brainstem features are described in Chapter 11. The immediate administration of massive doses of Vitamin B_1 will usually reverse the potentially lethal brainstem lesion but recovery of the memory disturbance is variable and always incomplete.

One very unusual and almost specific complication of alcohol abuse is acute auditory hallucinosis. In this condition a pure auditory hallucination, often musical in content is associated with paranoid thoughts.

Acute auditory hallucinosis and delirium tremens are alcohol withdrawal syndromes. Both conditions particularly tend to occur in alcoholics who have been admitted to hospital unless alcohol is being smuggled in to the patient to maintain the intake!

Delirium tremens often begins as a series of epileptic fits followed by severe confusion and agitation, sympathetic overaction and vivid visual hallucinations.

The condition is treated by heavy sedation with chlordiazepoxide or chlormethiazole and vitamin supplements. The majority of patients recover over a few days but the condition may be fatal.

Alcohol or sedative drug abuse should be suspected in any patient who has a fit after admission to hospital.

5. NEUROLOGICAL COMPLICATIONS ASSOCIATED WITH CARDIAC DISEASE

The most frequent cardiac disease is myocardial infarction. Because this is only one manifestation of diffuse vascular disease it is hardly surprising that some forty per cent of patients who suffer a cerebral vascular accident subsequently die of a myocardial infarct.

During and following acute myocardial infarction there are the immediate risks of impaired cerebral perfusion during the shock phase and the later risk of cerebral embolism when the circulation recovers and mural thrombus becomes detached from the damaged heart wall. In some series as many as thirty per cent of cerebral emboli were found to originate in the heart. Preventing these complications with anti-coagulants may lead to fatal subarachnoid haemorrhage. Fortunately anti-coagulants no longer play a major role in the management of myocardial infarction.

Congenital cardiac disease carries many risks. Coarctation of the aorta is associated with a high incidence of cerebral aneurysms almost certainly a direct consequence of the associated hypertension. The risk of subarachnoid haemorrhage is high and subarachnoid haemorrhage in children under 15 should always suggest this possibility.

Congenital cyanotic heart disease may cause complications due to chronic cerebral anoxia, polycythaemia or cerebral abscess as the blood bypasses the normal filtering effect of the pulmonary circulation.

Both congenital and acquired disease of the aortic and mitral valves predispose to subacute bacterial endocarditis. This may cause cerebral embolism, cerebral abscess or mycotic aneurysms.

Surgical treatment of valvular disease, although now much safer with cardiac bypass and an open heart approach, still carries the risk of operative or post-operative clot or air embolism with a tragic outcome in some instances with cortical blindness or hemiplegia.

Simple syncopal attacks always require careful auscultation of the heart to detect aortic or mitral valve lesions and in patients complaining of syncope occurring on exertion evidence of atrial septal defects and pulmonary valve disease should be sought. The stethoscope is an important part of a neurologist's diagnostic equipment.

6. NEUROLOGICAL COMPLICATIONS OF NEOPLASTIC DISEASE

The neurology of malignant disease is a subject in itself, and it is possible to make only some broad generalisations in the space available.

In spite of many extremely interesting but very rare remote

complications of malignant disease the fact remains that the majority of patients with malignant disease who develop a neurological disorder prove to have metastatic deposits.

These remote complications have been mentioned elsewhere and include peripheral neuropathy (Chapter 16), polymyositis (Chapter 17), Lambert–Eaton syndrome (Chapter 17), limbic encephalitis (Chapter 10) cerebellar degeneration (Chapter 12) and inappropriate secretion of A.D.H. (Chapter 26). A supposed relationship between motor neurone disease and visceral malignancy has not been substantiated.

Surprisingly, in view of their widespread nature and chronic clinical course, the malignant lymphomas produce few neurological complications other than by direct spread. Cord compression due to Hodgkin's disease and meningeal infiltration in the leukaemias are the main problem. Fungal meningitis due to cryptococcosis neoformans (cryptococcal meningitis) is occasionally encountered. An indian ink preparation of the C.S.F. is necessary to demonstrate the fungi. One of the rare complications of considerable interest is progressive multifocal leucoencephalopathy as there is now overwhelming evidence that this is due to an opportunist virus infection of the C.N.S. in patients with chronic diseases, particularly those leading to altered immune mechanisms. It produces a rapidly progressive illness in which brain stem and cerebellar signs are coupled with confusion and drowsiness. All patients with this condition have died, usually within a few months.

It should also be remembered that an altered immune state may predispose to the development of Herpes Zoster and herpes may complicate both malignant lymphomas, chronic lymphatic leukaemia and bowel carcinomas in particular.

In addition to metastasis (the source and location of metastases to the C.N.S. are described in Chapters 8 and 15), there are the additional problems posed by the neurological side effects of cytotoxic drugs (Chapter 24) and radiation damage (Chapters 14 and 18).

As a cautionary note it is important to remember that just because a patient has had malignant disease in the past it does not follow that any *new* disorder is necessarily a complication of that malignancy. An open mind is necessary until the diagnosis is established beyond doubt.

CASE REPORT

A 42-year-old female who had had a mastectomy for carcinoma of the breast four years previously developed diabetes insipidus and a bitemporal field defect. A metastasis seemed certain and steroids and other hormonal therapy were used without effect for several months. Further investigation and exploration were eventually undertaken and revealed a cystic craniopharyngioma which was successfully removed.

7. INFECTIOUS DISEASES AND THE NERVOUS SYSTEM

In general infection of the nervous system is a complication of infection elsewhere. For example, meningococcal meningitis can be regarded as a complication of meningococcal septicaemia, tuberculous meningitis is a complication of a breaking down tuberculous lesion or military tuberculosis and listeria monocytogenes or cryptococcal meningitis as opportunist nervous system infections in the presence of debilitating disease or altered immune status.

The meninges and subarachnoid space may be infected by viruses, bacteria, spirochaetes and fungi. The relative incidence of these causes varies enormously in different areas of the world and viral and bacterial infections sometimes show a seasonal variation.

A classical case of meningitis is unmistakable, but, as usual, there are many subtle presentations that may lead to a fatal delay in diagnosis. There are also several common disorders that can mimic "meningitis" to the extent that an immediate L.P. is desirable. These may include any febrile illness in childhood, acute influenza, a severe migraine attack or subarachnoid haemorrhage. There is also the very dangerous situation in which neck stiffness in a drowsy patient is due to coning. In these patients an L.P. may prove fatal (Chapter 25).

The diagnosis may prove difficult in infancy and senescence and the chronic types of meningitis may produce a "tumour-like" clinical picture in any age group.

In infancy the child may become unusually quiet or utter only occasional brief cries. Neck stiffness may be difficult to detect and one may be faced with a pyrexial, quiet, listless, limp infant. An epileptic fit is a common early feature of meningitis in infancy and may provide a clue to the diagnosis.

In senescence the features that may make the diagnosis difficult include an apyrexial course and neurological symptoms dominated by confusion, delirium or focal signs due to cerebral venous thrombosis, mimicking a cerebral vascular accident.

At any age focal inflammation of the brain, venous sinus thrombosis, cerebral arterial occlusions, blockage of C.S.F. circulation or cranial nerve palsies may lead to very focal presenting signs. If these complications develop later in the course of the illness, they may prompt reconsideration of the diagnosis and require definitive treatment in their own right. Many of these complications occur in incorrectly or inadequately treated meningitis.

Classical Features

In typical acute meningitis the features include a pyrexial

onset, considerable headache and photophobia and the development of neck stiffness and backache. The similarity to prodromal influenza is immediately obvious. If left undiagnosed and untreated drowsiness, vomiting and eventually coma may ensue. Different types of meningitis affect different age groups and produce some fairly specific features which may have diagnostic value.

Meningococcal Meningitis

Neisseria meningitides remains the commonest infecting organism, showing a seasonal variation (January to June) and an association with overcrowding. The illness invariably starts as a meningococcal septicaemia and this may prove to be the main problem and cause death. In some cases a chronic meningococcal septicaemia without meningitis may occur. The disease usually affects the under-12 age group and starts as an acute pharyngitis with fever which may rapidly worsen to include a petechial rash and in some cases a florid purpuric rash. In this group massive intravascular coagulation may occur with shock and circulatory collapse. This is known as the Waterhouse–Friderichsen syndrome and it has been suggested that Heparin may be of benefit. Previously steroids were used with little success, a use based mainly on the post-mortem finding of haemorrhagic necrosis of the adrenal glands. The onset of the meningitic component is usually fairly classical and is often associated with a herpes simplex eruption around the mouth. Metastatic infection of the eyes, joints and bones may occur and complicate the later course. From a neurological point of view late complications occur relatively rarely in correctly diagnosed and treated meningococcal meningitis.

Penicillin is the drug of choice although sulphonamide sensitive organisms are still responsible for the majority of cases in Great Britain. The dosage is 24–30 mega/24 hours in adults I.V. and 1 mega/Kg/24 hours in children I.V.

Haemophilus Influenzae Meningitis

Haemophilus meningitis occurs almost exclusively in children under five years of age. It tends to have a more benign onset and the signs of meningitis may be minimal. The child may be merely drowsy and febrile.

The special complication of haemophilus influenzae meningitis is the development of a subdural collection of pus. This may lead to an apparent relapse or the late development of focal neurological signs. In the writer's experience this is often the result of inadequate treatment with ampicillin.

Chloramphenicol remains the drug of choice in a dose of 75 mgm./Kg/24 hours for at least ten days. If ampicillin is

used very high dosage is necessary; 400 mgm./Kg/24 hours should be given by intravenous infusion.

Pneumococcal Meningitis

Pneumococcal meningitis is relatively uncommon. It is liable to occur when the dura is damaged or infected by a skull fracture, middle ear disease or sinus infections. The organism may also reach the brain via the blood stream in patients who have pneumococcal pneumonia. It is potentially the most lethal form of meningitis, a somewhat paradoxical situation considering that the organism is extremely penicillin sensitive. The danger arises from the rapid development of a thick basal exudate, cortical venous thrombosis and cerebral oedema. Total eradication may prove difficult and frequent recurrences may occur in patients with underlying sources of infection such as a basal skull fracture.

Penicillin in adequate dosage is the treatment of choice. The dose is 24–30 Megaunits/24 hours in the adult and 1 Megaunit/Kg/24 hours in children. Chloramphenicol is recommended in patients who are allergic to penicillin in a dose of 100 mgm./Kg/24 hours.

Other organisms

Other gram positive and gram negative organisms may cause meningitis. For this reason it has been traditional to use a triple therapy regime in those patients who do not have clinical evidence to suggest a specific organism and in those cases in which the gram stain of the C.S.F. is uncertain. The traditional regime included penicillin, chloramphenicol and sulphadiazine, all three drugs being used until the organism was identified. Recently regimes which include kanamycin and gentamycin combined with penicillin have been suggested and many use a wide spectrum antibiotic such as ampicillin. In the writer's view the old regime still has much to commend it.

The only important point in the management of meningitis is that once the diagnosis has been made an *adequate* dose of the *appropriate* antibiotic must be given. Many therapeutic failures result from the use of inadequate doses of specialised antibiotics such as cloxacillin or cephalosporin in the mistaken belief that the meningitis is due to a rare or antibiotic-resistant organism. Intrathecal therapy is rarely indicated in the treatment of meningitis. Therapeutic disasters have occurred as a result of intrathecal injections of antibiotics. The dosage of penicillin is 20,000 units in aqueous solution. This should be prepared by a pharmacist and no other dilution or diluent should be used. The intrathecal use of streptomycin is discussed in the next section.

Tuberculous Meningitis

Tuberculous meningitis is one of the most serious complications of tuberculosis. It results from the haematogenous spread of the organism.

Although tuberculous meningitis can occur at any age the peak incidence is between 2 and 5 years of age. The onset may be heralded by listlessness, lethargy, poor appetite and weight loss. The meningitic phase may occur very abruptly with acute extraocular nerve palsies, vomiting, headache, and epileptic seizures progressing to coma.

In the adult all these symptoms may occur but the onset can be extremely gradual and is sometimes dominated by intellectual and personality changes. Tuberculous meningitis should always be suspected in any vaguely ill patient with headache and personality change.

The diagnosis may be suggested by the C.S.F. findings. The fluid is usually mildly pleocytic, containing 50–300 cells, mainly lymphocytes, a slightly raised protein and a normal or slightly reduced glucose level. This type of fluid may occur in several conditions discussed below, but unless an alternative diagnosis can be established it is standard practice to start anti-tuberculous therapy on suspicion alone while the result of C.S.F. culture is awaited.

Streptomycin, P.A.S. and isonaizid are given in standard doses. Intrathecal streptomycin is rarely indicated. If the decision to use intrathecal therapy is taken the dose used is *only* 50–100 mgm. diluted in saline and C.S.F. and injected slowly. In severe cases the use of corticosteroid drugs has been recommended but this remains an extremely controversial topic.

Benign aseptic meningitis (Viral meningitis)

The enteroviruses and the mumps virus are the main causes of this condition.

The illness usually starts with an influenzal type of prodrome with fever, muscle pains and headache. The onset of neck stiffness heralds the meningitic phase. Clinically it is unusual for the patient to appear particularly ill although photophobia and malaise are prominent symptoms.

The C.S.F. usually contains between 30 and 300 cells almost all lymphocytes, although in the first twenty-four hours of the illness up to ten per cent of the cells may be polymorphs. The other constituents are usually normal and a significant increase in the protein or decrease in the glucose should raise serious doubt as to the diagnosis.

No specific treatment is necessary and the condition usually subsides within seven to ten days. With the exception of the variant known as lymphocytic choriomeningitis, recurrences are rare although a mild headache may persist for some weeks. Lymphocytic choriomeningitis is quite rare and is due to a virus transmitted by mice. It is characterised by a very high cell count which may rise to 5,000 lymphocytes and a rather more protracted course.

It is important that special care is taken with any patient who has a "sterile" meningitis, especially if the patient had been given antibiotics before admission to hospital.

If the C.S.F. contains any polymorphs, if the protein is significantly elevated or the glucose is low there are several other conditions that must be considered. These include; partially treated bacterial meningitis, tuberculous meningitis, cerebral abscess, cerebral tumour, cerebral vascular accident or malignant infiltration of the meninges. Fungal meningitis, which is extremely unusual in Great Britain, should also be considered especially in patients with malignant lymphomas.

The C.S.F. should always be cultured for tuberculosis and unusual organisms such as listeria monocytogenes, stained with indian ink for cryptococcus neoformans, and a cell block examined for malignant cells.

Careful follow-up is indicated and a repeat C.S.F. examination should be made before the patient is discharged. This is usually unnecessary in patients who have a typical aseptic meningitis although a convalescent serum should always be obtained in an attempt to identify the causal virus.

INDEX

A limited index is provided taking into account that the text is arranged in such a way that major topics are dealt with in one section or one chapter. Where necessary extensive coverage of different aspects of the same subject elsewhere is indicated in the text.

To avoid cross references in the index the major page numbers of each topic are entered under all possible similar reference words and the main sub-divided topics with only one main heading.

A complete list of eponymous neurological syndromes discussed in the text will be found indexed under "Syndrome".